Studies
in
Geriatric Psychiatry

Studies
in
Geriatric Psychiatry

Edited by
A.D. Isaacs and **F. Post**

The Bethlem Royal Hospital and The Maudsley Hospital
London

JOHN WILEY & SONS
Chichester · New York · Brisbane · Toronto

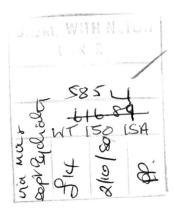

Copyright © 1978, by John Wiley & Sons, Ltd.

Library of Congress Cataloging in Publication Data:
Main entry under title:

Studies in geriatric psychiatry.

Bibliography: p.
Includes index.
1. Geriatric psychiatry. I. Isaacs, Anthony Donald. II. Post, Felix. [DNLM: 1. Geriatric psychiatry. WT150 S933]
RC451.4.A5S78   618.9'76'89   77-9990

ISBN 0 471 99550 9

Typeset by Computacomp (UK) Limited,
Fort William, Scotland
and printed by Unwin Brothers Limited,
The Gresham Press,
Old Woking,
Surrey,
England

CONTRIBUTORS

JULIAN DE AJURIAGUERRA, Professeur au Collège de France, Clinique Psychiatrique de L'Université, Bel-Air près Genève, Switzerland, 1225, Chêne-Bourg.

TOM ARIE, Professor of Health Care of the Elderly, University of Nottingham Medical School, Clifton Boulevard, Nottingham.

KLAUS BERGMANN, Consultant Psychiatrist, Newcastle General Hospital, Newcastle upon Tyne, NE3 6BE.

D.B. BROMLEY, Professor of Psychology, The University of Liverpool, 7, Abercrombie Square, Liverpool, 7.

EWALD W. BUSSE, MD, Associate Provost and Director, Duke University Medical Center, Durham, North Carolina, 27710, USA.

JEAN CONSTANTINIDIS, Professeur Assistant à la Faculté de Médecine, Médecin-chef à la Clinique Psychiatrique Universitaire de Genève, Bel-Air près Genève, Switzerland, 1225, Chêne-Bourg.

J.R.M. COPELAND, Professor of Psychiatry, The University of Liverpool, 7, Abercrombie Square, Liverpool, 7.

DANIEL T. GIANTURCO, Professor of Psychiatry, Duke University Medical Center, Durham, North Carolina, 27710, USA.

A.D. ISAACS, Consultant Psychiatrist, The Bethlem Royal Hospital and The Maudsley Hospital, Denmark Hill, SE5 8AX.

S. KANOWSKI, Professor of Gerontopsychiatry, Freie Universität Berlin, 1 Berlin 19, Germany, Ulmenallee, 40.

R. LEVY, Consultant Psychiatrist, The Bethlem Royal Hospital and The Maudsley Hospital, Denmark Hill, SE5 8AZ.

C.D. MARSDEN, Professor of Neurology, Institute of Psychiatry & King's College Hospital Medical School, De Crespigny Park, Denmark Hill, SE5 8AF.

FELIX POST, Consultant Psychiatrist, The Bethlem Royal Hospital and The Maudsley Hospital, Denmark Hill, SE5 8AZ.

D.M. PRINSLEY,   Professor of Gerontology and Geriatric Medicine, University of Melbourne, Mount Royal Hospital, Parkville, 3052, Melbourne, Australia.

JACQUES RICHARD,   Privat-docent à la Faculté de Médecine, Médecin-chef à la Clinique Psychiatrique, Universitaire de Genève, Bel-Air près Genève, Switzerland, 1225, Chêne-Bourg.

ANTONIA WHITEHEAD, PhD,   Lecturer in Psychology, University of Reading, Building 3, Earley Gate, Whiteknights, Reading, Berks. RG6 2AL.

CONTENTS

INTRODUCTION

This volume brings together contributions from workers engaged in practice, teaching, and research related to the psychiatry of late life. Contributors were invited to write about their own work and where appropriate to summarize that of others. Topics were chosen that are relevant to clinical work so as to provide some of the theoretical background to the practice of geriatric psychiatry. Because the range of topics is not fully comprehensive, however, in the following synopsis of the contents special reference has been made to some of those areas not covered in this volume, drawing the reader's attention to the relevant recent literature as a guide for further reading.

The book starts with an account of the mental health of a group of elderly non-patient volunteers followed up over a number of years. There have been similar studies in which patients developing mental disorders when young have been followed into old age, but it was not possible to include a detailed account of such work in the present volume. This is especially unfortunate as much of this work has been published in French and German, but the reader is referred to Ernst (1965) who followed neurotics into old age; to Müller (1957) more specifically for the long-term course of obsessional neurosis; to Ciompi (1965) for the fate of hysterics. Attention is drawn to Ciompi and Lai's (1969) monograph on depressives followed into old age. Monumental work concerning schizophrenia in late life has been reported by both Bleuler (1972) and Ciompi and Müller (1976). To summarize very briefly, the neurotic kinds of disorder tend to become less disruptive and disturbing as patients grow older (Müller, 1967). Patients with affective and with schizophrenic psychoses have a considerably increased mortality rate, so that there is a tendency for severe cases of illness not to survive into the senile period of life. Among survivors, depressions tend to be longer lasting but less severe, and once schizophrenic deterioration has continued for some five years it rarely worsens subsequently. In the case of schizophrenics, symptomatology becomes less disruptive or disappears altogether, but schizophrenics as a group tend to remain handicapped in their interpersonal relationships and social status.

Returning to the contents of this volume, a fresh look at the psychology of ageing is followed by an account of psychiatric disorders unrelated to structural brain changes. Disorders of mental functioning secondary to cerebral disease or deterioration are dealt with in two chapters, the first concerned with diagnostic procedures, and the second one with more general aspects of the dementias of late life and referring to some work so far unfamiliar to English speaking readers.

The pathophysiology of senile dementia and its pharmacological treatment is not considered in detail. This is a rapidly developing area, in which hypothetical speculations so far outstrip solid achievement. An exception is formed by the electrophysiology of dementia. The reader is also referred to Fenton's (1974) comprehensive summary of electroencephalographic researches in confusional states, in ageing, and in the dementias of late life with special reference to slowing and to the occurrence of abnormal wave patterns: the need for serial examinations is stressed. In contrast to the importance of endocrine and nutritional deficiences as well as of toxic factors for acute and subacute cerebral failure, progressive and irreversible failure (dementia) has not emerged as a regular and frequent result of deficiency of various substance such as vitamin B_{12} (Shulman, 1972) or folic acid, or of malnutrition in general (Department of Health and Social Security, 1972). However, senile dementia of Alzheimer type may be one of the abiotrophies of Gowers caused by an as yet unidentified defect of vital endurance leading to cellular death (Bowen and Davison, 1975; Bowen *et al.*, 1976). Other recent papers worth consulting concerning the biochemistry of senile dementia and related conditions are by Gottfries *et al.* (1969, 1974) and Crapper *et al.* (1973). There seemed little point, at present, to review critically the many publications reporting drug trials in the treatment of senile dementia, but an authorative statement can be found in an anonymous article (*Drug and Therapeutics Bulletin*, 1975).

Treatment by psychological methods is included in the chapter dealing with the clinical psychologist's contribution to work with elderly mental patients. There follows a cross-national comparison of diagnostic classification within psychiatry and in relation to geriatric medicine, and after this a geriatrician describes how he carries out the management of persistently confused patients.

The last two chapters of the book are more general in scope, but of highly practical importance: education in the psychiatry of late life and the planning and running of a psychiatric service for the elderly.

References

Bleuler, M. (1972) *Die schizophrenen Geistesstörungen im Lichte langjähriger Kranken- und Familiengeschichten*, Stuttgart, Thieme.

Bowen, D.M., and Davidson, A.N. (1975) Extrapyramidal disease and dementia', *Lancet*, **i,** 1199–1200.

Bowen, D.M., Smith, C.B., White, P., and Davison, A.N. (1976) 'Neurotransmitter-related enzymes and indices of hypoxia in senile dementia and other abiotrophies', *Brain*, **99,** 459–496.

Ciompi, L. (1965) 'Hysterie et vieillesse, étude catamnestique', *Congr. psychiat. neurol. franç.*, 69e session.

Ciompi, L., and Lai, G.P. (1969) *Depression et viellesse*, Berne, Stuttgart, Hans Huber.

Ciompi, L., and Müller, C. (1976) *Lebensweg und Alter der Schizophrenen*, Berlin, Heidelberg, New York, Springer.

Crapper, D.R., Dalton, A.J., and Krishman, S.S. (1973) 'Brain aluminium distribution in Alzheimer's disease and experimental neurofibrillary degeneration', *Science*, **180**, 511–513.

Department of Health and Social Security (1972) *Nutrition survey of the elderly*, London, HMSO.

Drug and Therapeutics Bulletin (1975) 'Drugs for dementia', *Drugs Therapeut. Bull.*, **13**, 85–87.

Ernst, K. (1965) 'Neurotische Langstreckenverläufe und ihre Beeinflussung durch Psychotherapie', *Z. Psychother.*, **15**, 185–194.

Fenton, G. (1974) 'The straightforward EEG in psychiatric practice', *Proc. Royal Soc. Med.*, **67**, 911–918.

Gottfries, C.G., Gottfries, I., and Roos, B.E. (1969) 'Homovanillic acid and 5-hydroxyindole acetic acid in CSF of patients with senile dementia, presenile dementia and Parkinsonism', *J. Neurochem.*, **16**, 1341–45.

Gottfries, C.G., Kjällquist, A., Ponten, U., Roos, B.E., and Sundbärg, G. (1974) 'Cerebrospinal fluid pH and monoamine and glucolytic metabolites in Alzheimer's disease', *Br. J. Psychiat.*, **124**, 280–287.

Müller, C. (1957) 'Weitere Beobachtungen zum Verlauf der Zwangskrankheit', *Psychiat. Neurol.*, **133**, 80–94.

Müller, C. (1967) *Alterspsychiatrie*, Stuttgart, Thieme.

Shulman, R. (1972) 'The present state of vitamin B_{12} and of folic acid deficiency in psychiatric illness', *Canad. Psychiat. Assoc. J.*, **17**, 205–216.

1

PSYCHIATRIC PROBLEMS ENCOUNTERED DURING A LONG-TERM STUDY OF NORMAL AGEING VOLUNTEERS

D.T. Gianturco and E.W. Busse

The Duke Longitudinal Study of Aging was initiated to investigate processes of ageing among a panel of non-institutionalized males and females 60 years of age and over, from the time of initial observation to death. All of the persons were volunteers who were initially considered reasonably well adjusted and living in the community. The study was conceived as exploratory and multidisciplinary and thus was organized to accumulate a wide range of observations from investigators with a variety of theoretical perspectives. The disciplines among project investigators included medicine, psychiatry, psychology, and sociology. The study was not guided by any single theory of ageing. Rather the focus has been on the generation and testing of hypotheses of interest to a variety of investigators who brought quite different theoretical perspectives to bear on the analysis of data. The aim of this longitudinal study was to identify social, psychological, and physiological factors influencing the behaviour of 'normal' elderly.

The study began in 1955 and more than four years were required to accumulate the basic panel of 264 volunteers on whom baseline determinations were made. Subsequent to this period, examinations were made approximately every two years until 1972. Thereafter the remaining volunteers were examined on a yearly basis. The tenth longitudinal observations were completed in July, 1975.

Design and sample

A snowball technique was used to create a panel of volunteers. The volunteers had to indicate a willingness to participate in the research and to complete a two-day series of interviews and clinical examinations. The selected methodological issues of sampling and panel maintenance in this study have already been discussed in detail (Maddox, 1962). The author, a sociologist, and an early participant in the formulation of the study, argued that the nature of the study and commitment it demands from the subjects presents no feasible alternative to the use of volunteers. He cites the difficulty in persuading subjects living in the community to come into a clinic for single examination, much less for a series of examinations. This difficulty is accentuated with elderly subjects (Cobb, *et al.*, 1957).

The decision to use volunteer subjects necessarily limits generalization from the data. Statements would be limited to data concerning the relationship among factors in the ageing process. Random sampling, itself, is not without its problems. Maddox points out that non-participation rates in such studies are often so high as to produce a sample which is essentially the equivalent of a collection of volunteers.

TABLE 1.1. Distribution of the sample at round one

	Male	Female	Total
White	85	88	173
Black	41	50	91
Total	126	138	264

The panel of 264 volunteers was drawn to reflect the age, sex, ethnic, and socioeconomic characteristics of the older population in Durham, North Carolina. Volunteers were offered a free physical examination as an inducement to co-operate. Initially, the median age of panellists was 70 and they ranged in age from 60 to 94 years. Most panellists seem to have been motivated by the medical examination provided at no cost at periodic intervals. An equally important factor in maintaining the panel has been the opportunity for participants to obtain satisfying social recognition regularly. This recognition takes the form of greeting cards on special occasions, telephone contacts, and solicitous attention during the examination.

TABLE 1.2. A summary of longitudinal observations

Medical history (original and interim)	Laboratory studies
Physical examination	Urinalysis
Neurological examination	Blood morphology
Mental status	Blood chemistry
Depression and hypochondriasis	Serologic test for syphilis
Dermatological examination	Cholesterol
Opthalmological examination	Urea nitrogen
Visual fields	Medical summary
Acuity	Psychological data
Colour perception	Rorschach
Depth perception	Aspiration level (TAT)
Colour photographs	Wechsler Adult Intelligence Scale
Audiometry	Reaction time
Pure tone	Social history and information
Speech threshold	Retirement data
Electroencephalogram	Activities
Chest X-ray	Attitudes

For each panellist, a series of observations were collected which included 738 pieces of information. Of these, 336 were medical; 109 psychiatric or neurological; 109 psychological, and 234 social. A summary of observations is found in Table 1.2. A summary rating of physical functioning was developed.

The psychiatric observations focus on aspects of mental status including affect, recent and remote memory, orientation, intellectual function, anxiety, and hypochondriasis. Particular attention was awarded the assessment of mood and other associated symptoms of depression. Later sections will review selected psychiatric findings from the initial data and then present a longitudinal analysis of follow-up data to clarify further the course of the initial psychiatric observations.

The prevalence of mental illness in late life

Evidence from hospitalization rates and community surveys demonstrate clearly that older age groups have a substantial amount of mental illness (Kay *et al.*, 1964). Prevalence rates of 10–20 per cent have been suggested (Shepherd *et al.*, 1966). These high rates among the aged, coupled with the fact that an extremely high proportion (50 per cent) of hospital and nursing home beds in the United States are filled with psychiatrically ill elderly people underscore the seriousness of this problem for the elderly (Stotsky, 1973). Psychiatric services have been largely confined to the institutionalized elderly, who now comprise two per cent of the 65–74 year age group and seven per cent of the 75 and over age group (Redick *et al.*, 1973). The numbers of aged in need of psychiatric services are expected to increase with the size of the elderly population at risk. Such high rates of illness have understandably stimulated research into the nature of mental illness in the later years. However, very little longitudinal research has been done on psychiatric problems of older people living more or less adequately in the community. Most research has been cross-sectional in nature which would be a satisfactory method if psychiatric disorders were fixed and immutable entities. The longitudinal method certainly has its own deficiencies, but it is an invaluable technique for the study of process. The nature and course of psychiatric disorders is one such example of 'process'.

Depression

A common clinical syndrome encountered in old age is 'depression'. A review of our own inpatient experience with geriatric patients at Duke Hospital indicated that in over one-half of the admissions in this age group, depression was the major disorder (Gianturco, 1974). There is indirect evidence that rates of depression, among elderly males at least, increase after the age of 65. One very impressive statistic in this regard is the data on suicides in white males. The base rate for white males aged 15 to 24 is 7·4 per 100 000. This rate increases steadily with age, so that for the 65 to 74 age group, the rate is 45·5 (Resnik and Kantor, 1970).

Many of the psychiatric investigations into the initial panel data focused upon the problem of depression in old age. Evidence was uncovered that indicates that

TABLE 1.3. Prevalence of depression

Number	I	II	III	IV	V	VI	VII	VIII	IX	X
						Round				
Evaluated	264	174	136	110	89	87	48	37	19	16
Not evaluated	6	24	12	8	14	4	7	6	10	6
Died/dropped out		72	122	152	167	179	215	227	246	248
Rated depressed	55 (21%)	38 (22%)	39 (29%)	17 (15%)	18 (20%)	20 (23%)	7 (15%)	9 (24%)	3 (21%)	4 (25%)

depressive episodes increase in frequency and depth in the advanced years of life. In one of the early investigations (Busse *et al.*, 1955), the researchers found that elderly subjects were aware of more frequent and more annoying depressive periods than they had experienced earlier in life. The subjects reported that during such episodes they felt so discouraged, worried, and troubled that they often saw no reason to continue their existence. However, only a small number admitted entertaining suicidal ideas, although a larger percentage did state that during such depressive periods they would welcome a painless death.

The vast majority of the subjects were able to trace the onset of most of these depressive episodes to specific stimuli. Previous research by Busse *et al.* (1954), related these depressions of old age to the loss of self-esteem which results from the aged individual's inability to supply his needs or drives (loss of narcissistic supplies) or to defend himself against threats to his security. The pathologic mechanism of introjection, or the turning inward of hostile impulses which are unacceptable to the super ego, is relatively common in the depression of younger adults, but seldom present, to the same degree, in elderly people. Thus, the depressions of old age may be relatively 'guilt free', with self-accusatory tendencies absent. Since these early studies additional data on prevalence of depression has accumulated and in the next section we should like to present those findings.

Longitudinal evaluation of depression

Table 1.3 presents an overall statistical summary of the prevalence of depression during the entire course of the study to date. These data document the high likelihood of depression throughout. With one exception the proportion of people rated depressed remained remarkably constant at approximately 20–25 per cent. These data demonstrate that depression is exceedingly common in well functioning elderly people living in the community. This point is further emphasized in Table 1.4 which summarizes the data according to the number of times the panellists were seen prior to death or drop-out. Since the surviving panel has had ten periods of evaluation it was decided to condense the Table into five categories for which the proportion rated depressed was enumerated. This clearly demonstrates the increasing proportion rated depressed over time. The cumulative effect is such that by seven or eight periods of evaluation, only 30 per cent of the people remaining had no depressive episode; 40 per cent had at least one such episode and 30 per cent had

TABLE 1.4. Frequency of depression

Number of depressive episodes	Number of times evaluated					
	1–2	3–4	5–6	7–8	9–10	Total
0	84 (66%)	26 (48%)	20 (47%)	10 (30%)	3 (43%)	143
1	39 (31%)	16 (30%)	23 (30%)	13 (40%)	1 (14%)	82
2 +	4 (3%)	12 (22%)	10 (23%)	10 (30%)	3 (45%)	39
Total	127	54	43	33	7	264

two or more episodes. This longitudinal analysis of data demonstrates rather clearly that very few, even well functioning, elderly people escape depression. The legacy of a long life appears to be a confrontation and struggle with the value of living. The issue for older people may well be not just survival but meaningful and purposeful existence.

Old age has been described as a 'season of loss', and depressive reactions are responses to losses. The theme of loss is cited by a number of authors (Pfeiffer and Busse, 1973; Shock, 1962; Kreps, 1969; Heyman and Gianturco, 1973), to include inevitable declines in physical vigour, mental agility, income, loss of loved one, and finally one's own impending demise. The ubiquitous nature of loss in this time of life may be one factor to explain the high frequency of depression.

The high prevalence of depression in old age is apparently not confined to the United States which is a culture that does not treat its elderly in a kindly fashion (Palmore, 1975). In a particularly noteworthy cross-cultural study utilizing participants from many countries with different cultural traditions, an extremely high incidence of depression in the 65 and older group was found (Zung, 1972). Loss of self-esteem was the predominant depressive factor uncovered. This study corroborates our findings and demonstrates that regardless of cultural attitudes, depression is the price that has to be paid for the privilege of survival.

Recurrent nature of depression

Table 1.5 classifies people according to whether they were depressed or not at round one and then whether they returned at least once more during a following round. The Table also presents the frequency of depression during later rounds for these two groups. Thirty-one people who were depressed at round one and 163 who were not depressed at round one were examined at least once more. For the sake of clarity the data is condensed into those seen two or three times and those seen four or more times. Table 1.5 clearly demonstrates that while there is a high frequency of depression for both groups, those rated depressed at round one had a much higher recurrence rate of depressive episode in the later rounds. The recurrent nature of depression is illustrated since almost 90 per cent of those depressed at round one had at least one other depressive episode. One cannot help but wonder if such recurrences may not be prevented with proper intervention. The extremely high recurrence rate mandates a strategy not only of treatment but of prevention.

TABLE 1.5. Recurrence of depression

Round	Depressed	
	Yes	No
I	31	163
II–III	6–16 (38%)	17–71 (24%)
IV–X	13–15 (87%)	49–92 (53%)

Age

Table 1.6 presents a cross-sectional analysis of all the depression evaluations based on age. All the data, regardless of when collected, were categorized by subject age. The number of patients rated depressed and not depressed were grouped into age decades.

TABLE 1.6. Depression and age

Age	Not depressed	Depressed
60–69	145 (74%)	51 (26%)
70–79	403 (81%)	96 (19%)
80–89	208 (78%)	58 (22%)
90 +	14 (78%)	4 (22%)
Total	770 (79%)	209 (21%)

There appears to be no relationship between the proportion of people rated depressed and age category within the elderly group. This suggests that depressive episodes are based upon other factors rather than simple chronological age. This finding is in agreement with a previous study on round one data. This early study tested the effect of age on the incidence of depression (Dovenmuehle and McGough, 1965). Age differences within the elderly group were not significant for incidence of depression.

Health and depression

The technique of stepwise multiple regression analysis was used to examine the correlation between a number of different variables and episodes of depression. The initial analysis on first round data related depression to financial situation and physical condition. However, analysis of the subsequent data in the following rounds made clear that there exists a sex difference in these related variables. Repeated episodes of depression in women is significantly associated with their financial state whereas in men physical function is the most significant variable. These findings do not mean that other variables such as age, sex, race, marital status, nearness to death, and education are not important but that no consistent pattern of association can be ascertained. The finding that there is an association between depression and the older person's health status (i.e. declining physical function is positively related to increased incidence of depression) is not a new observation.

In another previous study it was found that depressed subjects had significantly more physical pathology than normals (Busse and Dovenmuehle, 1959). This suggests that decline in physical function increases the likelihood of depression. Physical pathology often disrupts mobility which can lead to social isolation. It also interrupts many other pursuits and activities which ordinarily contribute to self-esteem (Pfeiffer and Busse, 1973).

Nowlin (1974) analysed the relationship between depression and health in the longitudinal population over a ten-year period of observations. He found an association between depression and limitation of activity, and lower self health ratings, concern about health, higher systolic blood pressure, and more abnormal cardiovascular ratings. He speculated that 'poor health with its attendant discomforts and limitations may invoke the feeling state of depression'.

It is tempting to speculate why such sex differences exist. Certainly the elderly men in the study grew up to manhood in a culture where performance, either in work or athletics, was highly valued among men. Decrements in physical abilities would be viewed as a greater threat to self-esteem. Also men have shorter longevity than women and decrements in health may be viewed with greater fears about survival. Women, on the other hand, may worry about finances since they do have a longer life span to look forward to. Both men and women place a high premium on their independence and such factors as poverty and ill health usually mean that to survive the older person must become more dependent. This is a prospect that all older people view with intense distaste.

Organic brain syndrome

The elderly are particularly prone to organic brain syndrome. The extensive epidemiological survey of old age mental disorders in Newcastle upon Tyne (Kay *et al.*, 1964), estimated that 5·6 per cent of all the elderly over age 65 have chronic brain syndrome. The increasing duration of life among the elderly raises the prevalence of this group of disorders, necessitating society to make increasing commitment to provide for the care of such persons.

What symptoms constitute an organic brain syndrome has been well defined. According to the Diagnostic and Statistical Manual of the American Psychiatric Association (DSM-II) these symptoms include: impairment of orientation; impairment of memory; impairment of intellect; impairment of judgment; and lability and shallowness of affect.

The technique of assessment for organic brain syndrome was the standard mental status examination. This method frequently revealed a discrepancy between the elderly person's subjective self-assessment of his abilities and the more objective 'tests'. Many elderly subjects will admit to memory decline or intellectual impairment, yet perform adequately on tests of these mental functions. For example, during the first series of observations, 26 per cent of the volunteers admitted to poor memory for recent events; six per cent said they had poor memory for remote events; and ten per cent considered themselves to have had a decline in intellectual function; yet, only 14 per cent of the volunteers had evidence of disorientation and just three per cent demonstrated confusion. This discrepancy may reflect the insensitivity of our 'tests' which were unable to discriminate the fine differences appreciated by the volunteers. Clearly our subjects complained more extensively about declining abilities than the objective testing could demonstrate.

Prevalence of organic brain syndrome

Table 1.7 presents a round by round tabulation of the prevalence of dementia in the community volunteers. Clinically, 26 per cent of these volunteers were judged to have a mild organic brain syndrome and three per cent were considered to have objective signs and symptoms severe enough to be diagnosed as organic brain syndrome of the moderate to severe extent in the first round. This latter figure is more similar to the prevalence of organic brain syndrome reported in the epidemiological literature (Kay et al., 1964).

TABLE 1.7. Prevalence of organic brain syndrome

Round		No disability	Mild disability	Moderate to severe disability
I	(n = 263)	71%	26%	3%
II	(n = 180)	78%	17%	4%
III	(n = 129)	79%	18%	4%
IV	(n = 106)	62%	33%	8%
V	(n = 89)	63%	29%	8%
VI	(n = 81)	60%	31%	9%
VII	(n = 45)	48%	46%	3%
VIII	(n = 37)	62%	30%	8%
IX	(n = 15)	77%	23%	
X	(n = 16)	50%	38%	12%

In eight of these impaired volunteers, there was an associated psychosis predominantly organic in origin (Busse et al., 1960). These eight subjects all had recent and remote memory defects. The finding that these subjects were maintaining a satisfactory adjustment in the community despite psychotic illness leads one to conclude that other factors which permit a person to maintain a satisfactory community role need investigation.

The proportion rated mildly disabled (less than 20 per cent disability) varies from a low of 17 per cent to a high of 46 per cent. There is a tendency, though not marked, for the percentage in this category to increase. This tendency is more apparent in the moderate to severe category of disability (greater than 20 per cent) where the increase is from three per cent in round one to twelve per cent in round ten. These figures indicate that dementia of varying degree is quite common among elderly persons living in the community. Since the average age of the sample gradually increases with each successive round, (average age 80 by round nine), there is a gradual increase in the prevalence of this disorder in our sample, though not so dramatic as to be obvious.

Course of organic brain syndrome

There were 76 people (26 per cent of total) who were rated impaired at round one. In the next round 32 of them were rated impaired. Sixteen were rated unimpaired, 18 were dead and ten did not return. Subsequent analysis revealed that there were an additional 39 subjects in the later rounds who received an impaired rating which were followed by unimpaired ratings. These findings reveal the high variability of the course of organic brain syndrome. Unlike the popular conception of this disorder as a fixed entity, organic brain symptoms are frequently characterized by varying degrees of remission and exacerbation.

This finding can be confirmed by clinical observation of impaired elderly individuals in institutions. Dramatic improvement of mental state can often be achieved when underlying physical problems are adequately treated, or the patient's milieu is altered so as to receive a satisfactory degree of interaction with others. Such programmes as reality orientation, occupational therapy, recreation, singing, and physical therapy are highly desirable alternatives to the usual practice of allowing brain syndrome patients to vegetate. Findings from the Duke Longitudinal Study of Aging support 'the activity theory' that the most satisfying pattern of aging is to maintain as high a level of physical, mental, and social activity as is consistent with the person's life style (Palmore, 1970).

Longitudinal analysis of all subjects revealed that 154 (59 per cent) of the subjects eventually received a rating of organic brain syndrome with disability prior to death or drop-out. This is a much higher frequency than any cross-sectional analysis of single round data on dementia (see Table 1.7). An episode of brain impairment can therefore be expected to occur in roughly half the elderly who survive their 65 birthday. This is a rather frightening prospect, particularly for the elderly, many of whom report they fear dependence and disability far more than death. Long term survival can be viewed as both a blessing and a burden. Life is sweet and enjoyable but the end of the road becomes increasingly fraught with perils of the worst sort.

Fortunately, despite the high prevalence of this syndrome in this sample, only one subject required hospitalization in a psychiatric institution. So, despite impaired brain function and the associated intellectual deterioration, these subjects were capable of living a community life. Clearly many factors other than brain impairment play a role in determining whether a person with organic brain syndrome may remain in the community. Adaptation to these changes as well as the stresses from the environment may play a crucial part in the psychological deterioration often associated with these disorders. Such complications as depression, regression, agitation, and paranoid symptoms may well be more determined by the person's personality and environment than the brain impairment. For this reason the clinical syndrome associated with this disorder has been described as a sociopsychosomatic disorder (Wang and Busse, 1970). The following example is illustrative of this view.

After the death of her husband, a 79 year old white female lived with her eldest daughter for two years. Over the last few months she manifested confusion, nocturnal restlessness, agitation, incontinence, and delusions of poisoning. The daughter was extremely devoted to her mother and painfully attentive to all her needs. She never displayed anger, irritation, or resentment over her enormous sacrifices of ministering to this elderly woman who required almost constant nursing. During her mother's hospitalization, the daughter refused to even consider placement and instead planned to take her mother home as soon as improvement could be effected. With the staff, the mother remained calm and collected, and even occasionally manifested periods of lucidity. She ate and slept well and was no longer incontinent. However, whenever the daughter visited, her behaviour quickly deteriorated. She would become visibly agitated, clutch at the bed rails and try to raise herself stating, 'I've got to get out of here'. Thereafter, she would spend a restless night and would wet the bed. The contrast in the woman's behaviour was most striking.

Related factors

The factors contributing to organic brain syndrome have been previously studied in this population of subjects (Busse and Wang, 1974). Many factors were found to be related including decompensated heart disease, low socioeconomic status, and inactivity. Mild elevation of blood pressure was positively correlated with preserved brain function. The authors speculated that the relatively high blood pressure may be necessary to maintain sufficient blood supply to the brain for adequate cerebral function.

There was no relationship found between the amount of social contacts and organic brain syndrome. This finding was confirmed by the San Francisco project (Lowenthal, 1965) where it was concluded that isolation may well be a consequence rather than a factor in organic mental illness of old age.

Much remains to be uncovered by future research. Promising research directions include studies of cerebral blood flow, neurochemical studies, effects of new drugs on mentation, and neuropathologic investigations.

EEG

An exhaustive review of the EEG findings during the longitudinal studies has recently appeared (Busse et al., 1973). The major findings are summarized as follows.

Progressive slowing of the dominant α frequency and the appearance of slow waves in the θ or δ range is characteristically found in organic brain syndrome (Wang and Busse, 1970). Furthermore, there is a highly positive correlation between EEG frequency and cerebral oxygen consumption or blood flow (Obrist et al., 1963). Focal abnormalities of the EEG, largely over the left temporal areas of the brain, have been repeatedly observed in a high percentage of apparently healthy older people (Busse et al., 1955). The origin of these foci and their significance is unclear. In any event the occurrence of focal EEG abnormalities have little or no prognostic or diagnostic value among the aged (Busse and Obrist, 1963), and are not related to transient ischemic attacks. An incidental finding, the significance of which is unclear, is that fast activity and temporal foci are much more common in elderly women than men.

Hypochondriasis

The neurotic disorder of hypochondriasis is defined by the Diagnostic and Statistical

Manual of the American Psychiatric Association (DSM-II) as 'a condition dominated by preoccupation with the body and with fear of presumed diseases of various organs. The fears persist despite reassurance and there are no losses or distortion of function'. This condition is encountered in many elderly people attending medical clinics and this pattern of illness frequently precipitates a request for psychiatric consultation. Such patients may be considered to have a psychotic disturbance if the hypochondriacal symptoms are of delusional quality or the functional incapacity is total.

Hypochondriacal reactions do occur in elderly people and interfere with their health and happiness. This category of reaction is usually considered to be a neurosis.

Psychoneurotic reactions were found to be extremely common among the volunteers. This group was found to differ markedly from the other elderly subjects (Busse et al., 1960). They had a much lower evaluation of their own happiness and contentment, fewer friends and fewer wholesome attitudes toward their friends. The authors pointed out that the vast majority of the severe neurotics were in fact hypochondriacs. Despite no difference in overall physical function, they showed a marked difference in health attitudes (a clear result of their neurotic concern with body functions). There was no discernible difference between the neurotic and normal groups in work attitudes. They argue that this may be an important finding since a socially acceptable attitude toward work may be one of the major factors in maintaining an individual in the community in spite of neurotic processes. These elderly differed from typical hypochondriacs in that they did not seek excessive medical attention.

The psychodynamics of hypochondriasis are considered to be a defensive operation against the loss of self-esteem by withdrawal from other persons and concentration on the self; the hypochondriacal symptoms may be viewed by the person as punishment and atonement for feelings of hostility; the symptom can serve the purpose of shifting anxiety away from interpersonal issues to less threatening concern with bodily function (Busse, 1975).

TABLE 1.8. Hypochondriasis

| Round II | Round I | | | |
	None	Mild	Moderate	Severe
None	103	14	5	2
Mild	8	16	13	8
Moderate	1	1	1	4
Severe	0	0	0	0

The longitudinal study has provided an opportunity to observe hypochondriacal tendencies in elderly subjects residing in the community. For the first six rounds of observations a global rating of hypochondriasis was made after the psychiatric interview. In the initial round 33 per cent were found to have hypochondriasis. This percentage declined over the course of the study to roughly half the initial percentage. Table 1.8 compares the ratings over the initial two rounds. The general direction is for hypochondriasis to remit. For example, the 14 people who were rated in the severe category initially, all received improved ratings in round two; 18 people rated moderate initially, improved. These findings indicate that hypochondriasis is not the constant tendency so frequently described in the literature as a life long pattern. Rather it appears to remit or exacerbate depending on numerous factors but most noticeably the phenomenon of depression. Statistical analysis revealed that there was no consistent pattern of association between hypochondriasis and sex, race, physical health, nearness to death, or financial condition. Depression appeared to be the only consistent associated variable. This is not surprising in view of the similarity in the psychodynamics of both disorders. The phenomenon of 'depressive equivalent reactions' are well known to clinicians—painful symptoms which express the person's underlying depressive state—yet conceal it since energy and attention are devoted elsewhere. This ailment is another example where hypochoncriacal tendencies and depressive reactions are interwoven in the same fabric.

Longitudinal analysis of the first six rounds of data reveal that ultimately over half the survivors receive a rating of hypochondriasis.

Terminal drop

The terminal drop hypothesis states that a decline in intellectual performance may be associated with impending mortality and that this decline may be detected several years prior to the death of the person (Kleemeir, 1962). This suggests that factors such as health deterioration are associated with intellectual decline rather than 'normal ageing'. Since the diagnosis of organic brain syndrome implies intellectual deterioration, an analysis of the survival patterns in the longitudinal study should provide a test of this hypothesis.

The test was completely negative and refutes the hypothesis of terminal drop. Statistical analysis of survival patterns after the onset of organic brain syndrome, controlled for age and sex, showed no substantive differences with other volunteers. The average survival time was roughly 120 months for both groups. This is a rather surprising result in view of the previously reported positive relationship between physical disability, particularly of the cardiovascular system, and organic brain syndrome (Busse and Wang, 1974). Several plausible explanations are possible. First, the number of volunteers in the study may have been too small to reveal the difference in mortality. Sound actuarial statistics are usually compiled from the mortality of thousands of persons. Secondly, it is entirely possible that the genuine difference in physical disability between the 'organic' and the 'non-organic' groups may have been too minimal to exert a deleterious impact on mortality. Thirdly, since the organically disabled volunteers remained in the community until their terminal illness, the favourable impact of supportive relationships and continued familiar physical surroundings may have been considerable.

The findings do agree with the previous report from the Duke longitudinal data. Utilizing Wechsler adult intelligence scores and distance from death (Eisdorfer and Wilkie, 1973), the authors found no significant correlation between IQ and death.

These findings are at variance with the Newcastle studies (Savage et al., 1973).

They found significant differences in mortality between community residents with organic brain syndrome and other elderly.

The terminal drop hypothesis has been recently reviewed by Siegler (1975). She conceptualized two components: the relationship between the level of cognitive performance with survival, and between the changes in cognitive performance and death. She cited five longitudinal studies in support of the hypothesis and three against. Clearly, the issue has not been resolved, but the author concludes that the concept has 'stimulated sharper evaluation of the effects of health status and correlates of survival into studies of cognitive functioning'.

Attitudes toward death

The final section of this chapter concludes with a review of the Duke longitudinal reports on age and death. Since attitudes toward death may have an effect on psychological adjustment in the later years, an exploration of the feelings and thoughts associated with physical death, either of the self or loved ones, is an entirely appropriate topic in a psychiatric paper.

During the first round of the study two questions about death were included. The responses contradicted the idea that most aged persons are fearful about death (Jeffers et al., 1961). Only ten per cent of the volunteers admitted to fear of death; 35 per cent said they had no fear; and the rest said no but with qualifications suggesting ambivalent feelings. Factors associated with no fear of death include frequent bible reading, belief in a future life, religious conceptions of death, less feelings of depression, and higher IQ scores. Seventy-seven per cent of the volunteers were convinced that a personal life after death exists. Very few denied such a belief outright (only two per cent).

A related investigation reported on the frequency of death thoughts in the volunteers (Jeffers and Verwoerdt, 1966). Most of the volunteers believed that people their age thought about death more often than in earlier years. Forty-two per cent stated that they thought of death daily, and seven per cent stated that death thoughts were a constant accompaniment to their life. Almost half thought that the enjoyment of life was marred by death thoughts. During the interviews the majority of subjects were extremely willing to speak about death and most did so with an accepting comfortable affect.

These findings can lead one to speculate that denial is an important mechanism for dealing with the anxiety associated with death. The mental mechanism of denial is therefore an important adaptive mechanism in personality adjustment associated with old age. This concept has recently received strong support from Becker (1975) who argues that 'terror of death is natural and is present in everyone'—the 'worm at the core' of man's pretensions to happiness. Man must therefore use defensive mechanisms—denial systems or else face overwhelming anxiety.

A discussion of death would not be complete without some comments on bereavement. Actually, while widowhood is one of the most significant events in life, the repercussions over time for the older person are not as dramatic as might be expected. Studies of the elderly persons who have been widowed during the course of the longitudinal study conclude that the normal elderly adapt to the death of the spouse in fashion characterized by (a) emotional stability supported by deep religious faith, and (b) relatively few life changes. Several women did show a trend in the direction of increased depressed feelings, and lowered feelings of usefulness (Heyman and Gianturco, 1973).

In addition to the factors enumerated previously the reasonable adaptation to bereavement in the elderly may be accounted for by 'death rehearsal'. This is an important psychologic mechanism, enabling people to prepare intellectually and emotionally for bereavement. The opportunity for death rehearsal permits gradual identification with widowhood role before the actual event. Such events as decline in health, a lingering illness, deaths of contemporaries, making of wills, reading the obituary column and frequent thoughts of death permit rehearsal at a leisurely pace.

References

Becker, E. (1975) *The Denial of death*, New York, Macmillan.

Busse, E. W., Barnes, R.H., and Silverman, A.J. (1954) 'Studies of the processes of aging: Factors that influence the psyche of elderly persons', *Am. J. Psychiat.*, **110**, 897–903.

Busse, E.W., Barnes, R.H., Silverman, A.J., *et al.* (1955) 'Studies of the processes of aging: X. The strengths and weaknesses of psychic functioning in the aged', *Am. J. Psychiat.*, **111**, 896–901.

Busse, E.W., and Dovenmuehle, R.H. (1959) 'Neurotic symptoms and predisposition in aging people', Paper read at the *Annual Orthopsychiatric Meeting*, San Francisco, April, 1959.

Busse, E.W., Dovenmuehle, R.H., and Brown, R.G. (1960) 'Psychoneurotic reactions in the aged', *Geriatrics*, **15**, 97–105.

Busse, E.W., and Obrist, W.D. (1963) 'Significance of focal electroencephalographic changes in the elderly', *Postgrad. Med.*, **34**, 179–182.

Busse, E.W., Schlagenhauff, R.E., and Corney, A.L. (1973) 'Round table discussion: EEG in gerontology moderated by Everts, W.H.' *Clin. Electroenceph.*, **4**, 152–263.

Busse, E.W., and Wang, H.S. (1974) 'The multiple factors contributing to dementia in old age', in *Normal aging II*, (Ed. E. Palmore), Durham, North Carolina, Duke University Press, pp. 151–159.

Busse, E.W. (1975) 'Aging and psychiatric diseases of late life', in *American Handbook of Psychiatry IV*, (Ed. M.F. Reiser) New York, Basic Books, pp. 67–89.

Cobb, S., King, S., and Chen, E. (1957) 'Differences between respondents and non-respondents in a morbidity survey involving clinical examination', *J. Chron. Dis.*, **6**, 95–108.

Dovenmuehle, R.H., and McGough, W.E. (1965) 'Aging, culture, and affect: Predisposing factors', *Internat. J. Soc. Psychiat.*, **11**, 19.

Eisdorfer, C., and Wilkie, F. (1973) 'Intellectual change with advanced age', in *Intellectual functioning in adults*, (Ed. L.F. Jarvik, C. Eisdorfer, and J.E. Blum) New York, Springfield.

Gianturco, D.T. (1974) 'The older psychiatric patient at Duke Hospital', in *Drug issues in geropsychiatry*, (Ed. W.E. Fann and G.L. Maddox) Baltimore, Williams and Wilkins, pp. 73–76.

Heyman, D.K., and Gianturco, D.T. (1973) 'Long-term adaptation by the elderly to bereavement', *J. Gerontology*, **28**, 359–362.

Jeffers, F.C., Nichols, C.R., and Eisdorfer, C. (1961) 'Attitudes of older persons towards death', *J. Gerontology*, **16**, 53–56.

Jeffers, F.C., and Verwoerdt, A. (1966) 'Factors associated with the frequency of death thoughts in elderly community volunteers', *Proc. VII Internat. Congr. Gerontology*, pp. 149–152.

Kay, D.W.K., Beamish, P., and Roth, M. (1964) 'Old age mental disorders in Newcastle upon Tyne, Part I: A study of prevalence', *Br. J. Psychiat.*, **110**, 146–158.

Kleemeier, R.W. (1962) 'Intellectual changes in the senium', *Proc. Am. Stat. Assoc.*, **1**, 290–295.

Kreps, J.M. (1969) 'Economics of retirement', (1969) in *Behavior and adaptation in late life*, (Ed. E.W. Busse and E. Pfeiffer) Boston, Little, Brown.

Lowenthal, M.F. (1965) 'Antecedents of isolation and mental illness in old age', *Arch. Gen. Psychiat.*, **12**, 245–250.

Maddox, G.L. (1962) 'Selected methodological issues', *Proc. Soc. Stat. Sec. Am. Stat. Assoc.*, **1962**, 280–285.

Nowlin, J. (1974) 'Depression and health', in *Normal aging II*, (Ed. E. Palmore) Durham, North Carolina, Duke University Press, pp. 168–172.

Obrist, W.D., Sokoloff, L., Lassen, N.A., *et al.* (1963) 'Relation of EEG to cerebral blood flow and metabolism in old age', *Elecetroenceph. Clin. Neurophysiol.*, **15**, 610–619.

Palmore, E. (Ed.) (1970) *Normal aging*, Durham, North Carolina, Duke University Press.

Palmore, E. (1975) *The honorable elders*, Durham, North Carolina, Duke University Press.

Pfeiffer, E., and Busse, E.W. (1973) 'Affective disorders', in *Mental illness in later life*, (Ed. E.W. Busse and E. Pfeiffer) Washington, D.C., American Psychiatric Association, pp. 107–144.

Redick, R.W., Kramer, M., and Taube, C.A. (1973) 'Epidemiology of mental illness and utilization of psychiatric facilities among older persons', in *Mental illness in later life*, Ed. E.W. Busse and E. Pfeiffer, Washington D.C. American Psychiatric Association, pp. 199–232.

Resnik, H.L.P., and Kantor, J.M. (1970) 'Suicide and aging', *J. Am. Geriat. Soc.*, **7**, 152–158.

Savage, R.D., Britton, P.G., Bolton, N. *et al.* (1973) *Intellectual function in the aged*, London, Methuen.

Shepherd, M., Cooper, B., Brown, A.C. *et al.* (1966) *Psychiatric illness in general practice*, London, Oxford University Press, pp. 1–21.

Shock, N.W. (1962) 'The physiology of aging', *Sci. American*, **206**, 100–110.

Siegler, I.C. (1975) 'The terminal drop hypothesis: factor artifact, *Exp. Aging Res.*, **1**, 169–185.

Stotsky, B.A. (1973) 'Extended care and institutional care: Current trends, methods, and experience', in *Mental illness in later life* (Ed. E.W. Busse and E. Pfeiffer) Washington, DC, American Psychiatric Association, pp. 167–178.

Wang, H.S., and Busse, E.W. (1970) 'Dementia in old age', in *Dementia* (Ed. C.E. Wells) Philadelphia, F.A. Davis, pp. 151–162.

✗ Zung, W.W.K. (1972) 'How normal is depression?', *Psychosomatics*, **13**, 174–178.

2

APPROACHES TO THE STUDY OF PERSONALITY CHANGES IN ADULT LIFE AND OLD AGE

D.B. Bromley

Introduction: contrasting approaches to the study of personality

The term 'personality' is sometimes used in psychology as a convenient and familiar label for a variety of characteristics such as 'neuroticism', 'life satisfaction', 'anxiety', or 'morale'—operationally defined and measured by standardized tests.

The term is also used in a vague, general way to refer to an ill defined area of psychology dealing broadly with (a) a range of behavioural differences between individuals and with (b) the study of persons as individual cases.

It would take too long to describe the history and current state of personality study—see Mischel (1976) for a comprehensive introduction. In any event personality in adult life and old age has not been well researched, and Mischel, for example, devotes less than one page to this aspect of personality study. There are several reasons which might explain the relative neglect of personality in middle age and later life. First, like other aspects of human ageing, it has not attracted many research investigators—see Neugarten (1968a, 1970, 1973). Second, most if not all the more widely used tests of personality were developed and standardized on samples of juveniles and young adults, reflecting, presumably, the pressures for assessment and guidance arising from education, employment, and mental health problems within these age groups. There has been some, but not much, effort devoted to extending these psychometric methods into middle age and old age, (see, for example, Savage, 1971; Pearson, Swenson, and Rome, 1965; Bolton and Savage, 1971; Rosen and Neugarten, 1960; Atchley, 1976) perhaps because the socioeconomic pressures for psychological research and its applications are correspondingly less. The growing numbers of patients in need of psychogeriatric services, however, can be expected to bring similar pressures for applied research on personality in later life. Third, some of the more interesting investigations into personal adjustment in adult life have used methods that (probably for the wrong reasons) are not favoured in mainstream personality research. I refer to case methods, incorporating interviews, life history data, direct observation, introspection, and projective (phantasy) tests, (for example, see Britton and Britton, 1972; White, 1975; Reichard, Livson, and Peterson, 1962; Pressey and Pressey, 1966). These and similar studies have avoided the danger of studying older persons *in vitro*, as it were (as if their personal qualities could be usefully ascertained without reference to their circumstances) and instead have tried to study them *in vivo* (not unlike the way one might study organisms in their natural habitat, but using methods appropriate to human subjects).

There have been a number of general metapsychological discussions of the problem of personality change through the lifespan (see, Livson, 1973; Looft, 1973). Longitudinal studies have provided a variety of relatively unrelated empirical findings, and they illustrate the difficulties of research into personality change with age (see, for example, Granick and Patterson, 1971; Angleitner, 1974; Haan and Day, 1974; Maddox and Douglas, 1974; Mass and Kuypers, 1975). Schwartz (1975) has provided a selected bibliography on psychological adjustment to ageing; Botwinick (1973), Bromley (1974), and Kalish (1975) describe the effects of ageing on personality in its wider context.

There are, no doubt, many other reasons why the study of personality in adult life has been neglected, but among the more important must be those concerned with methodological difficulties (see, for example, Gilmore, 1972). These difficulties include: statistical sampling and the validity of assessment methods for normative studies, the measurement of change in longitudinal studies, the confusing effects of secular trends, and so on. The whole problem of methodology in studies of ageing is discussed in Bromley (1974, pp. 330–371).

If one regards the study of personality as the psychometric study of 'individual differences' in traits, motives, values, and the like, then one is likely to see the remedy for our current ignorance about normal personality changes with age in the more systematic application of psychometric methods to representative adult age groups, on a longitudinal or cross-sectional basis. Indeed, as we have seen, this is the strategy that some research workers have adopted (see, for example, Heron and Chown, 1967; Pearson, Swenson, and Rome, 1965).

However, if one adopts a different point of view, and thinks of personality study in terms of the systematic study of 'individual cases', then one is likely to see the remedy for current difficulties in the application of case study methods to selected groups, namely, those which promise to reveal facts of some significance for the theory and practice of gerontology (see, for example, Townsend and Tunstall (1968) for a study of isolation and desolation).

Holt (1969) has written an elementary account of personality assessment which shows how psychometric methods can be incorporated into the study of individual cases.

The first approach uses normative psychometric methods and is well known, being the traditional and main stream of psychological research in personality. It could be argued that the psychometric approach is not very useful in dealing with individual cases, especially in psychogeriatrics. Personality tests may have little predictive or diagnostic value, and may be inappropriate for the investigation required. This is not to say, however, that such tests cannot be developed. The second approach uses 'quasijudicial' methods (see later) in the intensive study of selected individual cases; it attracts a small minority of research workers in psychology, but has close links historically and functionally with psychopathology and social work. In the author's opinion, case study methodology has been grossly neglected, to the detriment of personality study in general and to the study of late life personality changes in particular. For this reason, the main emphasis in this chapter is on processes and methods in the study of individual cases, with special reference, of course, to changes in personality and adjustment in adult life and old age. The more direct method of using testimony from competent and credible witnesses, e.g. a family member, by means of ordinary language and 'common sense' has been overshadowed by the less direct method of psychometric assessment.

The main conclusion towards which the arguments in this chapter are directed is simply that psychological case studies provide an appropriate scientific method for the study of personality changes in later life. By making systematic comparisons and contrasts between individual cases (and by engaging in the necessary kinds of conceptual analysis) it should be possible to establish a sort of psychological 'case law' in terms of which our knowledge and management of problems of adjustment in later life can be made more coherent and useful.

In one respect, therefore, this chapter is an exercise in counter propaganda. It is an attempt to promote the psychological study of 'individual cases' (rather than the traditional psychometric study of 'individual differences') as the primary method in the study of personality.

The thread running through the various sections is the attempt to show that our understanding of personality change in later life depends upon subjective psychological processes (within the investigator) as well as upon objective behavioural facts of human ageing.

There are two important reasons for choosing to study individual cases. The first is that it forces us to recognize that human behaviour is a function of the person and the situation he is in. This simple idea is sometimes lost in the psychometric approach to personality; it can be remembered easily by the following mnemonic equation: $P_i \times S_j \rightarrow B_{ij}$. Which means that an individual person, P_i, when faced with a given situation, S_j, will tend to behave in a particular way, B_{ij}. For example, a particular psychiatrist P_i who is favourably disposed towards Freudian psychology, when faced with a scientific report (S_j) describing poor results for a study of the effects of psychoanalytic treatment, tends (B_{ij}) to find fault with the report. This apparently simple example hides some extraordinary difficult conceptual and methodological problems in the study of personality. For example, how does one identify and assess the covert but relatively enduring dispositions (traits, motives, values, etc.) which appear to regulate the person's reactions across a wide range of situations? How does one identify and assess the covert but relatively short lived states of mind (feelings, moods, expectations, etc.) which appear to modify the person's reactions to any particular situation? How does one identify and assess which particular features or circumstances of a person's environment are psychologically (and behaviourally) significant for that particular person, i.e. those that influence his behaviour?

In general, since one can observe only overt actions, how can one justify one's conclusions about a person's covert qualities, states of mind, psychological defences, and so on? That is to say, how can one establish connections between the 'core characteristics' of personality and the 'peripheral characteristics' accessible to observation? (See Maddi, 1972.)

The relevance of these basic questions to the study of personality changes in adult life is easy to see, and we shall be looking at them more closely in this and subsequent sections.

The second important reason for choosing to study 'personality' through individual cases is that we come to recognize the importance of common sense and ordinary language in understanding other people even at a professional level and, indeed, in understanding ourselves (see Bromley, 1977). In view of the scientific status and the advanced technology of the psychometric approach to personality, this second reason requires some justification. Briefly, the history of personality study has been an attempt to develop objective measures of, i.e. normative standards for, traits (stable dispositions) by means of adjective check lists, rating scales, questionnaires and so on (see, for example, Cattell 1965, Gough 1965, Fiske 1971). The items in these various measures can be traced back to their origins in common sense and ordinary language. Over many years of test construction and elaboration, they have been refined and consolidated into various named tests with generally accepted levels of reliability, validity, and utility, e.g. Cattell's 16PF test, the MMPI, Gough's adjective check list, the California psychological inventory (see Lake, Miles, and Earle, 1973). These and other personality tests have been used for a variety of research and practical purposes, and it was claimed that they had revealed a great deal about the structure, dynamics, and correlates of personality characteristics. In recent years, however, these claims have been questioned (see Mischel, 1968). Briefly, Mischel argues that personality tests and ratings do not reveal stable traits, i.e. underlying psychological dispositions, and that their inter-relationships reveal more about the structure of common sense and ordinary language than they do about the realities of personality. For example, the intercorrelations between observers' ratings for familiar stimulus persons are similar to the intercorrelations between their ratings for strangers. Mischel has been criticized for overstating the case against personality tests and the concept of 'disposition' (trait) in personality study, and for understating the case against 'situationism'. Situationism attempts to account for human behaviour in terms of the shaping and controlling effects of environmental influences, i.e. rewards and punishments. I shall try to steer a course between 'situationism' and 'dispositionism', a course sometimes referred to as 'interactionism'. The differing emphases of these three approaches can be symbolized as follows:

$$
\begin{array}{llll}
\text{Dispositionism:} & \underline{\mathbf{P}} & \times & \text{S} \longrightarrow \text{B} \\
\text{Situationism:} & \text{P} & \times & \underline{\text{S}} \longrightarrow \text{B} \\
\text{Interactionism:} & \text{P} & \underline{\times} & \text{S} \longrightarrow \text{B}
\end{array}
$$

These mnemonic equations remind us that we are concerned with questions about 'persons in situations' and with the deep conceptual and methodological issues that lie behind them.

The criticisms that have been made of the psychometric approach to personality have been associated, in part, with the development of what is variously known as 'person perception', 'impression formation', 'social cognition', and 'understanding others'. This branch of psychology is closely related to the traditional study of personality in that it is concerned with what occurs in the mind of an observer when he is assessing another person. It drawn our attention to the fact that 'personality lies in the mind of the beholder'. This is a sobering thought, but by no means an unfamiliar one in scientific research. The problem is to disentangle the assumptions and ideas which guide our search for knowledge about other people from the tests and empirical observations by means of which we validate (or invalidate) our expectations.

A discussion, in the next section, of the relevance of person perception (or social cognition) to the study of personality in adult life and old age illustrates some of the concepts, methods, and findings to which I have alluded.

One's 'personality' can be described in terms of the consistencies and regularities which 'characterize' one's behaviour in a wide range of situations and over a reasonably long period of life. However, one's personality can also be described by any general fact that identifies one and distinguishes one from any other person. One's 'personality type' is defined by a fairly arbitrary characteristic or set of characteristics which one shares with others of the same class or type, the possession of which distinguishes one from those who do not have that characteristic or set of characteristics, e.g. 'extraverted', 'schizoid', 'authoritarian'.

The notion of 'personality change', therefore, presents something of a metapsychological puzzle, and in practice one uses this term either to refer to a drastic reorganization of the person's behaviour characteristics, e.g. in senile psychosis, or to refer to a relatively minor shift in one or more characteristic, e.g. increased depression, decreased anxiety, greater social participation. The major personality changes occur in the context of psychopathology, and so fall outside the scope of this chapter. The minor personality changes are interesting in their own way, but are of little practical significance in psychiatry, nursing and social work, unless, of course, they can be identified as sensitive indicators of the effects of treatment or as the precursors of more serious disorders. The problem here is to reliably determine which personality changes are psychologically significant and to distinguish them from the many random and irrelevant minor changes that occur over time.

The so called 'intrinsic' and 'pathological' effects of physical ageing on personality are sometimes difficult to distinguish from those effects which may arise as a consequence of disuse of functions, e.g. poor memory, social isolation, e.g. autism, and institutionalization, e.g. apathy.

Some studies, e.g. Neugarten (1968), Butler (1963), have suggested that more attention should be paid to the 'inner life' (i.e. the reflective awareness of thoughts, feelings, and desires) in middle aged and older people, since one's inner life may become more active and more important as one's mobility and social involvement decrease. Of particular importance is the individual's use, throughout adult and old age, of reminiscence and life review in reconstructing his life history, and, therefore, reconstructing his self concept. It might be possible, for example, to use psychological counselling to systematize a patient's reminiscences and thereby reinforce his sense of personal identity and his orientation to others.

The 'inner experience' of middle age has several interesting implications for personality change, for example with regard to the effects of time perspective, i.e. the growing awareness of how little time is left, and with regard to self–other comparisons in relation to self esteem (see Bromley, 1974, pp. 250–3).

One might have supposed that the substantial changes in appearance, in experience, in health and in functional capacity over the adult years would bring about substantial changes in the self concept (especially the 'body image'), and in 'personality' as assessed by objective methods. In fact, the evidence, such as it is, seems to reveal no such substantial changes for the average adult; common sense observation suggests that the essential features of the self concept particularly are resistant to change, in much the same way perhaps, as our impressions of other people are resistant to change. We focus on the important dispositional continuities or 'invariances' in ourselves and others, and ignore or de-emphasize the relatively superficial characteristics which change over time, attributing them, perhaps, to circumstances.

Part of the explanation for this apparent lack of personality change with age is that the various changes which do take place in the biological basis of our behaviour (and the changes which occur in our surrounding circumstances) are gradual, although cumulative and inter-related, so that there is usually plenty of time for the individual to prepare for, compensate for, and adapt to, these changes. In retrospect it may seem to us that we have changed little in our adult years.

Perhaps we tend to think of 'personality change' as something that is forced upon an individual through external stress or unavoidable psychological factors. Where the individual actively prepares for later life, compensates for the effects of ageing and continues to adapt to his new circumstances, we tend to regard him as relatively autonomous, self organizing and therefore unchanged.

Forming impressions of old people

It is common knowledge that, for many younger people, the physical appearance and behaviour of some aged persons, especially deteriorated patients in departments of geriatric medicine, have 'aversive' properties. (In saying this, of course, we must remember the very wide range of differences between elderly individuals in their physical appearance and behaviour.) The effects of these characteristics may be aggravated by the unpleasant features of an institutional environment. Aged people, in other words, are often perceived as unpleasant and frightening or, at best, as pitiful. Fear, disgust, rejection, and avoidance are not uncommon reactions. How can we explain such reactions? Why is it that aged impaired people do not usually evoke tenderness, pleasure, and a desire for physical proximity (as do children)?

One can speculate about the answers to these questions, but there is little in the way of evidence other than that available to common sense. Let us consider some of the ways in which ageing seems to change a person's expressive behaviour and the way he communicates with other people in non-verbal ways. This will help us to understand why first impressions of personality are important in social perception and social interaction, although they are by no means the most important aspect of the process of understanding other people. Our impression of a person we know reasonably well is a complex and fairly stable system of ideas and feelings; it guides our behaviour in relation to that person and can be expressed in the ordinary language of everyday life.

A little reflection on everyday social experience tells us that we are constantly communicating with other people, and they with us. We employ postures, gestures, facial expressions, and eye contacts, usually without much if any deliberation, to indicate interest or lack of interest, dominance or submission, agreement or disagreement, surprise, amusement, disbelief, and so on. We use a variety of accepted social signalling devices to acknowledge them, to greet them or to say goodbye, to pointedly ignore them, to foster or maintain intimacy or to keep one's distance, to suggest time is short or to say farewell. We use gestures and other forms of expressive behaviour to refer (by pointing), to emphasize (by thumping), and to demonstrate (by going through the motions). In addition, we can nod or shake our head, wink, smile, grimace, frown, glance, raise our eyebrows, wrinkle our nostrils, tap our fingers, and so on, through the whole gamut of non-verbal behaviour.

In all these non-verbal ways, then, we can attract another person's attention and hold it, or ward off his (or her) attention, or guide that person's behaviour and alter his state of mind, e.g. induce surprise or anxiety. These are a few of the many outward forms of behaviour by means of which we influence people and are influenced by them, and on the basis of which we form impressions of their personality, and they form their impressions of us. (I must add, if only in parenthesis, that the kinds of expressive behaviour and social signalling I have briefly listed occur not only in everyday life but also in psychiatric and social work settings with the elderly, and may affect the assessment made by professional workers without their being aware of the subtleties of the process.)

What happens to this sort of expressive behaviour and social signalling in later life, and how might it affect the impression we form of an aged person? Bearing in mind the wide range of individual differences, perhaps the most obvious change in later life is a decrease in mobility, responsiveness, and spontaniety as regards posture, gesture, facial expression, and eye contact. This relative lack of expressive behaviour and non-verbal signalling leads to difficulties in social interaction. Young people may feel that they are 'not getting through' to elderly people, and may not be able to register the psychological significance of their different and much reduced expressive behaviour. In addition, the elderly person may be unable to keep pace with the rapidity of the young person's expressive behaviour and social signals, and may also be unable to communicate his own lack of comprehension. The young person may be impatient with the aged person's slowness and lack of response, he gets too little

24

'feedback' and is left puzzled, wondering whether he has communicated successfully or not.

It is well known that the normal effects of ageing lead to some impairment in mental speed and in the so called 'fluid' intellectual abilities (see Bromley, 1974, pp. 178–210). Such effects are bound to lead to changes in 'personality', in the sense of altering the person's self concept, and his modes of adjustment to his environment. For example, as regards social interaction, the old person's slower mental reactions, poorer perceptual and cognitive processes, poorer attention, and so on, must reduce his sensitivity to social signals. Moreover, if social habits and expectations have become entrenched this may make him unreceptive to helpful people whose unfamiliar appearance and styles of behaviour do not provide him with the sorts of social signals he understands, e.g. those with different ethnic origins and cultural backgrounds.

As we have seen, non-verbal signalling is a relatively primitive, but nevertheless effective, means of communicating in social encounters of a basic sort. It is used in attracting and holding another person's welcomed attention, e.g. a nurse or a visitor, as well as in warding off or terminating encounters with unwelcome people. Some research has been done on sex differences and social class differences in 'bodily communication' as it is sometimes called (see Argyle, 1975). The effects of adult age changes in social perception and communication, however, have not been well researched. Nardi (1973) has discussed person perception research in ageing from a rather different point of view from that taken in this section.

The apparent reduction in later life in strength of feelings and desires would also help to explain the reduction in frequency, amplitude and diversity of expressive behaviour. Moreover, poorer vision and hearing—the main distance receptors—bring an increased dependence on closer, even direct physical, contact, e.g. holding hands, touching and stroking, passive movement (to guide action or attention), for communication purposes, and a decreased ability to 'signal at a distance' (see Figure 2.1).

The elderly person's reduced physical mobility and sitting posture drastically reduce the range of his expressive actions and non-verbal signals. In particular, the elderly person has less freedom to choose his interpersonal distance and position relative to others in social encounters. The study of this aspect of non-verbal interaction is called 'proxemics' or 'spatial behaviour' (see, Argyle, 1975; Sommer, 1970; Lawton, 1970; Scheflen and Scheflen, 1972). It deals with the relationships (distances, orientations, postures) of people in social encounters, and their psychological significance, for example, in courtship, conflict, and negotiation. We have seen that the elderly person seems to have less control over social encounters.

It is not very surprising that the younger person's aversion to the elderly, coupled with the elderly person's greatly reduced capacity for social interaction and communication, should lead to the segregation of the aged, especially the elderly infirm. Such segregation may also be fostered by implicit prejudice in the 'social distance' and 'professional detachment' characteristic of some staff in institutions. Segregation and downgrading are also fostered by separate and different living arrangements and other facilities, by a tendency on the part of some people to adopt

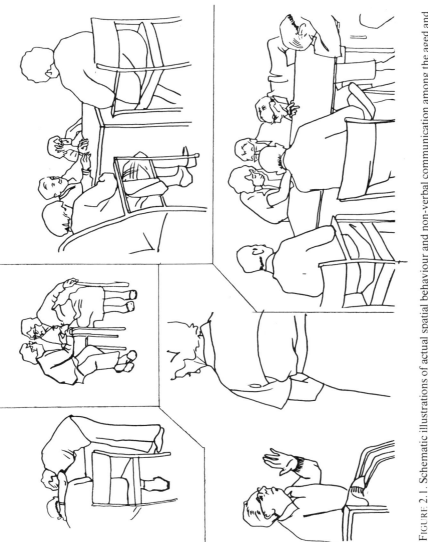

FIGURE 2.1. Schematic illustrations of actual spatial behaviour and non-verbal communication among the aged and staff of residential institutions

condescending and paternalistic attitudes, and even, unfortunately, a tendency to enforce dependency, to tease, to deny privacy, and to curtail personal freedom.

A person who is engaged in the daily care of patients in departments of geriatric medicine, a nurse for example, faces difficult problems of social interaction. The work often calls for close intimate contact, for example with regard to feeding, physical support, and care of the body. But, as we have seen, patients not infrequently exhibit unpleasant physical and behavioural characteristics, which may lead to aversion, rejection and neglect. Indeed the 'personality impressions' formed by a nurse of patients will contain, as salient features, these negative attributes. It has been suggested that in order to reinforce the nurse's sympathy with, understanding of, and concern for, such patients (and to offset what I shall call, with some hesitation, a 'natural' aversion) there should be material and social incentives, as well as special training to cultivate scientific understanding, favourable attitudes, and congruent values. This would also follow for community workers and family members who work with the aged. There are, however, risks in offering material incentives for looking after the aged. First, the rewards for specific behaviour may not improve behaviour in general and, second, the work may come to be seen as even more unattractive (otherwise why should it be specially rewarded?). The rewards, whatever they are, should somehow reflect the value of the social role.

This brief statement of the less desirable aspects of social interaction between the elderly infirm and younger people may seem harsh, but it helps us to appreciate the relevance of person perception (social cognition) to the study of personal adjustment in adult life and old age. Perhaps the most disturbing possibility is that younger adults may not actually perceive patients as 'persons' in the accepted sense, especially if they are grossly impaired mentally and behaviourally, and physically repulsive. If we tend, unwittingly, not to see patients as 'persons', i.e as human beings, then we shall be inclined to treat them as 'objects', and to dehumanize them in ways that are only too familiar.

One reason for our changed perception of some geriatric patients (and aged normal persons) is that they have lost a number of highly valued human attributes: an acceptable physical appearance, behavioural competence, autonomy, expressive spontaneity and social responsiveness. In the crude cost—benefit terms of social exchange theory, which provides an interesting and useful framework for the analysis of human social relationships, the elderly patient may seem to have little or nothing to give in exchange for any services rendered by a younger person, and he is costly for the younger person to interact with. Thus, in general, social interaction with an aged person gives rise to a poor 'cost—benefit ratio' for a young person, especially in comparison with the available alternatives. In addition, social interaction between young and old tends to be reduced or less compatible because of demographic and social factors, e.g. geographical separation and differences in values and attitudes. Such factors may contribute to the gradual development of misunderstandings, disagreements and rejection within families.

One interesting and important aspect of social interaction concerns what animal ethologists would call 'bonding behaviour'. This refers to the process whereby two or more individuals provide close intimate services, usually multilaterally but sometimes unilaterally. For example, in the case of elderly people, this could be mutual help in dressing and grooming or help given by a nurse in feeding or locomotion. In ordinary daily life, such mutual servicing fosters positive mutual regard—with its various social and psychological benefits. In old age, however, illness and death reduce the availability of same-age companions, and the adverse cost–benefit ratio referred to above reduces the availability of younger people willing and able to provide intimate services. Lack of physical contact, and lack of emotional stimulation and intimate personal services, however, are likely to aggravate the adverse effects of social isolation, contributing, perhaps to depression and apathy. The notion of 'desolation' (Townsend and Tunstall, 1968) is perhaps relevant to this issue.

The aversive properties of old age, which became particularly potent in the appearance and behaviour of mentally impaired geriatric patients, may lead, as we have seen, to rejection and neglect on the part of young people, unless inhibited by countervailing feelings of affection and pity. Thus, we do not have to look far for an explanation of the social neglect of the aged, for the frequent identification of elderly women as witches in former times, for the lack of interest in geriatric medicine on the part of medical students and nurses. Aged, infirm people have lost some essential stimulus properties as human beings. Hence, we tend not to see them quite as persons like ourselves. They seem to fall outside the range of the concepts and methods we normally employ in perceiving and understanding other adults. A similar failure of understanding may also occur in respect of 'social deviants' and 'insane people' and others, e.g. strange or primitive people, whose appearance and behaviour cannot be assimilated to our 'normal' frame of reference for understanding human nature. Prejudice, social stereotyping and segregation provide means for dealing with the aged and other people who fall outside our normal range of understanding; the other alternative is to acquire new knowledge of a scientific and professional sort which will extend the range of common sense so that it can account for, and help us to come to terms with, the worst features of old age.

The aversive and unpleasant characteristics of old age depend to some extent on cultural and historical factors. Anthropologists have described some societies in which the aged make a useful contribution through their special knowledge and skills, and so are held in high esteem. Esteem may also derive from the high status achieved by the aged in areas such as ritual, religion, and magic. However, people in such societies may hold a very different conception of human nature from that which is prevalent in modern industrial society. In such simple societies, the spirits of dead ancestors are thought to exercise an important controlling influence, by supernatural means, on the welfare of the living; and, moreover, a belief in reincarnation blurs the distinction between the living and the dead, and between self and others (Shelton, 1969). It is not surprising therefore that in societies like these, the aged might be treated with considerable reverence in spite of their aversive appearance and behaviour. The early history of man's beliefs about ageing and death shows the power of animism in primitive thinking (Bromley, 1974, pp. 33–50).

The foregoing account argues that our perception of aged people is rooted in our basic conception of human nature, which is, of course, a social construction, i.e.

relative to our culture and historical period. The origins of our implicit assumptions about human behaviour have not yet been fully explored by psychologists, but it seems likely that they lie in the infant's early encounters and experiences with other people. The infant's world is largely a human world; so that it is not surprising if, at first, he attributes human characteristics—thoughts, feelings, desires, and actions— to physical objects and events. He has to learn that some aspects of his environment are not alive and do not have thoughts, feelings, and desires, and are not autonomous and reactive in the way that human beings are. It takes several years for the average child to shed animistic forms of thought, and indeed he may never shed them if the society to which he belongs incorporates animistic beliefs in its social construction of reality, e.g. in religion and magic. Religious and moral codes incorporate prescriptions and practices designed to inculcate respect for and obedience to the elders in society, especially parents and grandparents. In view of current research into the evolution of altruism, one might speculate that some kinds of social evolutionary pressures are at work in intergenerational relationships—some favouring positive regard for the aged, some favouring neglect and rejection.

An aged person who has lost some of the essential stimulus attributes of human beings constitutes a strange sort of 'stimulus person', and the ordinary observer must experience some ambivalence, at least until he has had extensive experience with the elderly and has developed a more comprehensive conception of human nature, i.e. one that enables him to recognize humanity and personal identity in spite of change and decay.

I have argued that there may be a fundamental difference between the way we perceive a 'normal' adult and the way we perceive an impaired geriatric patient or 'aged' person. The segregation of the aged from other members of society emphasizes the difference, in at least two ways. Firstly, because we then encounter them less often, and the contrast with the 'normal' human adult, when it occurs, is even more marked. Secondly because segregation itself 'labels' the aged and assigns them the status of 'discarded person'; people, as it were, who cannot be fully human, otherwise they would not have been discarded, and therefore who need not be treated as such.

Thus, one important and interesting aspect of personality change in old age is the change that occurs in the observer's perception and understanding when he considers aged people as compared with 'normal' younger people. Personality, I have said, lies in the eye of the beholder.

One of the factors affecting social interaction between elderly residents in institutions is their tendency to identify an object or place, e.g. a chair, as belonging to them personally (Sommer, 1970). This sort of 'territoriality' and personal ownership, however, is by no means confined to the elderly but can be found in all age groups. In fact, it reflects an important aspect of personality, namely, the tendency to extend one's conception of oneself so as to incorporate a wide range of objects and other persons. Similarly, we tend to think of another's personality not merely in terms of his physical existence and behaviour but also in terms of what that other person regards as part of his self. Thus one's house, spouse, child, diary, pen, even political party, have what Allport (1955) called 'ownership peculiarity'.

We feel that they belong to us personally, that they are part of one's self and we have strong feelings about them. Thus, even our perception of physical objects is, at times, imbued with feelings and meanings associated with the personality of their owners.

The impression we form of another person, i.e. our assessment of his personality, usually includes some account of the more important objects and relationships over which that person's sense of ownership and influence extends, and in relation to which his adjustment is assessed. At least, this is so if we use common sense and ordinary language, since formal methods of psychometric personality assessment omit this important facet of personality.

In a residential home or hospital for the elderly, the sense of personal ownership, the sense of the self extending into the world of physical objects, affects a patient's attitude towards his immediate personal belongings, his bed, his room, his chair, or place in the lounge. It is likely that the presence of familiar personalized objects in his environment helps the aged person to maintain a sense of personal identity. Failure to establish individualized environments for patients, e.g. a personal laundry service, may lead to confusion and conflict because of competing claims for the personal use of communal resources. This failure hinders the establishment of personal routines and hinders the development of self-fulfilling activities beyond those associated with personal security.

This aspect of personal adjustment in later life highlights yet another facet of person perception. Elderly infirm people become dependent upon others, and are obliged to accept restrictions on their freedom and intrusions into their privacy, e.g. by having to share communal facilities in a residential home, and by being unable to 'ward off' unwelcome people because of impaired social communication. Our society values personal freedom, privacy, and autonomy; but the elderly lose these characteristics, to some extent at least, and hence are held in lower esteem. Moreover, the elderly themselves, in so far as they are capable of recognizing the limitations on their behaviour, will hold themselves in lower esteem, because they are likely to share the values and attributes prevalent in the larger community to which they belong. In our kind of society, 'bourgeois' values and attitudes are unsuited to communal living and probably contribute to feelings of inadequacy and frustration among the elderly in residential homes or hospitals. Fortunately, there is much that can be done to reconcile individual and communal interests given trained staff and reasonable financial resources.

The establishment of individualized, i.e. 'personalized', environments for the elderly, even in a communal setting, is by no means difficult. Indeed, nowadays it could be regarded rather as a basic requirement. Research has been carried out on individualized assessment and treatment programmes (Brody et al., 1971) in an attempt to eliminate 'excess disability', i.e. functional incapacity greater than that warranted by objective assessment of the patient's physical and mental condition.

An interesting incidental finding from research into individualized treatment for geriatric patients is that the patients who seem to derive most benefit are those with rather selfish and aggressive personalities (Kleban et al., 1975). We are thus reminded that the decline with age in emotional expressiveness and social responsiveness makes it more difficult to establish or to maintain friendly relationships, and that a person who is in any case characteristically phlegmatic, melancholy, shy, or introverted will be further disadvantaged in comparison with the more active, extraverted, assertive, stimulus seeking individual. Perhaps the value of self-seeking in old age is that it delays the loss of dominance, and the respect and benefits that accompany dominance in social relationships.

Although I have described a sorry state of affairs concerning the effects of old age on social behaviour and concerning the socially undesirable impression created by the aged stimulus person, yet it would be wrong to adopt a nihilistic attitude and suppose that little or nothing could be done to improve this state of affairs. The first and most obvious step would be to educate the public in general, and geriatric staff in particular, in order to achieve a better scientific understanding of, and better professional methods for dealing with, the aged. The second step would be to train staff to be more sensitive to, or have greater empathy with, the aged. Exercises in role playing have been shown to be useful in improving nurses' attitudes towards, and understanding of, dying patients. Role playing might be useful in sensitizing staff to the importance of non-verbal communication. The third step would be to give more attention to grooming and cosmetic care for the elderly to help improve their physical appearance; this might have beneficial side effects on the patients' self-esteem, and increase the opportunity for 'bonding' through the exchange of intimate personal services. The fourth step would be to develop social skills training, as a sort of preventive treatment, for the aged; the aims would be to improve both verbal and non-verbal communication, and to increase the extent of self-help (in the interests of autonomy, privacy, and self-esteem). Behaviour modification procedures would undoubtedly be effective in shaping the behaviour of elderly patients towards self-help, mutual help, and greater expressiveness, although it is likely that the beneficial effects would soon wear off in the absence of a sustained treatment programme. Perhaps the most important step would be to reduce the institutional and management factors which appear to foster the undesirable characteristics we have identified, poor physical condition and appearance, apathy, deviant behaviour.

Adaptive behaviour: strategies and tactics

The previous section dealt with the immediate or initial impressions of personality formed in response to physical appearance, expressive behaviour and social signals. Such impressions are largely implicit (non-verbal) and often have a strong emotional tone (like or dislike). However, since we encounter some people repeatedly and establish strong personal relationships with a few, there is ample opportunity to develop deeper and more extensive 'impressions' of other people. We are able to integrate a wide range of experiences and information relevant to understanding these other people, we can reflect on these ideas and organize them rationally, and eventually we can express them in ordinary language in the form of opinions or even quite lengthy personality descriptions. Common sense and ordinary language thus provide the normal framework for understanding other people (and ourselves); scientific knowlege and professional skills build on this infrastructure or 'tacit understanding' of human nature.

There appears to be no evidence that the normal processes of ageing produce sudden or substantial changes in personality, i.e. in the individual's identity, traits, values and so on. There are, of course, many gradual and cumulative effects, e.g. changes in intelligence, shifts of interest, alterations in appearance and in physical health and mobility. These are well-known and do not present serious problems as far as personality assessment is concerned. Their relevance to personality study lies in the alterations they bring about in the relationships between the person and his environment. Changes in vision and physical stamina, for example, lead to changes in occupational activities and leisure pursuits; changes in material assets and social roles (associated with living arrangements and marital status) lead to changes in the activities of daily living and to the adoption of age-appropriate values and attitudes.

Thus the overall effects of normal ageing could be described as 'adaptive' in the sense that the individual gradually evolves a lifestyle or overall strategy of adjustment by means of which he 'comes to terms' with life. The conditions governing this changing lifestyle include the satisfactions and dissatisfactions (rewards and punishments) experienced by the individual in his encounters with other people and in relation to his material environment. Some forms of conduct are reinforced whereas other forms are not. The person's intentions are governed by his feelings and expectations, by pleasure and hope, or by pain and disappointment. In this way the person's patterns of adjustment throughout life are shaped, in part, by the contingencies of reinforcement operating in his environment.

There is obviously a considerable amount of variation and chance in the way our patterns of adaptive behaviour evolve during the lifespan as a whole. Human responses vary somewhat from one occasion to another even for what seems to be the 'same' situation. Spontaneous variations can lead, in a trial and error fashion or in a creative problem solving fashion, to the emergence of new forms of conduct. Also, human beings frequently engage in exploratory and 'stimulus seeking' activities, by means of which they extend the range of their behaviour and the scope of their environment or 'habitat', e.g. in making new friends, and in adopting different foods, styles of dress, and leisure activities.

The environment does not offer unlimited scope for individual action, nor does the individual have at his disposal an unlimited range of personal resources. The individual is, to some extent, a creature of circumstance bound by the conditions which nature and society impose on him. He is also bound by the physical and psychological characteristics of his own nature, characteristics which, as we have seen, change gradually and cumulatively with age in all kinds of ways, and affect his inclinations and the outcome of his attempts to satisfy these inclinations.

A convenient and useful way of describing and analysing the gradual evolution of a person's adaptation to his environment over the long period of adult life and old age is to distinguish (a) the relatively short term, even brief, 'tactical adjustments' to particular situations as and when they arise, from (b) the relatively long term 'strategic adaptations' to the familiar, well defined, regular circumstances which constitute the individual's 'normal' environment. (The environment, of course, includes other people.)

The term 'personality' can be used to refer to those stable patterns of adjustment which make up the individual's long term strategic adaptations. Thus, in the classical study by Reichard *et al.* (1962), five fairly distinct strategies of adjustment were identified, making it possible to classify aged people according to their personality type as 'constructive', 'dependent', 'hostile', 'self-hating', or 'defensive'. This work is well known and needs no elaboration here; a similar set of strategies has been described by Neugarten (1973).

The term 'personality' can also be used to refer to the person's basic psychophysiological dispositions, e.g. his outgoingness, aggressiveness, and quickness, which seem to direct and limit his behaviour, and to enable him, with experience, to acquire adaptive skills and routines.

Personal adjustment, in the sense of evolving an effective long term adaptation to one's environment seems to demand at least three basic achievements: the resolution of conflicts (both within the person, and between him and his environment), the fulfilment of his potential, and the elimination of inconsistencies and contradictions in his behaviour and experience. These are the so called 'core characteristics' in human nature (Maddi, 1972). We cannot deal with this interesting concept here, except to say that these 'core characteristics' persist into later life and express themselves in a variety of ways, e.g. in the conflict between autonomy and dependency or in the conflict with the younger generation, in the attempt to fulfil social obligations and personal aims, and in the processes of life review and reminiscence associated with the attempt to make sense of the story of one's life (Butler, 1963).

The discussion so far confirms the importance of the 'interactionist' approach to personality symbolized by the mnemonic equation $P_i \times S_j \rightarrow B_{ij}$. It also confirms the importance of ecological and evolutionary concepts in the analysis of personality change in adult life. We can think of the individual person as occupying an 'ecological niche', i.e. as having established a place for himself in the world and in relation to other people which enables him to live a particular style of life. From time to time, because of age changes in his physical and psychological make-up, and because of changes in his environment which are outside his control, e.g. technological innovations, accidents, political events, he feels the need to evolve new ways of coming to terms with life because the old ways are no longer sufficiently satisfying. In addition, from time to time, through his own efforts or through chance he is provided with opportunities to improve and extend his 'ecological niche', e.g. by marriage (or divorce), by a change of employment, by finding new friends or leisure activities. At other times, in other ways, his behaviour is constrained and frustrated.

In this section so far, we have dealt in rather general terms with the conditions governing the normal range of adaptations required in adult life and old age. This account needs to be qualified in two ways. In the first place, it does not follow that a normal adult will necessarily evolve the best lifestyle available. On the contrary, it could be argued that most adults and old people fail to maximize their potential and fail to seek out the most congenial and rewarding environments. Some people get locked into a comparatively unrewarding style of life without realizing what other possibilities life holds. Other individuals evolve singularly unrewarding and maladjusted, e.g. neurotic, lifestyles, for reasons which lie in the individual's life history.

The notion of cost–benefit analysis, to which we have referred in another context, provides a useful conceptual framework for describing and comparing different lifestyles. For example, the process of psychological counselling, e.g. marital and retirement counselling, or rehabilitation counselling, incorporates an attempt to get individuals to re-examine their hopes and fears, their satisfactions and dissatisfactions, so that they can weigh the pros and cons (the benefits and costs) of alternative courses of conduct and alternative environments. The general aim is to help the individual to establish a physical and social environment, a 'personal habitat', that is more congenial and rewarding (less stressful and less damaging) than the one he currently occupies. An essential point to remember is that success in counselling depends not only on changing the person's dispositions and behaviour, but also on changing his circumstances and improving the balance of costs and benefits which help to change or maintain new patterns of adjustment.

In the second place, as we have seen, personal adjustment in adult life sometimes calls for tactical adjustments to unforeseen circumstances, i.e. adjustments which cannot be made by recourse to familiar and habitual reactions. The main point of a 'strategy' of adjustment is to minimize unforeseen problems and to facilitate the achievement and maintenance of long term rewards by means of actions designed to prevent, to circumvent, or to cope with the various problems and obstacles that are expected to arise.

Among the more important sorts of tactical adjustment in adult life are those associated with what have been called 'psychosocial transitions' (Neugarten, 1970; Parkes, 1971) e.g. bereavement, illness, retirement. One of the most striking features of adulthood and old age is the unpredictability of life events. Whereas the juvenile period is characterized by a relatively orderly and systematic programme of developmental stages, carefully nurtured in a regular sequence of domestic, educational, and social settings, the adult period is characterized by a relatively disorderly and unsystematic series of breakdowns which interact to produce diverse and cumulative impairments of functional capacity, often in the absence of remedial and supportive settings, consider, for example, physical disability and isolation, depression and suicide.

An adult's environment is normally arranged in such a way as to minimize stresses and to avoid pushing the individual close to the limits of his functional capacity. However, other people form a major part of the individual's 'personal habitat'; so that, in later life particularly, there are unpredictable changes in his physical and psychological capacities—brought about by disease and damage, and equally unpredictable changes in the physical and psychological capacities of other people upon whom his personal adjustment depends. Thus, the ageing individual is constantly having to readjust his changing capacities and inclinations to changes in his environment, especially his social environment. These readjustments are initially 'tactical adjustments', in the sense that the individual cannot put into operation an effective prearranged course of action (having had little or no experience of such problems); so he has to resort to short term measures which reflect his basic psychological resources, e.g. optimism, intelligence, confidence in people, and his weaknesses, e.g. dependency, jealousy, casualness.

The distinction between 'long term strategies' and 'short term tactics' in the analysis of adult personality and adjustment is not unlike the distinction between 'crystallized abilities' and 'fluid abilities' in the study of adult intelligence (Bromley, 1974, pp. 178–210). Long term strategies and crystallized abilities are the products of experience; they are largely acquired forms of knowledge, disposition and skill, of a general sort, which enable the individual to deal quickly and effectively, i.e. routinely, with a range of familiar and recurrent situations. Short term tactics and fluid abilities, on the other hand, largely reflect natural endowment, i.e. native intellectual capacity, temperament (emotional make-up), and fundamental human needs. They comprise the individual's basic psychological resources and provide the initial means whereby he learns to cope with and to explore his environment (and, subsequently, to acquire strategies and skills).

The psychosocial transitions of adult life and old age provide good evidence relevant to the description and analysis of personality. The way the person copes with a transition (his tactical adjustment) reveals his basic psychophysiological resources and make-up, i.e. his basic personality. The sort of new long term strategy of adjustment (lifestyle) he evolves to cope with his changed circumstances reveals other aspects of his personality, such as his habits and daily activities, his social relationships, his sources of satisfaction, and his orientation towards the future.

Before we move on to consider a systematic framework for the description and analysis of personality in adult life and old age (including a method for the assessment of individual cases), let us consider the relevance of the discussion so far to psychopathology and social work. Serious abnormalities of personality arising from organic or functional disorders are, by definition, outside the range of common sense and ordinary language, and outside the scope of our analysis. But, in fact, many of the maladjustments of adult life and old age arise as a consequence of relatively normal psychophysiological impairments and common sorts of environmental stress (Lowenthal and Chiriboga, 1973).

The 'personality changes' in such disorders can often be described in terms of a breakdown in the individual's strategies of adjustment caused by psychophysiological impairments, and stresses arising from his social and physical environment. In other words, the person's 'ecological niche'—his 'personal habitat'—is no longer satisfactory; he is under immediate psychological pressure to make some kind of tactical and temporary adjustment to the transitional situation until he is able to evolve an adaptive longer term strategy to the new conditions of life, as in retirement, bereavement or disability.

The implications of this analysis for psychiatry and social work are obvious. First, preparatory education and training are needed, so that people are not completely unprepared for the stresses, transitions and restrictions of later life. Such preparatory education has been developed in respect of retirement, but is still in a rudimentary stage as regards, for example, the menopause, bereavement, mid- and later-life illness, and chronic infirmity. It is apparent, for example, that many patients undergo medical treatment, surgery for example, without adequate information and guidance on the physical and psychological consequences of treatment.

Second, individualized assessment and counselling could be used not only to remedy the 'excess disabilities' of patients in residential care, but also to improve the 'ecological niche' of elderly normal people in the community. This would require a substantial investment in social and psychological treatment; although greater use might be made of television, radio, and other media, to educate people, to influence the behaviour of the elderly, and to increase self help and mutual aid. Various voluntary and statutory bodies are fully aware of how much more might be done to improve the lifestyle of the aged as a class, and are actively engaged in social welfare services. The problem, as we have seen, is not only to retard and remedy disabilities arising from within the ageing person but also to improve the supportive framework of his social and physical environment. As we have seen, his personal adjustment (B_{ij}) is a function of the interaction between the aged person himself (P_i) and his circumstances (S_j).

A framework for the description and analysis of individual cases

For reasons which are not immediately obvious, the study of individual cases has not been vigorously pursued as a legitimate scientific method in psychology, in spite of the revolutionary, though now debatable, ideas arising from its use in psychoanalysis. Paradoxically, the same revolutionary ideas forestalled the development of systematic case methods appropriate to social work.

I have argued that the traditional psychometric methods have not yet been sufficiently developed to deal with the psychological problems of ageing, and that they may not be appropriate anyway. Individual case study methods, by comparison, seem to offer more immediate practical benefits and possibly longer term theoretical advances in understanding personality and adjustment.

The neglect of systematic case study methods in psychology and social work, coupled with an excessive concern for quantification and laboratory controls in personality study, means that we have almost lost sight of the fact that judicial and natural history methods are capable of dealing rationally with empirical data and are respectable scientific procedures.

The essential feature of a psychological case study is that it focuses upon the 'person in a situation'; it does not attempt to study the personality as a whole (an impossibility) but to study this or that specific problem of personal adjustment. The case study method, in other words, is a way of solving problems—human problems.

Formulating the human problem correctly is important because it directs the investigator's subsequent thoughts and actions. For example, what at first looks like a problem of disturbed sleep may prove to be basically a problem of interpersonal conflict. Systematic inquiry should lead eventually to a sensible provisional account of what the problem is, how it arose, and what remedies seem feasible. It is usual for the simple, obvious explanations to be tested first; if they prove to be false, then the investigator must collect further evidence relevant to his hypothesis about the nature of the problem. Problems of personal adjustment in late life, of course, are likely to be multifaceted, and so require more extensive inquiries and a longer follow-up than might be needed for problems earlier in life.

A brief life history is usually incorporated in a case study as background material to help show how the problem arose and to indicate possible interpretations and remedies. But the main emphasis in a case study is on the contemporary situation. The difficulty of researching and of writing a condensed account of an aged person's life history must be dealt with rather than evaded, otherwise important lines of inquiry may be missed (Jarvik *et al.*, 1973).

By using his imagination and experience, and by testing his reasoning against the relevant empirical evidence, an investigator can gradually narrow down the number of possible interpretations of the individual's predicament. Eventually, if things go well, he is left with one interpretation which fits all of the evidence and is contradicted by none.

In a psychological case study, the investigator is free to search for relevant evidence wherever he can find it—he is not restricted to a particular personality test. Nor is he, in his reasoning, restricted to any particular theory of personality. Sources of evidence include: the testimony of the person under investigation; direct and indirect observation by the investigator and his assistants; personal documents and official records; medical reports and the results of psychological tests or ratings; the testimony of friends, family and others directly acquainted with the subject of the inquiry. The psychological case study, therefore, is a 'quasi-judicial' method of investigation (modelled on the procedures of jurisprudence and historiography) tailored to meet the requirements for a scientific method. It is obvious that the psychological case study is analogous to the medical (especially psychiatric) case study; the underlying logic is the same. The difference is simply that the psychological case study does not yet have the benefit of an agreed systematic conceptual framework in terms of which evidence (data) can be organized and interpreted.

How can a case study describe and analyse personality? A person can be described in terms of a number of facets or aspects of his existence. I shall list a number of the main facets—a more detailed account can be found in Bromley (1977). The list is not exhaustive; even so, a particular case study may not require information under all of these headings, only information which is relevant to understanding and dealing with the person's problem need be included.

Aspects of personality which might be described in a psychological case study are as follows:

life history and present predicament; critical incidents; material circumstances; routine activities of daily living; physical and mental health; psychological attributes, i.e. general traits, specific traits, expressive manner, motives, abilities and attainments, attitudes, moral values, self concept; social attributes, i.e. social roles, family relationships, friendships and loyalties, interpersonal attitudes and reactions, comparisons with other people; relationships with the investigator(s) and informant(s); ethical status (where appropriate); prospects for the future.

The information contained in a case study does not take the form of a simple list or catalogue of facts, but is organized into a series of related arguments, so that a 'pattern of meaning' is imposed on the evidence. One's conclusions and recommendations, of course, have to be suitably qualified, depending upon the nature of the evidence and the psychological theories one is using again. See Bromley (1977) for a fuller account of the logic of psychological case studies.

It is of interest to note that the sorts of information listed above are typically found in personality descriptions written by adults in the ordinary language of daily life and based on common sense notions of human nature. Even the language of personality descriptions used by professional psychiatrists, psychologists, and social workers differs only in degree, if at all, from that of common sense and ordinary language. Even the technical language of the psychopathologist and psychometrician depends, fundamentally, on the infrastructure of common sense and ordinary language.

It is also of interest to note that the language of personality descriptions is much the same for self descriptions and descriptions of others. That is, we tend to think of ourselves in much the same way as we think about others. The self concept, therefore, is easily integrated into a personality description or case study. The normal effects of ageing on the self concept during adult life have not been intensively researched—see Bromley (1974, pp. 240–1) for brief comments on this topic in the context of a general review of personality and adjustment in middle age and old age. The author is currently investigating normal age differences in the self concept using the methods of content analysis on self descriptions in ordinary language.

It has been suggested that exhaustive case studies are not necessary in psychological and social work with the aged because the resources for individualized treatment or management are not available. According to this line of argument, all one needs to do is to establish simple criteria to determine whether an aged person is or is not likely to benefit from one or other of a limited range of available resources. Although this may state the realities of the present situation, it is not relevant to questions about personality changes in late life, except in the very narrowest sense. Nevertheless, we must ask whether there is any advantage to be gained by studying personality in late life in this narrow sense. This brings us back to the question of whether there are any significant effects of age on personality characteristics which can be 'measured' by means of valid and reliable tests. I have argued (Bromley, 1974, pp. 330–71) that there are serious methodological problems in standardizing tests for older age groups, and that it is doubtful whether tests developed for younger adults measure equivalent functions in older adults. However, this does not affect the argument that if a personality characteristic, e.g. depressive mood, extraversion, optimism, can be shown to discriminate well between those who will benefit from an available treatment and those who will not, then there are grounds for trying to develop adult norms and standards for psychological screening tests—on the analogy of medical screening tests. However, just as one would not confuse a medical screening test with a systematic and comprehensive medical assessment, so one must not confuse a psychological screening test with a systematic personality appraisal. There is no personality test which provides a comprehensive personality appraisal—such an appraisal is possible only by means of a rigorous and systematic case study, in which personality tests may play a small part, or no part at all.

I have argued that the psychological case study promises to be a useful method in dealing with the practical problems arising as a consequence of adverse personality changes in later life. It might be asked whether any theoretical advances are likely to ensue from the more extensive use of this method. I think the answer would be 'yes', because one could develop a systematic body of 'case law'—based on comparisons and contrasts between individual cases—which would constitute the empirical generalizations and rational principles required for an objective (inter-subjective) science of personality study. Indeed such 'case law' is already in existence, mostly informally and unsystematically, in many areas of professional work with people, including psychogeriatrics.

Acknowledgements

I wish to thank Dr A.D.M. Davies, Dr A.J.J. Gilmore, Dr P. Ley, Miss M. Marshall, and Dr C. Powell, whose comments on an earlier draft I have tried to take account of in this final draft. Naturally, I must be held responsible for any misconceptions, factual errors and blemishes that remain. My thanks are due to Mrs D. Southern, Miss E. McTear, Mrs M. Thompson, and Miss M. Thomas for typing the manuscript, and to Miss P. Snaith and my wife Roma for the schematic illustrations in Figure 2.1.

References

Allport, G.W. (1955) *Becoming: basic considerations for a science of personality*, New Haven, Connecticut, Yale University Press.

Angleitner, A. (1974) 'Changes in personality of older people over a 5-year period of observation', *Gerontologia*, **20**, 179–85.

Argyle, M. (1975) *Bodily communication*, London, Methuen.

Atchley, R.C. (1976) 'Selected social and psychological differences between men and women in later life', *J. Gerontology*, **31**, 204–11.

Bolton, N., and Savage, R.D. (1971) 'Neuroticism and extraversion in elderly normal subjects and psychiatric patients: some normative data', *Br. J. Psychiat.*, **118**, 473–4.

Botwinick, J. (1973) *Aging and Behavior*, New York, Springer.

Britton, J.H., and Britton, J.O. (1972) *Personality changes in aging*, New York, Springer.

Brody, E.M., Kleban, M.H., Lawton, M.P., and Silverman, H.A. (1971) 'Excess disabilities of mentally impaired aged: impact of individualized treatment', *Gerontologist*, **11**, 124–33.

Bromley, D.B. (1974) *The psychology of human ageing*, Harmondsworth, Penguin.

Bromley, D.B. (1977) *Personality description in ordinary language*, London, John Wiley.

Butler, R.N. (1963) 'The life review: an interpretation of reminiscence in the aged', *Psychiatry*, **26**, 65–76.

Cattell, R.B. (1965) *The scientific analysis of of personality*, Harmondsworth, Penguin.

Fiske, D.W. (1971) *Measuring the concepts of personality*, Chicago, Aldine.

Gilmore, A.J.J. (1972) 'Personality in the elderly: problems in methodology', *Age and Ageing*, **1**, 227–32.

Gough, H.G. (1965) *Adjective check list manual*, Palo Alto, California, Consulting Psychologists Press.

Granick, S., and Patterson, R.D. (Ed.) (1971) *Human aging II. An eleven-year followup biomedical and behavioral study*, Rockville, Maryland, US Department of Health, Education and Welfare.

Haan, N., and Day, D. (1974) 'A longitudinal analysis of change and sameness in personality development: adolescence to later adulthood', *Internat. J. Aging Hum. Develop.*, **5**, 11–39.

Heron, A., and Crown, S.M.(1967) *Age and function*, London, Churchill.

Holt, R.R. (1969) *Assessing personality*, New York, Harcourt Brace Jovanovich.

Jarvik, L.F., Bennett, R., and Blumner, B. (1973), 'Design of a comprehensive life history interview schedule', in *Intellectual functioning in adults; psychological and biological influences*, (Ed. L.F. Jarvik, C. Eisdorfer, and J.E. Blum) New York, Springer, pp. 127–36.

Kalish, R.A. (1975) *Late adulthood: perspectives on human development*, Monterey, California, Brooks–Cole.

Kleban, M.H., Lawton, M.P., Brody, E.M., and Moss, M. (1975) 'Characteristics of mentally-impaired aged profiting from individualized treatment', *J. Gerontology*, **30**, 90–96.

Lake, D.G., Miles, M.B., and Earle, R.B. (1973) *Measuring human behavior*, New York, Teachers College Press.

Lawton, M.P. (1970) 'Ecology and aging', in *Spatial behavior of older people*, (Ed. L.A. Pastalan and D.H. Carson) Ann Arbor, Michigan, The University of Michigan–Wayne State University, Institute of Gerontology, pp. 40–67.

Livson, N. (1973) 'Developmental dimensions of personality: a life-span formulation', in *Life-span developmental psychology, personality and socialization* (Ed. P.B. Baltes and K.W. Schaie) New York, Academic Press, pp. 97–122.

Looft, W.R. (1973) 'Socialization and personality throughout the life-span: an examination of contemporary psychological approaches', in *Life-span developmental psychology, personality and socialization*, (Ed. P.B. Baltes and K.W. Schaie New York, Academic Press, pp. 25–52.

Lowenthal, M.F., and Chiriboga, D. (1973) 'Social stress and adaptation: toward a life course perspective', in *The psychology of adult development and aging*, (Ed. C. Eisdorfer and M.P. Lawton) Washington, DC, American Psychological Association, pp. 281–310.

Maddi, S.R. (1972) *Personality theories: a comparative analysis*, (rev. ed.), Homewood, Illinois, The Dorsey Press.

Maddox, G.L., and Douglas, E.B. (1974) 'Aging and individual differences: a longitudinal analysis of social, psychological and physiological indicators', *J. Gerontology*, **29**, 555–63.

Mass, H.S., and Kuypers, J.A. (1975) *From thirty to seventy: a forty-year longitudinal study of adult life styles and personality*, San Francisco, Jossey-Bass.

Mischel, W. (1968) *Personality and assessment*, New York, John Wiley.

Mischel, W. (1976) *Introduction to personality* (2nd ed.), New York, Holt, Rinehart, and Winston.

Nardi, A.H. (1973) 'Person perception research and the perception of life-span development', in *Life-span developmental psychology, personality and socialization*, (Ed. P.B. Baltes and K.W. Schaie) New York, Academic Press, pp. 285–301.

Neugarten, B.L. (Ed.) (1968a) *Middle age and aging*, Chicago, University of Chicago Press.

Neugarten, B.L. (1968b) 'The awareness of middle age', in *Middle age and aging*, (Ed. B.L. Neugarten) Chicago, University of Chicago Press, pp. 93–98.

Neugarten, B.L. (1970) 'Dynamics of transition of middle age to old age. Adaptation and the life cycle', *J. Geriat. Psychiat.*, **4**, 71–87.

Neugarten, B.L. (1973) 'Personality change in late life: a developmental perspective', in *The psychology of adult development and aging*, (Ed. C. Eisdorfer and M.P. Lawton) Washington, DC, American Psychological Association, pp. 311–338.

Parkes, C.M. (1971) 'Psycho-social transitions: a field for study', *Soc. Sci. Med.*, **5**, 101–15.

Pearson, J.S., Swenson, W.M., and Rome, H.P. (1965) 'Age and sex differences related to MMPI response frequency in 25,000 medical patients', *Am. J. Psychiat.*, **121**, 988–95.

Pressey, S.L., and Pressey, A.D. (1966) 'Two insiders' searchings for the best life in old age', *Gerontologist*, **6**, 14–16.

Reichard, S., Livson, F., and Peterson, P.G. (1962) *Aging and personality: a study of eighty-seven older men*, New York, John Wiley.

Rosen, J.L., and Neugarten, B.L. (1960) 'Ego functions in the middle and later years: a thematic apperception study of normal adults', *J. Gerontology*, **15**, 62–7.

Savage, R.D. (1971) 'Psychometric assessment and clinical diagnosis in the aged', in *Recent developments in psychogeriatrics*, (Ed. D.W.K. Kay and A. Walk) *Br. J. Psychiat., Spec. Publ. 6.*, Ashford, Kent, Headley Brothers, pp. 51–62.

Scheflen, A.E., and Scheflen, A. (1972) *Body language and the social order*, Englewood Cliffs, New Jersey, Prentice Hall.

Schwartz, A.N. (Ed.) (1975) *Psychological adjustment to aging: a selected bibliography*, Los Angeles, Ethel Percy Andrus Gerontology Center, University of Southern California.

Shelton, A.J. (1969) 'Igbo child-rearing, eldership, and dependence: a comparison of two cultures', in *The dependencies of old people*, (Ed. R.A. Kalish) Ann Arbor, Michigan, The University of Michigan–Wayne State University, Institute of Gerontology, pp. 97–106.

Sommer, R. (1970) 'Small group ecology in institutions for the elderly', in *Spatial behavior of older people*, (Ed. L.A. Pastalan and D.H. Carson) Ann Arbor, Michigan: The University of Michigan–Wayne State University, Institute of Gerontology, pp. 25–39.

Townsend, P., and Tunstall, S. (1968) 'Isolation, desolation and loneliness', in *Old people in three industrial societies*, (Ed. E. Shanas, P. Townsend, D. Wedderburn, H. Friis, P. Milhøj, and J. Stehouwer London, Routledge and Kegan Paul, pp. 258–87.

White, R.W. (1975) *Lives in progress* (3rd ed.), New York, Holt, Rinehart, and Winston.

3

NEUROSIS AND PERSONALITY DISORDER IN OLD AGE

K. Bergmann

Introduction

Growing old seems to most people a sufficient cause for depression and fear and perhaps this has inhibited the search for neurotic disorder in this period of life. Maudsley (1895) in speaking of involutional depressive illnesses said 'He who has been content to know, begins henceforth to believe that he must die. Life has to be lived without relish and the energy which made it worth living'. He continued to describe various losses experienced in ageing and concluded, 'Obviously there is in such circumstances the sufficient reason for mental collapse when a character has not been so moulded by previous good discipline'.

Is neurosis in old age a problem, how frequently is it found and where must the search be made? Shepherd and Gruenberg (1957) investigated the age specific incidence and prevalence of neurosis using records of hospital admissions and discharges and also of 'new cases' registered with a health insurance plan under the title of 'Service for psychoneurosis'. They demonstrated a peak onset of neurosis in early maturity followed by rapid decline in prevalence from the 40s onwards. Their results tended to suggest that neuroses do not constitute a major problem in old age. However, they themselves cast doubt on this proposition and put forward several hypotheses that might explain the results; for example, that neurosis may lessen in severity, that patients may complain less or that physicians may be less responsive to neurotic disorder in elderly people. Whichever of the above explanations is correct their work suggested that the hospital clinic was not the place where the elderly with neurotic disorder could readily be found.

General practice studies by Bremer (1951), Primrose (1962), and Watts and Watts (1952) did not suggest a decline in the prevalence of neurotic disorder in old age. The comparison between outpatient figures and recordings of psychiatric morbidity from general practice records (Kessel and Shepherd, 1962) though confirming the decline in the prevalence of neurotic disorder among elderly outpatients in hospital did not show similar decline of neurotic disorder in old age in the practice samples. A survey of psychiatric illness in general practice, Shepherd et al. (1966) showed that although patient consulting rates per 1000 at risk for psychiatric illness did not decline steeply, and chronic cases indeed rose, the consultation rates for new psychiatric cases after the age of 55 declined very steeply indeed.

Surveys in the community present a different picture and studies in Scandinavia (Essen-Möller, 1956; Nielson, 1962) confirmed a high prevalence of neurotic and personality disorder, though Scandinavian diagnostic terminology makes direct comparison with other studies difficult. A true stratified random sample in the city of Newcastle upon Tyne (Kay *et al.* 1964a, b) demonstrated that elderly community residents do suffer from neurotic and personality disorders and those of at least moderate severity represent about 12·5 per cent of the population. Furthermore, five per cent of the elderly community residents appeared to have neurotic illnesses starting after the age of 60 years with no evidence of earlier neurotic disorder and could be considered to represent new neurotic illness in old age. A later study (Bergmann, 1971) which focused more specifically on neurotic disorder in old age, especially that of late onset, indicated that eleven per cent of this sample of 300 elderly community residents over the age of 65 appeared to have neurotic disorder, of at least moderate severity, manifesting itself after the age of 60 years.

The discrepancy between surveys which show neurosis in the elderly, often appearing to begin in old age, and practice and clinic studies which show a decline in new cases reported requires some explanation. A re-examination of Williamson's study (Williamson *et al.*, 1964) in which general practitioners awareness of psychiatric disorder was directly compared to the prevalence ascertained in their practices sheds some light on this problem. Psychiatric conditions are listed according to the percentage of cases remaining undetected by the general practitioner (see Table 3.1). It can be seen that dementia in the community remains very much undetected, depression and affective disorders coming second and neurosis third. Conditions that are readily detected include severe alcoholism and paranoid states. It would appear therefore that 'nuisance value' is an important factor in bringing cases of psychiatric disorder to light and that certainly some forms of neurotic disorder in old age fail to reach a critical level in this respect.

TABLE 3.1. Percentage of patients not known to general practitioners

	Alcoholism
25%	Paranoid states
61%	Neurosis
71%	Depression
87%	Dementia

Adapted from Williamson *et al.* (1964).

Problems in defining 'neurotic illness'

It is perhaps worth speculating about how patients with neurotic disorder in general become a 'case'. Goldberg (1972) discusses this in some detail and he points out that the severity of symptoms is not necessarily directly related to the degree of incapacity for or interference with day-to-day life. Furthermore, both interpersonal factors and external social factors may determine 'whether a given set of symptoms is taken to a doctor'. Shepherd *et al.* (1966) emphasize that there is no clear dichotomy between 'cases' and normals where neurosis is concerned. They go on to suggest that there is no agreed stringent criterion for a case definition and suggest that 'it may be predicated that social as well as purely medical parameters will enter into their definition'.

Perhaps the pathway to becoming an established psychiatric case may begin with a failure to fulfil a variety of adult role expectations including marital, occupational, and social roles. Susser and Watson (1971) state 'role expectations exist in all societies together with the sanctions to ensure compliance with the expected behaviour'. When sanctions therefore are threatened overtly or implicitly this may lead to the assumption of a sick role and where physical sickness and appropriate treatment cannot be instituted then patients may be deemed to be amenable to or requiring psychiatric investigation and care. This leads to several questions; what is the role of the elderly in society, what demands are made of them and when are they not fulfilling them?

Certainly on the negative side extremes of behavioural disturbance and antisocial habits are outside the remit of the normal elderly person and as a minimum requirement the elderly are expected not to commit a nuisance, not to break down their families or immediate neighbours with excessive and unreasonable demands nor to transgress against the basic social norms of cleanliness, hygiene, and safety. If this be the case then it is perhaps not surprising that neurotic disorder is infrequently referred for psychiatric care and the low referral rate on new cases of neurotic disorder in old age may also be related to the allied phenomenon of 'low social visibility' of psychiatric disorder in the elderly, which has been described in the San Francisco studies comparing hospital and community samples (Simon, 1968). Is neurosis significant in old age or a minor phenomenon, which if it cannot be ignored, can at least be given a very low priority in psychiatric thinking? The significance of neuroses and personality problems in old age may perhaps be judged by their relationship to some of the major difficulties encountered in later life. Perhaps the most important being personal suffering, physical health, social stresses, threats to independence, and the quality and enjoyment of life experienced by the elderly person.

Physical health

There is a strong association between physical ill health and neurotic and affective disorder arising in old age. The relationship between ill health and neurotic disorder in old age will be discussed more fully in the section which deals with the aetiology of neurotic disorder in later life. The higher mortality of elderly patients with neurotic disorder has been demonstrated (Kay and Bergmann, 1966) and this does suggest the possibility that the onset of neurotic disorder in later life may, at least, in some cases be an indicator of life threatening or serious occult physical ill health especially in elderly men. Kerr *et al.* (1969) found this to be true for atypical depressive illness occurring in middle aged men.

It might therefore be safest to consider all neurotic illness beginning in later life as a sort of 'organic body syndrome' (Lewis, 1966, personal communication) until a thorough medical history, examination, and appropriate investigations refute this assumption.

Do elderly people 'suffer' from neurotic disorder?

Suffering is an essentially subjective phenomenon and of itself has never appeared to be a great determinant of whether a patient receives psychiatric help. Implicit in much writing about elderly people is the assumption that neurosis and personality problems in the aged are just neuroses from earlier life, diminished, damped down, and no longer of great significance. Certainly some support for this view comes from Ernst's catamnestic study *Die Prognose der Neurosen* (1959). Though anxiety states were found to be intractable other conditions ameliorated over a period of years and hysteria, for instance, did not appear to persist for more than about five years, the behavioural disturbances shifting to a series of complaints. Neurotic illness became mild in old age and this was assumed to be because of reduced drive. This view of old age neurosis as a chronic long standing condition is held by Diethelm and Rockwell (1943) and is summarized by Cameron (1956) in the following statement: 'Although we have insufficient data upon which to base a final statement it is possible that most ageing persons who develop neurotic symptoms have similar maladaptations under stress when younger'.

The opposite view, however, has also been held for sometime (Abraham, 1920; Clow and Allen, 1951; Straker, 1963). These authors all describe patients whom they recognize as having a neurotic illness which began in later life. They suggest that apparent adjustment in earlier life is not uncommon and submit that in spite of their age such persons should be considered as suffering from acute neurotic illness. Perhaps one difficulty in gauging the suffering of such patients is the fact that they have 'adequate' precipitating causes; including bereavements, real health problems, and worries over finance, retirement, moving into a strange environment, and loss of status, which in themselves require help regardless of the symptomatology or psychic disturbance.

A comparison of elderly persons without neurotic symptoms, those with longstanding symptoms and those in whom neurotic symptoms appeared to start in later life was carried out and reported (Bergmann, 1971) (see Table 3.2) and when comparing the problems and maladjustments of old age it became evident that the elderly person with late onset neurotic disorder suffered more from loneliness and greater difficulty caring for themselves and were less likely to have active hobbies or holidays. By contrast the elderly person with longstanding chronic neurotic

TABLE 3.2. Significant features differentiating normal elderly community residents from those with late onset and chronic neurotic disorders

Diagnostic groups	Events in childhood and family history	Problems in adult life	Stresses in old age	Problems in old age
Late onset neurosis (LON) *vs* Chronic neurosis (CN)	Childhood neurotic traits (CN) Poor relationship with parents (CN) Later in birth order (CN)	No significant differences	Cardiovascular disease (LON) Severity of physical disability (LON) Poor mobility (LON) Lower income (LON)	Loneliness (LON) Impaired self care (LON) No hobbies or holidays (LON)
Late onset neurosis *vs* Normal	No significant differences	Marital disharmony Psychiatric disorder in children Late marriage, or single Lower social class	Cardiovascular disease Severity of physical disability Gastrointestinal disease More occupied than normals Impaired mobility Isolation	Hypochondriasis (CN) Hypochondriasis Impaired self care
Chronic neurosis *vs* Normal	Childhood neurotic traits Poor relationship with parents Psychiatric disorder in siblings	Psychiatric disorder in children Poor club attendance before 6 y Estrangement from children	Gastrointestinal disease More occupied than normals	Hypochondriasis Loneliness

46

symptoms was little different from the normal elderly person apart from the prominent symptom of hypochondriasis, which by itself accounted for nearly three-quarters of the variance between the two diagnostic groups. It is also of interest to know that chronic neurotic elderly people complained more of hypochondriacal symptoms than those with neurotic reactions manifested themselves in later life. It would appear that apart from physical ill health the main problems associated with neurotic disorder coming on in later life are the problems of loneliness, impairment and difficulty in self care, and a lower level of recreational activity.

Loneliness

Distinctions between loneliness and isolations have been drawn by Lowenthal (1965) who demonstrated that isolation of itself i.e. few social contacts, is of little psychopathological significance. Townsend (1957) maintains a similar distinction between isolation and 'desolation' in many ways analogous to loneliness. A factor analytic study on a random sample population of community residents (Garside *et al.*, 1965) derived an isolation factor which was also independent of a general illness factor, psychiatric diagnosis factor, and socioeconomic factors. Tunstall (1966) also emphasized the distinction between loneliness and isolation and in his sample only a quarter of isolated old men and women were 'often lonely'. He pointed out that there were a smaller total number of 'often lonely' than isolated people. The overlap

TABLE 3.3.

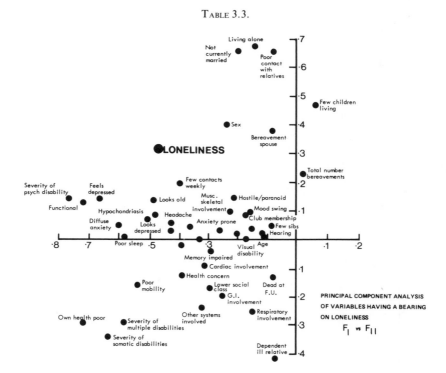

between the lonely and the isolated is not to be denied, however, and old people who lived alone were much more likely to be lonely. Though loneliness is difficult to define it is possible to assign people, on their own categorization, into various groups such as those who see themselves as not lonely, sometimes lonely or often lonely.

TABLE 3.4.

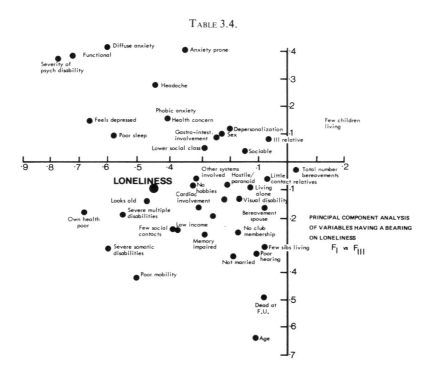

A study carried out on 300 community residents (Bergmann, 1971) also gave an opportunity to examine the question of loneliness in more detail as all subjects were asked to state to what degree, if at all they were lonely. A factor analytic study was then carried out which included variables covering physical ill health, social and economic status, psychological state, personality traits and objective measures of contacts with significant relatives and friends as well as less intimate day-to-day social contacts, (see Tables 3.3 and 3.4). The first three factors derived were identified as:

(1) An illness factor on which both neurotic, anxiety, and depressive symptoms and physical ill health were highly loaded.
(2) A low degree of personal or intimate contact with relatives or friends, the general measure of contacts based on that of Townsend (1957) did not appear to be highly loaded in this factor.
(3) An ageing factor indicative of the vicissitudes of life connected with increasing old age.

48

The variable 'loneliness' lay between factors (1) and (2) indicating the possibilities of an admixture of isolation and ill health or the possibility that different types of elderly lonely subjects could be distinguished.

T ABLE 3.5.

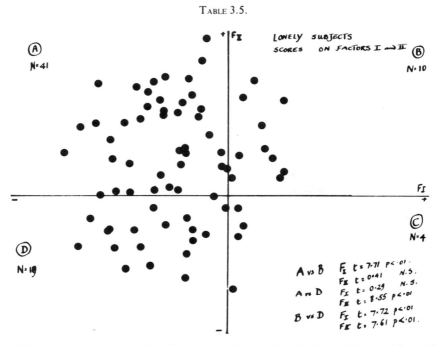

All lonely subjects were therefore plotted for the distribution of factors (1) and (2) (see Table 3.5). The types of lonely old people so described might be enumerated as follows:

(1) Essentially well elderly people without gross physical psychiatric illness but with the loss of intimate relationships and contacts, (high loading on factor (1) in quadrant A).
(2) Elderly persons with adequate social and intimate contacts but suffering from marked degree of physical and psychiatric disability, in the latter depression and anxiety figured prominently, (high loading on factor (2) in quadrant D).
(3) Elderly persons in whom factors (1) and (2) seemed to be represented together to a significant degree.
(4) A very small group of elderly persons who while not unduly isolated from intimate contacts nor yet physically or psychiatrically disturbed admitted to feeling lonely. Such a group could not be defined any further by the variables included in the study but were possibly a group who admitted to some form of 'existential' loneliness of a more subtle type, (quadrant B).

Identification of the significance of the two factors described in these various types of elderly lonely persons would perhaps give help in deciding whether an appropriate response to the plea of loneliness was the psychiatric treatment of anxiety and depression, medical treatment to improve mobility and general health or social intervention such as visiting or befriending of various types. Loneliness is a condition which is often complained of by elderly persons; general practitioners and health visitors often mention loneliness when they refer patients for psychiatric care, but it takes careful thought, consideration, and clinical acumen to decide on the appropriate intervention and the part, if any, that the psychiatrist has to play.

Impairment of self care

Kay et al. (1973) reported on a random sample of 477 elderly subjects seen in the community. These elderly people were divided into recipients of services, those at risk, i.e. showing impairment of the ability to cope with day-to-day life, and subjects not in need of services nor at risk. Subjects at risk had a significantly higher proportion of elderly with functional psychiatric disorder (87 per cent with neurotic disorder with at least moderate severity). Goldberg (1970) in investigating the needs of the elderly and the efficacy of various types of social work intervention found that 32 per cent of her sample, initially selected as being referred for social need to the welfare department suffered from depression ranging from a rating of above average severity to severe. Only one per cent was judged to be suffering from an actual depressive illness. This author notes how few patients were receiving psychiatric treatment and how the general practitioner, on the whole, did not seem to be aware of their psychiatric needs. A further study of a consecutive series of patients admitted to day hospital care from the community and suffering from functional psychiatric disorder (Bergmann *et al.*, 1975) show that these patients attracted a higher level of care with regard to meals on wheels, home help, than did those patients suffering from organic psychiatric illnesses; this difference could not be accounted for by differences in the initial social situation nor by the fact that more functional patients were known to the local authority social services department, (see Tables 3.6 and 3.7). Furthermore, after full multidisciplinary assessment patients with functional psychiatric disorder (78 per cent suffering from neurotic or personality disorder) did not require a significant increase in the level of services though they certainly did require a considerable amount of psychiatric and medical treatment. A review three months later suggested some reduction in services, such as social work and health visitor supervision, a lesser reduction in home help and meals on wheels, had taken place. The majority of elderly patients with moderately severe neurotic disorder appear to have their social needs recognized at least in an area where there is a comprehensive local authority social services department, but perhaps the response to psychiatric needs for the relief of depression and anxiety is expressed in terms of increasing social worker and health visitor contact, and providing home helps and meals. In some of these cases the major need may be for treatment of psychiatric and physical ill health to improve the capacity for socialization and an independent life rather than laying on an ever increasing number of supportive services. It is disappointing, however, that psychiatric care given to day patients did not appear to

TABLE 3.6.

COMMUNITY SERVICES RECEIVED ON REFERRAL (Percentages)

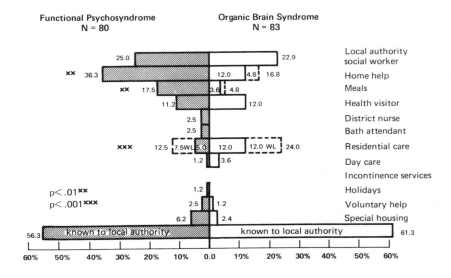

TABLE 3.7.

ADDITIONAL SERVICES RECOMMENDED (Percentages)

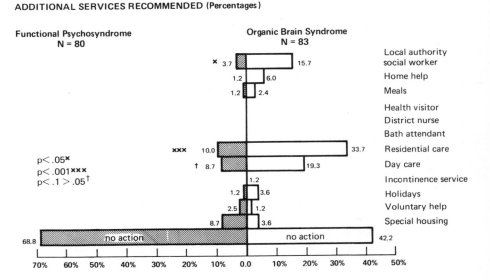

reduce drastically the need for domiciliary services and perhaps it should be pointed out that when the need for services is once acquired or the habit of independence and self help once broken an irreversible process may have been triggered off and that the preventative effects of psychiatric care and psychotherapeutic rehabilitation requires implementation at an early stage before expensive and unnecessary services become fixed as an immutable feature of the elderly persons' lifestyle.

The psychopathology of neurotic disorder in later life

As Ernst has pointed out (1959) anxiety neurosis is the most persistent. Other long term studies such as those by Schapira *et al.* (1972) would confirm these findings. The rarity of persistent hysterical illness manifesting itself in old age has also been noted both by Ernst and by Diethelm and Rockwell (1943). Severe obsessional states rarely begin in old age (Pollitt, 1957) and in a random sample survey (Bergmann, 1971) no case could be found which would fulfil the strict criteria of an obsessional neurosis. However, phobic anxiety is noted as occurring in old age both in the persistence of longstanding, symptomatically florid, chronic phobic anxiety states, often without a high level of free floating anxiety, and also in the form of acute attacks of phobic anxiety beginning in later life. Such attacks may be quite dramatic and are often in response to the impact of severe physical ill health especially myocardial infarction and of operative surgical intervention such as the removal of cataracts. It is easy in old age to miss phobic illnesses and to confound them with the disability which has precipitated these states. This results in medical attendants creating neurotic invalidism in their patients and influencing families in such a way that they unwittingly and unnecessarily rob the elderly of their independence. In late onset neurotic disorder the depressive symptoms are commonly found. Seventy-five per cent of respondents with late onset neurotic reactions of moderate severity were considered to be suffering from neurotic depression.

McDonald (1967b) distinguishes between 'affective' neurotics and others in a sample of elderly patients and suggests these be grouped as suffering from 'affective illness' rather than neurosis. The catamnestic and symptomatic grounds justifying such a distinction are not clear.

In the catamnestic review of neurotic disorder by Ernst (1959) the syndrome of hysteria and its stability and persistence were examined. In the neurotic population followed up, hysteria, strictly confined to dissociative or conversion disorders and arising as a primary illness, rarely persisted for more than five years. Such patients did not, after five years, convert suddenly to a picture of positive mental health but changed their acting out behaviour to one in which complaints became a major feature. How is one to view the manipulative and demonstrative behaviour, hysterical paralyses, and ataxias, bizarre functional disturbances of consciousness, and other hysterical symptoms not infrequently seen in elderly patients?

It is best to assert dogmatically the primary hysterical illness does not begin in old age. Even when lifelong hysterical personalities experience a recrudescence of their earlier hysterical behaviour or symptoms this should not be accepted with complacency. An underlying functional psychosis, often depressive, early organic psychiatric disorder and sometimes silent but serious physical disease may coexist. Silent carcinoma of the lung has been responsible for several presenting pictures of 'hysterical' illness in cases known to the author. In such cases the hysterical symptoms can be seen as a primitive communication of a disease of which the patient is not more directly aware.

Hypochondriacal symptoms have been seen as being of particular importance in the neurotic reactions of the aged and Pfeiffer and Busse (1973) list hypochondriasis first in considering the neurotic reactions of old age. They consider hypochondriacal neurosis as a separate condition and cite its inclusion in the second edition of the Diagnostic and Statistical Manual on Mental Disorders of the American Psychiatric Association (DSM-II) as a distinct nosological entity. Hypochondriasis, they consider is frequent among elderly patients particularly elderly women and that the dynamic function of such a neurotic illness is to escape from feelings of personal failure: retirement from work, loss of social prestige or financial security may be considered as contributing to such feelings. Their view can, however, be disputed especially as the initial theoretical work on which it is based was drawn from a volunteer sample which might indeed be biased towards hypochondriasis as a free exhaustive, not to say exhausting, physical examination and investigations were included among the fringe benefits of their study. D'Alarcon (1964) in investigating hypochondriasis in relation to depressive illness in elderly patients found strong links between hypochondriasis and depression and in 29 per cent of his series it was the first symptom of a depressive illness and indicative of an increased suicidal risk. A study of the people judged to be hypochondriacal regardless of psychiatric diagnosis in a random sample of elderly community residents (Bergmann, 1971) showed a strong relationship between various psychiatric symptoms, depressive, phobic and hysterical, and the level of hypochondriacal complaints. A past history of psychiatric breakdown was also a significant factor in discriminating between hypochondriacal subjects and others. Furthermore, Kay et al. (1966) demonstrated that a patient's own complaints of physical ill health, rather embarrassingly, were a better indicator of mortality four years later than the initial medical assessment. Three general conclusions might therefore be drawn:

(1) Hypochondriasis is an important sign.
(2) Lifelong hypochondriacal tendencies combined with personality disorder ought to be distinguished from hypochondriacal complaints arising in later life.
(3) Where hypochondriacal complaints appear to rise in later life it may be an important indicator not only of depression and an increased risk of suicide but also of serious and perhaps unrelated underlying physical disease of which the patient is not otherwise aware.

Psychological measures of neuroticism of ageing

Parsons (1965) employed the Maudsley personality inventory (MPI) as a measure of neuroticism and found this to be satisfactory with a random sample population of elderly respondents seen in Swansea. The gradations of his neuroticism scores matched in a reasonable and clinically appropriate manner the diagnostic assessments of the severity of the disorder. McDonald (1967a), however, found that the MPI did not hold against his clinical assessment whereas the appropriate section of the Cornell medical index did so. Britton and Savage (1966) established normative values for the Minnesota multiphasic personality inventory data (MMPI) applied to a subsample of community residents studied by the present author. Though the data showed considerable deviations from the standardization population originally employed, appropriate age corrected norms could be worked out and a comparison with the data of Swenson (1961) showed that the profile patterns contained in both samples was similar. Britton *et al.* (1967) compared the MMPI findings with psychiatric clinical diagnosis and the conclusions were drawn that psychiatric status correlated most with the scales on the MMPI labelled 'hysteria', 'hypochondriasis' and 'depression'. The majority of cases in this study had a formal psychiatric diagnosis of neurotic depression or diffuse and phobic anxiety states.

Intellectual function and neurotic disorder in the elderly

It is a common clinical observation that elderly people with early mild dementia present with neurotic symptoms. Manipulative, dissociative, and hysterical behaviour, sudden anxiety symptoms, and depressive reactions may all mask a subtle early dysmnestic syndrome and the beginning of mild generalized intellectual impairment. It is an easy step from this to suggest that neurotic disorder in the elderly is to be seen as a predromal phase of a dementing illness. The concept of a central old age disease with different types of psychiatric colouring is a most persistent one.

The evidence of clinical studies in hospital populations points more strongly towards the establishment of separate syndromes than to a unitary old age psychosis. Elderly people with functional psychiatric disorder have been shown to have a very different clinical course and prognosis as to life from those originally diagnosed as suffering from organic psychiatric diseases (Roth, 1955). It has also been demonstrated with the use of actuarial data that patients with functional and organic psychiatric disorder differ very significantly from each other in their expectation of life, the former approximating closely to the expectation of life of the population in general. However, the mild and less clear cut neurotic and personality disorders might be considered to follow a very different pattern.

Bergmann and Eastham (1974) in following up the Newcastle community sample of elderly subjects over an average period of three years (range 18 months to four and a half years) noted that only 4·8 per cent of those with functional disorders (mainly neurotic disorder) developed dementia and this did not differ significantly from the percentage (4·5 per cent) developing dementia in the sample as a whole.

McDonald (1967a) examined the relationship between the Inglis paired associate learning test (PALT) which he used as a measure of the presence of brain damage with the scores on the M–R scale of the Cornel medical index, indicative of neuroticism. His results did not support the hypothesis that neuroticism in old age is associated with brain damage.

Though intellectual impairment of an organic type does not seem to be significantly related to the onset of neurotic disorder in later life it is not unreasonable to inquire about the effects of lifelong low intelligence in facing the stresses of old age. Evidence has accummulated from the Newcastle studies of a community random sample of the aged (Britton *et al.* 1967) that elderly persons with functional disorder (usually neuroses) had a relatively low score on the Wechsler adult intelligence scale. The survivors of this population were reassessed six years later and medical, psychiatric, and psychometric data were obtained (Nunn *et al.*, 1974) and evidence was found that 'below average intelligence is one of several factors which independently contribute to the development or persistence of neurosis in old age'. It is suggested that the capacity to adapt to the altered circumstances of old age may explain the significance of low intelligence, whether this be due to innate factors or cultural and educational deprivation.

The aetiology of neurosis in old age

Neurotic disorder in old age, whether it arises *de novo* or whether it be an exacerbation of a longstanding condition, has always to be seen as a combination of personal predisposition, life experience and the stresses met in later life.

Those elderly persons who have weathered the stresses of earlier life successfully may yet succumb to what in some cases, must seem an overwhelming collection of losses of social status, economic security, close ties of blood and friendship, and physical health and bodily integrity. To a younger observer the life of elderly people seems to be full of so many unacceptable and unpalatable occurrences that when symptoms of anxiety, phobias, obsessional, and hypochondriacal preoccupations, and depressive reactions arise they are more than sufficiently explained and so perhaps little interest or systematic exploration of the causes of neurosis in old age carried out. It is very simple to list the factors that accompany neurotic disorders and reactions in old age or even to record those perceived by elderly persons as being the cause of their symptoms. Such a list would take into account physical illness, adverse home environment, bereavement, compulsory retirement, financial difficulties, and other social circumstances. Such statements volunteered by elderly persons attending a clinic were offered as 'causes' of neurotic disorder in old age (Cowan, 1969).

These experiences, however, can also be seen as the inevitable concomitants of ageing. Moreover, 75 to 80 per cent of elderly persons do not suffer from neurotic reactions of any severity, cope adequately with the vicissitudes of later life and face poverty, socioeconomic loss, and changed circumstances with flexibility and courage. The elderly who successfully cope with ageing and severe stresses must cast strong doubts on the standard and somewhat stereotyped view, which assumes an inevitable and increasing rigidity in the personality structure of the elderly person. Studies of elderly patients seen in hospital inpatient and outpatient samples with neurotic disorder do not answer the doubts of queries raised in the preceding paragraphs. The experiences of doctors, nurses, and social workers is with 'patients' or 'clients'. Even when the elderly are not overtly selected for neurotic qualities there is considerable evidence for the existence of emotional distress (Goldberg, 1970) but these studies cannot answer questions as to which life events and stresses appear to be most critical and which personalities are the most vulnerable to them. Indeed reports from doctors and social workers are based on elderly persons selected in the first instance for vulnerability and incapacity to cope.

A 'normal' control sample is therefore desirable and necessary; preferably the neurotic sample should also be community resident and broadly comparable to the normals. It also seems necessary in the interests of simplicity to exclude those people who developed or appeared to develop their neurotic reactions in later life. A study of such a random sample population (Bergmann, 1971) permitted this comparison to be made.

TABLE 3.8.

Variables considered to have a bearing on the aetiology of neurotic reaction in later life

ysical Disability	Personal predisposition	Social stresses
reasing Age	Abnormal Personality insecure rigid	Poor health of spouse
verity of main disability		Recent bereavement sibs/children
in disability somatic	Abnormal Personality anxiety-prone/hysterical	Recent bereavement spouse, etc.
in system involved Cardiac		Few visits neighbours
in system involved Respiratory	Abnormal Personality Paranoid hostile	Infrequent visiting by rels.
in system involved Musculo-Skeletal		Recent decrease in contacts
in system involved Gastro-intestinal	Abnormal Personality inadequate	Recent fall in income
in system involved Others		Lack of occupation
aired mobility		Low income
derate or severe secondary		Difficulty in self-care
ability		Social class
		Not currently married

TABLE 3.9. 'Best' ten variables, of aetiological significance, which discriminate between late onset neurotic and normal groups

	β	r	% P.V.
Abnormal personality anxiety/hysteria	0·28	0·37[3]	26·5
Main system cardiac	0·20	0·29[3]	14·8
Severity of main physical disability	0·17	0·32[3]	13·9
Female	0·16	0·29[3]	11·8
Abnormal personality insecure/rigid	0·18	0·21[2]	9·6
Main system gastrointestinal	0·14	0·19[1]	6·4
Bereavement siblings/children	0·13	0·18[1]	6·3
Bereavement spouse	0·12	0·14NS	4·3
Impaired self care	0·05	0·26[3]	3·3
Isolation	0·05	0·21[2]	2·6

$R^2 = 0.39$; $R = 0.63$ ($p < 0.01$); $F = 13.2$ (df 10 and 210); $F_d = 1.44$ N.S; β = standardized partial regression coefficient; r = product moment correlation coefficient; PV = predicted variance; R = multiple correlation; F_d = F ratio of the difference between 29 and 10 variables.
[1] $p < 0.05$
[2] $p < 0.01$
[3] $p < 0.001$

The more common vicissitudes of ageing such as increasing poverty, loss of income, low socioeconomic status, bereavements, poor contact with neighbours and relatives, lack of a spouse, and difficulties in carrying out the day-to-day tasks were listed. Some of the major abnormal personality traits were also included and also general and more detailed estimates of various types of physical disability were recorded (see Table 3.8). In order to get some indication of the 'causes' of neurotic disorder in the elderly the most important question to ask seemed to be, which factors best discriminated between elderly community residents showing evidence of late onset neurotic reactions and those who could be classified as 'normal'? A multiple regression was employed using the diagnostic dichotomy as the dependent variable in order to carry out discriminant function analysis (Table 3.9). It can be seen that social factors play a surprisingly small part and that personal vulnerability and physical health appear to be major considerations. It is therefore proposed to consider the problem of personal vulnerability, the effects of physical ill health and the place and position of social stress in the following sections.

Personal vulnerability

The consideration of personality and adjustment in ageing lends itself to alternative approaches representing psychiatric and sociological orientations. The first is an attempt to define clinically abnormal personality characteristics which militate against successful ageing and especially those which are more prominent in later life. Secondly there exists a developmental view of personality in which patterns of successful and unsuccessful ageing are identified. The latter view, perhaps, is characterized by two apparently opposed theories of successful ageing, the disengagement theory (Cumming and Henry, 1961) which notes the decrease in social interaction and the process of withdrawal by the ageing person now suggests that these are adaptive responses to the vicissitudes of ageing. The more commonly held theory perhaps corresponding to the popular idea of adjustment in old age is the activity theory which, to quote Havighurst (1968): 'Implies that except for the inevitable changes in biology and in health older people are the same as middle aged with essentially the same psychological and social needs ... the older person who ages optimally is the person who stays active and who manages to resist the shrinkage of his social world'. The attempts to test these two theories in a longitudinal study of elderly community residents in Kansas City indicate that neither the activity nor the disengagement were adequate to account for the observed facts. These types of personality study based judgements on both life adjustment and life satisfaction ratings and complex definitions were defined by Neugarten and her coworkers (Neugarten, 1964) including such divisions as between integrated and unintegrated, dependent or autonomous, and engaged or disengaged, according to the level of activity. There is certainly a completeness and wholeness about these definitions emphasizing, as they do, the positive features of personality but there is also circularity in which a successful personality and a successful definition of adjustment and satisfaction are confounded.

Reports on personality changes in old age are longstanding and well established and these include increased introversion (Eysenck, 1957) increased rigidity in old age, the components of which were investigated by Chown (1962).

Savage (1973) in a comprehensive review on personality measurement in old age suggests that the 'development of more adequate personality assessment procedures by Cattell, Eysenck and others give hope for the future but one cannot help but be disappointed by the small amount of research in this area on old people'. He further mentions that no normative data on Cattell's 16PF can be presented though some studies which include within the spectrum elderly subjects suggest (Saley, 1965) that elderly men and women become more depressed and gloomy, more adventurous and outgoing, more unconventional and more tough minded with age. However, without both fairly extensive cross sectional testing and longitudinal studies in which the relationship to psychiatric outcome is examined the connection between such personality factors and vulnerability to neurotic disorder in old age cannot be determined.

TABLE 3.10.

SIGNIFICANT PRODUCT MOMENT CORRELATIONS WITH ANXIETY PRONE PERSONALITY TRAITS

Early experience, family and personal history

	r	
Early marriage	0.15	*
Marital disharmony	0.15	*

Current Social Factors

No significant correlations

Physical Disability

Poor mobility	0.15	*

Complaints

Poor sleep	0.27	***
Sees own health as poor	0.18	**
Hypochondriasis	0.16	*

Psychiatric Symptoms

Psychic tension	0.36	***
Lifelong tendency to worry	0.33	***
Autonomic overactivity	0.30	***
Depression	0.24	***
Endogenous depressive features	0.22	**

Diagnosis of late onset neurotic reactions 0.37 ***

In clinical practice the categorization of personality is not easy. The Scandinavian classification developed by Sjöbring was employed in community survey by Essen–Möller (1956) but would not find acceptance or be readily employable by psychiatrists outside the Scandinavian area. Vispo (1962) listed 36 traits with which he assessed functional psychotic patients whose illness started at the age of 60 and compared them with a normal group drawn from the random sample provided by

58

TABLE 3.11.

SIGNIFICANT PRODUCT MOMENT CORRELATIONS WITH INSECURE RIGID PERSONALITY TRAITS

	r	
Early experience, family and personal history		
History of poor relationship with parent(s)	0.22	**
Loss of parent before 15 years of age	0.17	*
Psychiatric disorder in children	0.16	*
Late in birth order	0.14	*
Current Social Factors		
Few children alive	0.22	**
Physical Disability		
No significant correlation		
Complaints		
Poor sleep	0.14	*
Loneliness	0.14	*
Psychiatric Symptoms		
Obsessional symptoms	0.34	***
Autonomic overactivity	0.32	***
Psychic tension	0.27	***
Phobic symptoms	0.18	**
Hysterical symptoms	0.17	*
Endogenous ("vital") depressive features	0.16	*
Depressive symptoms	0.14	*
Diagnosis of late onset neurotic reactions	0.21	**

Kay *et al.* (1964). He found that five classes could be derived consisting of sociability, dysthmia, a tendency to anxiety, obsessive, paranoid, and hostile traits. A study by the author (Bergmann, 1971) followed this basis but separated those traits that were basically an unfavourable self report of personality such as poor sociability, health concerned into a separate group from those that were also based on a critical evaluation of the respondents account of their feelings and behaviour, in relation to a semistructured review of their life history. The personality traits selected included anxiety proneness and dissociative or conversion symptoms, the type of personality that could be described as rigid and insecure (including also the anankastic subject without any symptoms) and the paranoid hostile personalities. In addition clinical experience with a pilot sample indicated that in spite of the unsatisfactory nature of the description a further category of 'inadequate personality' had to be employed. This latter group consisted of persons who were isolated throughout their lives, barely coped with the day-to-day problems of getting a living, rarely gained their independence from their family, had few meaningful contacts, interests, or social outlets and who in spite of these findings appeared to show no other gross features of neuroticism.

TABLE 3.12.

SIGNIFICANT PRODUCT MOMENT CORRELATIONS WITH PARANOID HOSTILE TRAITS

	r	
Early experiences, family and personal history		
Poor relationship with parent(s)	0.24	**
Childhood neurotic traits	0.20	**
Marital disharmony	0.14	*
Current Social Factors		
Poor work record	0.18	*
Physical Disability		
No significant correlations		
Complaints		
Hypochondriasis	0.22	**
Psychiatric Symptoms		
No significant correlations		
Diagnosis of late onset neurotic reactions		
No significant correlations		

It was noted that the anxiety prone and hysterical personality traits seemed to indicate the most vulnerability to the development of neurotic and reactive depressive syndromes in old age (see Table 3.10). In earlier life anxiety prone subjects tended to marry early and show evidence of marital disharmony. The traits associated with an insecure, rigid, and anankastic personality (see Table 3.11) also seemed to be significantly associated with late onset neurotic disorder and affective reactions in old age. These subjects tended to give a history of poor relationship with parents, early parental loss, a history of psychiatric disorder in the children, and tended to be late in the birth order. On the other hand patients with paranoid personality traits and those labelled from their lifelong pattern as 'inadequate' (see Tables 3.12 and 3.13) showed no significant correlation with late onset neurotic disorder in spite of the fact that certainly those respondents with paranoid hostile traits had significantly worse relationships with parents, more frequent reports of childhood neurotic traits and were more likely to give a history of marital disharmony in earlier life than normal subjects. Those defined as inadequate showed more frequent evidence of marital disharmony in their life, a poor work record and a poor attendance at social gatherings or clubs before the age of 60 than normal subjects.

TABLE 3.13.

SIGNIFICANT PRODUCT MOMENT CORRELATIONS
WITH INADEQUATE PERSONALITY TRAITS

Early experiences and family history	r
Marital disharmony	**0.22 ****
Current Social Factors	
Poor work record	**0.32 *****
Poor attendance at clubs before aged 60	**0.14 ***
Physical Disability	
Main system involved gastro-intestinal	**0.25 ****
Increasing age	**0.15 ***
Complaints	
No significant correlations	
Symptoms	
Endogenous features	**0.18 ****
Depression	**0.15 ***
Diagnosis of late onset neurotic reactions	
No significant correlations	

The evidence of this study seemed to suggest that anxiety traits were less frequently related to early life experiences than were the anankastic ones and genetic factors have to be considered.

Slater and Shields (1969) review studies which show evidence for the hereditary components of anxiety especially with regard to the autonomic response to stimuli, clinical studies although presenting more difficulties of definition tended to confirm the evidence of genetic factors in anxiety traits especially as demonstrated in twin studies. They conclude, 'twin studies of man have shown variation in autonomic function to have hereditary components. Psychometric questionnaires given to normal MZ and DZ twins tend to show the same thing as regards the dysthymic aspects of neuroticism with which anxiety may be closely connected'.

With regard to the vulnerable aspects of insecure and anankastic personality traits the author's studies suggest that early experience may have a significant bearing and the review of psychodynamic models of anxiety in relation to the stresses of ageing is of interest. Freud (1933) viewed the development of psychoanalytic concepts of anxiety, retraced his steps from the first model whereby anxiety was considered as a deflection of sexual libido, through the developments which emphasized the importance of castration fears and finally to the fear of loss of love which he supposed to be 'obviously a continuation of the fear of the infant at the breast when it misses its mother'. Schilder (1940) considered that the threat of injury to any part of the body could in later life represent an equivalent to the castration fears of earlier life and certainly although this view is somewhat simplistic it might be said to relate well to the great importance of physical ill health in the neurotic reactions of later life. Butler (1968) saw the central problem in the psychopathology of ageing as the problem of facing death and arising out of this the resolution of the problem of guilt, a useful formulation but far from a sufficient one. Such psychodynamic models and explanations of personal vulnerability have an unsatisfactory ring when some of the more puzzling clinical cases of neurotic breakdown in old age are considered. It is difficult, on the surface, to explain why a person with some anxiety and anankastic traits often copes with life's vicissitudes and is a model citizen, rears a stable family, obtains promotion and is in no way seen in earlier life by the family, friends or medical attendants as 'neurotic'. These people have often weathered hard and deprived childhoods, poverty stricken adult lives, world wars and unemployment; yet they decompensate with anxiety, phobias, depressive reactions, and obsessional symptoms in old age. What is the predisposition to breakdown which is potently activated in old age and which can be traced back to early experience? Bowlby (1969) presents an attractive model. He argues cogently for the concept of anxiety as a response to the loss of 'affectional bonds' which in their turn led to an attachment behaviour for the protection of the young of the species from their predators. He argues further that this protection allows the young infant to respond to alarm stimuli in a realistic and adaptive manner rather than with generalized or sometimes inert fear responses. It is not unreasonable to suppose that the fear reactions and genuine threats to existence in old age produce alarm responses which require a very adequate or perhaps even superior basis of attachment and learning in earlier life in order to permit coping behaviour in old age.

Coping and adequate behaviour in the face of the very real threats of old age is of importance in avoiding depression and anxiety. Seligman (1975) has argued cogently for the deleterious effects of personal helplessness and unpredictable situations in the genesis of depression and anxiety. His 'symptoms' of helplessness have a direct relevance to the problems of coping with stress in later life, especially lowered initiation of voluntary responses; 'animals and men who have experienced uncontrollability show reduced initiation of voluntary responses and negative cognitive set'; 'helpless animals and men have difficulty learning that responses produce outcomes'. Such concepts appear to extend the understanding of the psychopathology of depression and anxiety in old age and in addition provide at least some basis for the general management and more special psychotherapy of the aged with neurotic and affective disorders (see below).

Deviant personalities without neurotic disorder

Among the elderly some can readily be identified, who in earlier life failed to live up to the standards of society. Their work record, marital history, ability to develop interests, and socioeconomic self-sufficiency is rated as 'inadequate'. Others can be identified who have refused to conform to social expectations, reject offers of friendship, refuse services from others, as well as denying their own obligations.

They tend also to have hostile and extra-punitive traits and are called 'paranoid' personalities. The position of the paranoid and alienated personality is a matter which has been considered by several authors. It has been suggested (Birren *et al.* 1963) that there may be elderly people who show 'an adaptive use of schizoid mechanisms in coming to face the problems of ageing'. Also socially inadequate extreme isolates, paranoid, hostile personalities have been described by Lowenthal (1968): 'They are almost without exception single males, low socioeconomic status who lived alone, often worked hard at sheer survival, they spoke without emotion, of having left home at a very early age or sustaining no contacts with parental or extended family, of battling against the world, earning a living by strenuous efforts, they called themselves with apparent pride "lone wolves" ... yet they never complained of loneliness, they ranked about as high as anyone else on our morale scales and they were no more likely to be hospitalized for mental illness than were their more sociable peers'. Providing such people remain fit, strong and capable of carrying out their strategy they survive well in the community. The author's studies (Bergmann, 1971) bear this out and both paranoid and inadequate personalities appear to make their own but separate adjustments. The inadequate person provides a focus for help for family, for friends, and even sometimes for quite casual contacts. They show gratitude, their dependency and lack of achievement allows them to fit in to the setting that many people with more normal pride and self respect would find most uncongenial. On the other hand the fighting stance of the hostile paranoid personalities keeps them intact, failure is never their own, ill health could be remedied if only the doctor gave adequate treatment etc. The world, at large, has to be taken on in single combat; life presents a very busy and diverting struggle against the dangerous and hostile forces from without and there is little time for despair, depression, fear, and anxiety.

It could be asked whether in a Western industrial civilization where only the nuclear family remains as the main supporting unit and there is a devaluation of the position of the aged in society, that extreme poles of behaviour, i.e. fighting to death or abject surrender, may not sometimes provide a more effective strategy than the modes of adjustment to which our social values are more likely to award the label of 'normal'.

Physical ill health and neurotic disorder in old age

The association between physical ill health and affective disorders beginning in old age has frequently been demonstrated (Roth and Kay, 1956; Post, 1962). Those elderly patients in whom affective disorder presents as a recurrence of earlier manic depressive disease have no more risk of physical ill health than would be expected by chance, whereas those elderly persons whose affective disorder begins in old age have a significantly increased prevalence of physical ill health and disability. Studies of outpatients and office patients have noted physical ill health as one of the major adequate external causes recognized both by the patients and their physicians (Clow and Allen, 1951; Straker, 1963). Random samples of community residents (Kay *et al.*, 1964b) demonstrate a strong association between neurotic and affective disorder and measures of physical disability and disease.

The longitudinal follow-up of community residents with predominantly neurotic and affective disorder (Kay and Bergmann, 1966) demonstrated a significantly increased mortality of elderly persons with functional disorder and this difference was most marked among male subjects. Nevertheless, the issue is not simple or straightforward, for elderly persons with quite severe physical illness cope without developing neurotic disorder and also people can be identified who develop neurotic or affective disorder in association with physical ill health who improve from their depression and anxiety while their physical health continues to deteriorate.

It is of interest to consider the reciprocal interaction of physical ill health and neurotic disorder and some of the hypotheses that have been advanced:

(1) That physical ill health always causes neurotic disorder and therefore there is little remarkable about this association to require discussion.
(2) There is little genuine association between neurosis and physical ill health in old age and therefore complaints of ill health are likely to be part of a hypochondriacal neurotic reaction masquerading as genuine ill health or exaggerating the extent of physical disability.
(3) That neurotic disorder itself has a deleterious effect on physical health and makes an independent contribution to morbidity and mortality in old age.

It is evident that not all ill persons develop neurotic reactions in response to their physical ill health and in the random sample examined by the author about 32 per cent of 'normal' respondents were judged to be suffering from moderate or severe physical disability. Though nearly twice that number of late onset neurotics suffered from moderate or severe ill health, the normals with physical ill health represented an important subgroup. It has been observed that a significant proportion of people with continuing physical ill health recover from late onset neurotic disorder (see above) and this suggests that the physical ill health is not by itself both a necessary and sufficient cause for the neurotic state. Further support for this view can be drawn from acute medical ward samples of elderly patients (Bergmann and Eastham, 1974) in which it was evident that among acutely ill elderly only 29 per cent reacted with neurotic or affective disorders to any appreciable extent. It would seem therefore that some consideration needs to be given as to why elderly people with physical ill health even sometimes during the recovery or convalescent phase may develop neurotic reactions and others with comparable disability do not. The psychological effects of physical ill health are difficult to delineate but several factors would appear to be operative. First at the most obvious level perhaps is that illness in later life is more likely to be seen as life threatening, leading to death, or at least giving intimations of mortality. Physical disability may also disturb the elderly person's fragile balance and adjustment. This is especially true with obsessional personalities who have kept a sense of unworthiness and guilt at bay by being tidier, harder working, and more self sacrificing than others. Physical ill health prevents these important props to self esteem and personality and Butler (1968) has pointed out how in some elderly people 'counterphobic' overactivity can reach extreme and grotesque levels in an effort to keep realization of death at bay. Those elderly persons who by chance or on account of their previous personality structure do not have close family ties and who rely more on physical activity and outings may also specially be affected by illness limiting their mobility and range of activities. To sum up, physical ill health and a sense of worthlessness may often go hand in hand in persons in whom there is not a strong central core of personal value and integrity ('Ego-integrity versus despair', Erikson, 1959).

The elderly are said to be more hypochondriacal and studies on 'healthy' volunteers by Busse *et al.* (1960) certainly emphasize the importance of hypochondriasis and find little significant relationship between neurotic disorders in old age and physical ill health. This finding at first seems very much at variance with European work but may perhaps be explained by the fact that they worked with community volunteers tempted by the offer of a free physical examination in an era before Medicare was available. Neither the findings of the present author (Bergmann, 1971) or earlier studies by d'Alarcon (1964) bear out the idea that elderly people are universally hypochondriacal and hypochondriasis where it does exist is more often associated with genuine depression and anxiety and sometimes with underlying and severe physical ill health of a system other than that complained of by the patient.

The question of whether neurotic disorder in the aged affects and exacerbates physical ill health is not easy to answer. If one examines the types of physical ill health most commonly associated with neurotic and affective disorder then cardiac disease must be very prominent. Studies of hospital samples (Dovenmuehle and Verwoerdt, 1963) show the great importance of cardiac disease and the frequency of reactive depressions among elderly people experiencing this condition. These authors found that the most significant correlate with affective disorder was the severity of the physical ill health rather than neurotic personal predisposition. However, a random community sample (Bergmann, 1971) showed the highly significant association of cardiac disorder, independently of the severity of the disability, with late onset neurotic reactions. It has been suggested (Bull, 1969) that autonomic overactivity may, in conjunction with basic atherosclerotic pathology, have a deleterious effect on the long term prognosis of cerebrovascular and ischaemic heart disease. There is also some evidence to suggest that regardless of diagnostic category, acutely ill elderly people with reactive affective disorder require longer to recover from their physical ill health than do patients not suffering from reactive neurotic and affective disorder (Bergmann and Eastham, 1974). It would perhaps be fruitful to examine the possibility of recognition and treatment of neurotic and emotional upset in the acutely ill elderly and the hypothesis could be tested that psychiatric treatment speeds up recovery and reduces mortality in non-demented elderly persons.

The psychiatrist also has a part to play in advising general practitioners and physicians dealing with the elderly of the psychological aspects of treating physical ill health, the emotional benefits that small therapeutic successes may bring and the despair and helplessness arising in elderly patients in response to any therapeutic nihilism in the physician.

Social stresses

Undoubtedly, the elderly person is at a disadvantage both socially and economically. Statistical returns collected on a national basis (*Social trends*, 1975) indicate that pensioner households show a significantly lower weekly income than households in general and the expenditure on various items is also consistently lower. The overall household expenditure is on average £39·43 and that of households where the head is aged 65 or over only £21·95. Financial deprivation is a source of worry to many elderly persons and there can be little dispute that their range of choices is restricted by this. Also elderly persons often congregate in the deteriorating inner city residential areas, when others have moved out to newly built suburban development. Isolation from friends and neighbours who have moved and fears of vandalism and other depredations are common.

Bereavement with consequent loss of old friends, relatives as well as the loss of husband or wife is an increasingly common occurrence and survivors into extreme old age may have to cope with grief and mourning from the deaths of their children.

It was therefore somewhat surprising to find that social stresses did not seem to have any strong correlation with a tendency to develop neurotic disorder in later life. That is not to say that depressed and anxious elderly persons were not found in situations of great poverty, deprivation, and isolation but to suggest that many elderly experiencing such conditions coped without developing neurotic or affective disorders. Doctors and social workers who work with elderly patients and clients, tend to exaggerate and generalize the significance of social stress from the base of their experience of a specially selected and vulnerable population of elderly persons. They obtain a picture of neglectful families, miserable and poverty stricken elderly persons, and in general such a gloomy atmosphere surrounds the world of the elderly that it becomes impossible to accept that there might be elderly persons who are happy, well adjusted, adequately provided for, and not suffering from neurotic or affective disorder.

Valuable corrective work has, of course, been done by Townsend (1957) even where the elderly persons move into the less warm intimate atmosphere of suburban London, support and family connections still hold up well (Wilmot and Young, 1960). Retirement which is dreaded by many and seen as a very potent stress both for physical and mental ill health certainly seems more the result of ill health where retirement is optional (Richardson, 1956) and a sociological review on the position of retirement (Susser and Watson, 1971) suggests that 'general attitudes towards retirement are becoming more favourable and accepting, and a growing number of men who retire (about two out of every three wage and salary workers) say they retired by their own decision (Palmore, 1964)'.

The question of isolation which is often cited as one of the major causes of emotional upset of the elderly requires examination. Lowenthal (1964, 1965) examined the problem of isolation in old age and its connection with mental illness though not specifically in her case, with neurotic illness. She did not consider people who had led a lifelong isolated existence as being psychiatrically vulnerable. In a random sample of community residents (Garside *et al.*, 1965) isolation also emerged as an independent factor which was orthogonal to the psychiatric illness factor. In the author's own study, although isolation correlated highly with late onset neurotic disorder it did not, after due allowance for its relationship to physical ill health and poor mobility, make a very significant independent contribution.

Bereavement is seen as a self-evident 'cause' of neurosis in old age but, here again, contrary to public expectation, the role of bereavement in the genesis of neurotic and affective reactions of later life is not at all clear cut. The study by Parkes (1964) suggests that bereavement as a cause of mental illness becomes less significant with increasing age. Though, of course, where strong personal predisposition in terms of a previously dissociative and denying personality are evident, often abnormal mourning reactions occur. Mysterious anniversary reactions are not uncommon, strange symptoms may occur mimicking the lost person's terminal illness and distortion and limitation of social life of the elderly person may lead to self-imposed isolation, lack of interests or purposeful activity. Difficulties and failures in self care and a change to negative behaviour in the surviving family member have all been noted. However, it has to be said that these reactions are minority reactions and that in a representative sample of the elderly in the community a very large majority cope adequately with loss, grief, and the resolution of mourning.

It can be argued that elderly persons with the most social stresses are selectively removed from the community into hospitals and institutions but in Britain, where 95 per cent of the elderly remain outside institutions, selective removal must have only a limited effect on the picture.

Psychotherapy of neurotic disorder in old age

The classical psychoanalytic treatment for neuroses was not considered by Freud (1905) to be applicable to patients in later life. Such patients were thought to be too rigid for the requisite personality shifts to occur. In general dynamic psychotherapy for elderly patients has come late on the scene. A notable exception was Abraham (1920) who undertook psychotherapy with elderly persons. In his paper entitled 'The applicability of psychoanalytic treatment to patients at an advanced age' he stated that there were a certain group of patients who did well even when they were of an older age than was usually recommended as suitable for psychotherapy. He defined this group as follows: 'the prognosis in cases, even at an advanced age, is favourable if the neuroses has set in, in its full severity, only after a period has elapsed since puberty and if the patient has enjoyed for at least several years a sexual attitude approaching the normal and a period of social usefulness'. This passage seems to suggest the recognition by Abraham of a late onset neurotic group with a relatively good previous adjustment of personality and an approach of, at least some, therapeutic optimism.

Some models for psychotherapy with elderly people do not have a greatly different structure from those developed in the dynamic psychotherapy of patients in earlier life. They emphasize the importance of transference, instinctual drives, and gratifications and look for the reactivation of earlier problems. Such a view is presented by the review of Blau and Berezin (1975). To such psychotherapists what is of particular importance is to trace the connection with, and the reactivation of childhood psychopathology in the present situation.

Rockwell (1956) in an earlier review of 'Psychotherapy in the aged individual' prefers a Meyerian approach 'the technique of distributive analysis and synthesis'. Perhaps nowadays the assets of this psychobiological method are a part of any good general psychiatric multifactorial approach and certainly form the centre of ordinary care with elderly persons whether they be in a medical geriatric unit or in a psychiatric unit.

Psychotherapeutic techniques and models developed to help individuals during adolescence, courtship, marriage, career struggles, child bearing, and child rearing seem less relevant to elderly people. Perhaps predominantly intrapsychic factors such as transference and dependence, castration fears, and regression have to be reviewed along side very significant external factors such as the approach of death to friends and oneself, the loss of physical independence, the helplessness and lack of choice which poverty and poor housing induce, and the actual rejection, tyrannical treatment, and loss of respect which elderly people often encounter. What is normal adjustment in the aged? How does a normal elderly person cope with the stresses and vicissitudes of ageing, these questions are rarely asked and unsatisfactorily answered. The social and psychological studies of Neugarten and her associates based on the Kansas City studies have produced typologies which label successful adjustment in age in terms of integration, activity, engagement or disengagement and dependency verses autonomy (Neugarten, 1964).

It is, however, difficult to link these types of personality and strategies described, very clearly with the major tasks faced by elderly people. An attempt can be made to sum up these tasks as follows:

(1) An acceptance of the increasing imminence and reality of death.
(2) Coping with genuine, sometimes painful, severe disabling physical ill health.
(3) Co-ordinating the necessary dependence on medical, domestic, and family support and making an accurate estimation of the available independent choices that can still be made in order to achieve maximum satisfaction.
(4) To give and obtain emotional gratification from friends and relatives.

Perhaps these issues relate to the ones that Erikson (1959) summarized in his view of the central issue of old age 'Ego-integrity versus despair'.

Coping with death

The most systematic and perhaps helpful review of the question of facing death and the psychotherapeutic approach to elderly people concerning this is that put forward by Butler (1968). He sums up his approach as follows: 'Put succinctly, the psychotherapy of old age is the psychotherapy of grief and of accommodation, restitution and resolution inside the "coming to terms with", bearing witness, reconciliation, atonement, construction, reconstruction, integration, transcendence, creativity, realistic insight with modifications and substitutions, the introduction of meaning and of meaningful useful and contributory efforts. These are among the terms that are pertinent of therapy with older people'. He lays particular emphasis on the need for life review, for a recognition of how to function as an elderly person and how to gain strength from the survival and adaptation which has already been experienced.

Physical ill health and hypochondriasis

Coping with severe physical ill health can never be easy and the general malaise and difficulty of carrying out tasks of day-to-day living sometimes seems insuperable to the elderly person. Pfeiffer and Busse (1973) deem hypochondriasis to be one of the most important neurotic reactions of the aged.

They consider that elderly persons are especially liable to escape from 'personal failure into the sick role' and consider that a hypochondriacal complaint is a distress signal which requires a significant gesture of caring on behalf of the therapist with later insight into underlying neurotic complaints. However, other workers (Kay *et al.*, 1966) have found that the patients' estimate of their own health is, all too often, a better predictor of subsequent death than that of the physician. Nevertheless some patients cope with disabling physical ill health in a realistic and effective manner while others do not. Inability to cope effectively with physical ill health may be determined by two major psychological causes. The presence of guilt and loss of self esteem may be a major feature to be found in intrapunitive personalities and anger, resentment and a deep sense of injustice in extrapunitive ones. Guilty feelings are not at all uncommon among physically ill elderly people. They do not only relate to the obvious burdens that are caused to friends and relatives but also to the loss of ability to carry out tasks in the home, to be cleaner than anyone else, to be harder working, to be more tidy, to be more self-sacrificing, to always do things for other people that characterize those who require many props to their fragile and unstable self esteem. These patients require psychotherapy to adopt a less poor idea of themselves and support in reviewing their lives and sharing with the therapist a more optimistic kindly and positive view of their achievements and abilities.

Those elderly persons who feel angry, resentful, and wish to protest against the way they have been treated by fate or their physicians are in a difficult situation. They are helpless. Their anger may lead to reprisals and, of course, this is not an unrealistic fear as unpleasant and 'paranoid' elderly people find themselves disposed of rapidly.

The therapist's task may be to explore their sense of injustice, permit expression of anger in safety and without reprisals and establish a link if there is one to be established with earlier and persistent feelings of injustice that may date back to childhood. The transformation of the drive behind such anger into obtaining just deserts and better treatment has also to be considered because anger and the resentment are not always ill-founded and may represent a better view of reality than smiling and uncomplaining acceptance. Nevertheless, the elderly person has to be helped to harness this feeling into a productive use of medical, nursing and other help in order to avoid rejection.

The problem of dependency

Dependency is a 'bad' word in psychotherapy with younger neurotic patients. Ideally it must not be fostered, overt reassurance and support are to be avoided, and analysis of regressive dependent transference relationships then permits a more 'adult' method of coping. Psychotherapy in old age has to take cognizance of a different situation and an analysis of the problems of dependency in the elderly and its relevance to psychotherapeutic intervention has been carried out by Goldfarb (1968). He reviews the multiple causes of decline in later life with the attendant losses of resources, decreased mastery, increased feelings of helplessness and fear and the consequent search for aid. He defines the basic dichotomy between a 'healthy' and 'unhealthy' response as that between a rational search for skilled aid and an irrational search for a parent substitute or significant other, accompanied by regressive behaviour. He includes in the neurotic search for aid displays of helplessness, hypochondriasis, depressive and paranoid reactions, and exploitative and manipulative behaviour.

Among the treatment aims are the possibility of helping the patient to become less helpless or to feel less helpless by providing an 'illusion of strength' in their power to influence the therapist and by trying to recognize from their pattern of searching for aid what type of personal relationship the patient seeks and what kind of person he thinks he needs. He also discusses the problem, encountered by any psychiatrist who has worked with elderly people, of the 'pseudo-independent' behaviour which often renders a person intolerable because of their failure to accept help, advice and relief, and points out that such a person can only be helped by establishing, 'even in a disguised form ... some dependence in a protective relationship'.

The psychopathological model of anxiety described by Bowlby (1969) provides a good basis for the psychotherapeutic use of the dependent relationship. The therapist has to accept dependent attachment and 'affectional bonds' and use these feelings to guide and encourage the other person to face external threats in an adaptive and realistic way. In many patients these bonds have to be transferred to other persons or institutions (e.g. day centres, clinics or health visitors, and practice nurses) and maintained, however tenuously, for the rest of the patient's life. Such a prosthetic bond allows stresses and threats to be faced with courage, help to be sought realistically, and can be maintained on an economical and viable basis. Reduction of 'learned helplessness' (Seligman, 1975) and the clarification of areas of choice available to the patient are important. Later in the therapeutic transaction a certain hardness in confronting the elderly patient with the choices he must make becomes a significant ingredient in diminishing learned helplessness and furthering the psychotherapeutic process. Perhaps it is not too fanciful to liken the whole process to infancy, childhood, adolescence and maturity especially when one confronts the extremely regressed and child-like behaviour often met in the elderly patients with severe neurotic and physical disabilities.

The elderly patient's interpersonal relationships

Interpersonal relationships and the gratification to be derived from them is one of the important motivations for staying alive and functioning independently in old age. Most elderly persons are in contact with their family or at least some close friends, but neurotic and maladaptive relationships frequently disrupt the opportunities for contact and giving and receiving love. Post (1958) has described a particularly frequent problem situation which he terms the 'mother–daughter' syndrome. This occurs in closely attached dependent women who remain with their mothers, turning to them for advice and avoiding outside relationships. The mother, in such a situation, retains the gratification of her sense of power and control while the daughter assuages her fears and insecurities. Reversal of this situation with loss of power by the parent and increasing demands placed on the child bring frictions and tension, and ultimately anxiety and depression accompanied by manipulative behaviour in the parent and stirrings of anger, hatred, and revolt in the child. Psychotherapeutic intervention must aim at giving, at least, the child some insight into the situation and it may, in fact, be the only measure which can avoid numerous recurring crises and accidents often leading to frequent admissions to various hospital departments. Other constellations can be recognized though little systematic work has been carried out on the need for and effects of systematic dynamically orientated family therapy in helping elderly persons and their families to cope with life at home.

One such constellation is not uncommon and has been observed by the author and his coworkers and requires prompt recognition and help.

This syndrome might be called 'power reversal' in the family hierarchy. The elderly patient has typically been a well thought of, conforming member of the family. They are often shy, unassertive, obedient, conformist and with a strong need to be 'good'. In such people self assertion and the overt expression of demands and needs has been muted for many years. They may be seen by the family to be less 'bright', less enterprising or less driving and thus justify their subordinate and lowly position in the family.

A life threatening illness in the patient supervenes sometimes, such illnesses as cancer, severe obstructive airway disease with marked cyanosis and heart failure, malignant hypertension and ischaemic heart disease, or at other times perhaps a depression or repeated falls and agitation or inexplicable exaggerated pains, or persistent and severe anorexia and weight loss may be seen as a new and sinister life threatening condition.

The family, somewhat guilty and ashamed, responds with warm concern, close support and desires and wishes are gratified almost before they are spoken. Such power is irresistible and childish, demanding, hypochondriacal and sometimes violent and dictatorial behaviour ultimately leads to recurring crises and finally rejection and extrusion of the patient either into a psychiatric unit or under the care of a puzzled physician who can find no change in the physical state to account for the current crisis.

An understanding of family dynamics is important and the relatives have to receive help in learning to cope with a shift of power which in part may be legitimate and yet has to be contained and limited and not rewarded any more. Legitimate self-assertion and reduction of helplessness have to be encouraged but regressive and manipulative power seeking behaviour has to remain unrewarded even when blackmail includes the explicit or implicit threat of suicide. The need for institutional care is the admission of failure on both sides but may have to be frankly accepted and realized.

Other constellations in which power shifts occur can also be described and are perhaps not so complex. For instance, the 'fallen dictator' a powerful husband and father with a subservient wife and children reacts very strongly to the loss of physical strength and financial dominance. Such losses may necessitate neurotic, hysterical and manipulative behaviour to control and maintain dominance in the family.

In general these situations concern themselves with shifts of power and dependency which upset the equilibrium of the family and prevent the exchange of good feelings which elderly people need from their relatives. It is to be emphasized that the lifelong 'isolate' though deemed 'abnormal' by case-workers, doctors and nurses does not figure in this section, as they have made an adjustment which does not require close or intimate exchanges of feeling in earlier life, as dependency of some type is central to all the situations (Goldfarb, 1968).

Conclusion

This review of neurotic disorder may arouse in the reader a commonly occurring response: Why bother with this when there is so much misery due to organic psychiatric disorder in the elderly, surely consideration of the neuroses is a luxury we cannot afford?

The treatment of neurotic disorder within the health service setting is certainly still a matter for argument. Nevertheless, cogent reasons have been put forward for the inclusion of psychotherapy of some type as a provision for younger patients within the health service (Wolff, 1973).

Epidemiological study suggests that neurotic reactions to the stresses of ageing exist and cause suffering to elderly persons and would appear to justify at least comparable resources to those deemed necessary for younger people. Arguments are advanced that in old age somehow patients do not 'suffer' from their neuroses but only enjoy the best of neurotic ill health. The facts do not bear out this view and the suffering found by elderly persons is at least as severe, though not always as readily recognized, as in earlier life. Other arguments put forward against treating neurotic disorders in old age are that fundamental cure is no longer possible in elderly patients and that therefore they ought to receive a lesser priority than younger ones. Such an argument seems neither scientifically nor morally tenable. The prime consideration for all age groups seems to the author to be the relief of suffering. Economic arguments would perhaps permit the claim that the elderly are unproductive and therefore psychiatric help must be given in the first instance to those working in industry, vital services and in rearing children. This argument ignores the 'negative productivity' of those elderly, unhappy and disturbed persons whose effects on neighbours, children and even grandchildren can be measured (Grad and Sainsbury, 1968).

Finally it needs to be said that many patients with organic psychiatric disorders present with disruptive crises related to the psychodynamic interactions between the elderly person and their family circle. The lack of a body of knowledge, expertise and understanding of the neuroses and personality problems of the elderly robs us of one of the few therapeutic possibilities in treating and preventing the breakdown of the supporting network which keeps brain damaged elderly people viable in the community.

References

Abraham, K. (1920) 'The applicability of psychoanalytic treatment to patients at an advanced age', in *Selected papers of Karl Abraham*, trans. D. Bryan and A. Strachey (1927), International Psychoanalytical Library, No. 13, London, Hogarth, pp. 312–317.

d'Alarcon, R. (1964) 'Hypochondriasis and depression in the aged', *Geront. clin. (Basel)*, **6**, 266–277.

Bergmann, K. (1971) 'The neuroses of old age', in *Recent Developments in Psychogeriatrics*, (Ed. D.W.K. Kay and A. Walk) *Br. J. Psychiat.*, Spec. Pub. 6, pp. 39–50.

Bergmann, K., Kay, D.W.K., Foster, E.M., McKechnie, A.A., and Roth, M. (1971) 'A follow-up study of randomly selected community residents to assess the effects of chronic brain syndrome and cerebrovascular disease', *Proceedings of Vth Congress of Psychiatry, Psychiatry, Part II*. pp. 856–865.

Bergmann, K., and Eastham, E.J. (1974) 'Psychogeriatric ascertainment and assessment for treatment in an acute medical ward setting', *Age and Ageing*, **3**, 174–188.

Bergmann, K., Foster, E.M., Justice, A.W., and Matthews, V. (1975) *Reversible functional disorders—the significant factors in multidisciplinary management*, paper presented to the World Congress of Gerontology, Jerusalem, June, 1975, (Abstract).

Birren, J.E., Butler, R.N., Greenhouse, S.W., Sokoloff, L., and Yarrow, M.R. (ed.) (1963) *Human aging: a biological and behavioural study*. Public Health Service Publication, No. 986. Washington, DC, Government Printing Office.

Blau, D., and Berezin, M.A. (1975) 'Neuroses and character disorders', in *Modern perspectives in the psychiatry of old age*, (Ed. J.G. Howells) New York, Brunner/Mazel, Ch. 9, pp. 201–231.

Bowlby, J. (1969) 'Psychopathology of anxiety: the role of affectional bonds', *Br. J. Psychiat.*, Spec. Pub. 3, 80–86.

Bremer, J. (1951) 'A social psychiatric investigation of a small community in northern Norway', *Acta psychiat. neurol. (Kbh.)*, Suppl. 62.

Britton, P.G., Bergmann, K., Kay, D.W.K., and Savage, R.D. (1967) 'Mental state cognitive functioning, physical health and social class in the community aged', *J. Geront.*, **22**, 517–521.

Britton, P.G., and Savage, R.D. (1966) 'The MMPI and the aged—some normative data from a community sample', *Br. J. Psychiat.*, **112**, 941–943.

Bull, G.M. (1969) 'A comparative study of myocardial infarction and cerebral vascular accidents', *Geront. clin., (Basel)*, **11**, 193–205.

Busse, E.W., Dovenmuehle, R.H., and Brown, R.G. (1960) 'Psychoneurotic reactions of the aged', *Geriatrics*, **15**, 97–105.

Butler, R.N. (1968) 'Towards a psychiatry of the life cycle: implications of sociopsychologic studies of the aging process for the psychotherapeutic situation', in *Aging in modern society*, (Ed. A. Simon and L.J. Epstein), Washington DC, Psychiatric Research Reports of the American Psychiatric Association, Ch. 20, pp. 233–248.

Cameron, N. (1956) 'Neuroses of later maturity', in *Mental disorders in later life*, (Ed. O.J. Kaplan) 2nd ed. London, Oxford University Press, Ch. 8, pp. 201–243.

Chown, S.M. (1962) 'Rigidity and age', in *Social and psychological aspects of aging*, (Ed. C. Tibbitts and W. Donahue) Columbia, Columbia University Press, pp. 832–835.

Clow, H.E., and Allen, E.B. (1951) 'Manifestations of psychoneuroses occurring in later life', *Geriatrics*, **6**, 31–39.

Cowan, N.R. (1969) 'Early diagnosis—the Rutherglen experiment', in *Vol. I. Abstracts of Symposia and Lectures, 8th International Congress of Gerontology Proceedings*, Washington, DC.

Cumming, E., and Henry, W.E. (1961) *Growing old: the process of disengagement*, New York, Basic Books.

Diethelm, O., and Rockwell, F.V. (1943) 'Psychopathology of aging', *Am. J. Psychiat.*, **99**, 553–556.

Dovenmuehle, R.H., and Verwoerdt, A. (1963) 'Physical illness and depressive symptomatology. Part II: Factors of length and severity of illness and frequency of hospitalization', *J. Geront.*, **18**, 260–266.

Erikson, E.H. (1959) *Identify and the life cycle. Selected papers*, Psychological Issues, Vol. 1, No. 1, Monogr. 1, New York, International Universities Press.

Ernst, K. (1959) *Die Prognose der Neurosen*, Monogr. Neurol. Psychiat., No. 85, Berlin, Springer.

Essen-Möller, E. (1956) 'Individual traits and morbidity in a Swedish rural population', *Acta Psychiat. neurol. scand.*, Suppl. 100.

Eysenck, H.J. (1957) *The dynamics of anxiety and hysteria*, London, Routledge and Kegan Paul.

Freud, S. (1905) 'My views on the part played by sexuality in the aetiology of the neuroses', in *Complete psychological works of Sigmund Freud*, (trans. J. Strachey), London, Hogarth, Vol. 7, p. 271.

Freud, S. (1933) *New introductory lectures on psycho-analysis*, (translated W.J.H. Sprott), London, Hogarth Press.

Garside, R.F., Kay, D.W.K., and Roth, M. (1965) 'Old age mental disorders in Newcastle upon Tyne. Part III: A factorial analysis of medical, psychiatric and social characteristics', *Br. J. Psychiat.*, **111**, 939–946.

Goldberg, E.M. (1970) *Helping the aged a field experiment in social work*, London, Allen and Unwin.

Goldberg, D.P. (1972) *The detection of psychiatric illness by questionnaire*, Institute of Psychiatry, Maudsley Monographs 21, London, Oxford University Press.

Goldfarb, A.I. (1968) 'Clinical perspectives', in *Aging in modern society* (Ed. A. Simon and L.J. Epstein) Washington, American Psychiatric Association, Ch. 12, pp. 170–178.

Grad, J., and Sainsbury, P. (1968) 'The effects patients have on their families in a community care and a control psychiatric service—a two-year follow-up', *Br. J. Psychiat.*, **114**, 265–278.

Havighurst, R.J. (1968) 'Personality and patterns of aging', *Gerontologist*, **8**, 20–23.

Havighurst, R.J., Neugarten, B.L., and Tobin, S.S. (1964) 'Disengagement, personality and life satisfaction in later years', in *Age with a future*, (Ed. P.F. Hansen) Copenhagen, Munksgaard, pp. 419–425.

Kay, D.W.K., Beamish, P., and Roth, M. (1964a) 'Old age mental disorders in Newcastle upon Tyne. Part I: A study of prevalence', *Br. J. Psychiat.*, **110**, 146–158.

Kay, D.W.K., Beamish, P., and Roth, M. (1964b) 'Old age mental disorders in Newcastle upon Tyne. Part II: A study of possible social and medical causes', *Br. J. Psychiat.*, **110**, 668–682.

Kay, D.W.K., and Bergmann, K. (1966) 'Physical disability and mental health in old age', *J. Psychosomatic Res.*, **10**, 3–12.

Kay, D.W.K., Bergmann, K., Foster, E.M., and Garside, R.F. (1966) 'A four-year follow-up of a random sample of old people originally seen in their own homes: A physical, social and psychiatric enquiry', Excerpta Medica International Congress Series, No. 150. *Proceedings of the IVth World Congress of Psychiatry*, Madrid; Amsterdam, Excerpta Medica.

Kay, D.W.K., Foster, E.M., and Bergmann, K. (1973) *Indications for domiciliary services*. Paper presented to World Psychiatric Association, Psychogeriatric Section Meeting, Institute of Psychiatry, London.

Kerr, T.A., Schapira, K., and Roth, M. (1969) 'The relationship between premature death and affective disorders', *Br. J. Psychiat.*, **115**, 1277.

Kessel, W.I.N., and Shepherd, M. (1962) 'Neurosis in hospital and general practice', *J. Ment. Sci.*, **108**, 159–166.

Lowenthal, M.F. (1964) 'Social isolation and mental illness in old age', *Am. Soc. Rev.*, **29**, 54–70.

Lowenthal, M.F. (1965) 'Antecedents of isolation and mental illness in old age', *Arch. gen. Psychiat.*, **12**, 245–254.

Lowenthal, M.F. (1968) 'The relationship between social factors and mental health in the aged', in *Aging in modern society*, (Ed. A. Simon and L.J. Epstein), Washington, American Psychiatric Association, Ch. 14, pp. 187–197.

Maudsley, H. (1895) *The pathology of mind: a study of its distempers, deformities and disorders*, London, Macmillan.

McDonald, C. (1967a) 'Measures of neuroticism in the elderly', *Aust. N.Z.J. Psychiat.*, **1**, 44–47.

McDonald, C. (1967b) 'The pattern of neurotic illness in the elderly', *Aust. N.Z.J. Psychiat.*, **1**, 203–210.

Neugarten, B.L. (1964) 'Personality types in an aged population', in *Personality in middle and late life*, (Ed. B.L. Neugarten *et al.*), New York, Atherton, Ch. 8.

Nielson, J. (1962) 'Geronto-psychiatric period-prevalence investigation in a geographically delimited population', *Acta psychiat. scand.*, **38**, 307–330.

Nunn, C., Bergmann, K., Britton, P.G., Foster, E.M., Hall, E.H., and Kay, D.W.K. (1974) 'Intelligence and neurosis in old age', *Br. J. Psychiat.*, **124**, 446–452.

Palmore, E. (1964) 'Retirement patterns among aged men: findings of the 1963 survey of the aged', *Soc. Sec. Bull.*, **27**, 3–10.

Parkes, C.M. (1964) 'Recent bereavement as a cause of mental illness', *Br. J. Psychiat.*, **110**, 198.

Parsons, P.L. (1965) 'Mental health of Swansea's old folk', *Br. J. Preve. Soc. Med.*, **19**, 43–47.

Pfeiffer, E., and Busse, E.W. (1973) 'Mental disorders on later life—affective disorders; paranoid, neurotic and situational reactions', in *Mental illness in later life*, (Ed. E.W. Busse and E. Pfeiffer) Washington, American Psychiatric Association.

Pollitt, J. (1957) 'Natural history of obsessional states', *Br. Med. J.*, **i**, 194–198.

Post, F. (1958) 'Social factors in old age psychiatry', *Geriatrics*, **13**, 576.

Post, F. (1962) *The significance of affective symptoms in old age*, Maudsley Monograph No. 10, London, Oxford University Press.

Primrose, E.J.R. (1962) *Psychological illness: a community study*, Mind and Medicine Monographs, London, Tavistock.

Richardson, I.M. (1956) 'Retirement: a socio-medical study of 244 men', *Scot. Med. J.*, **i**, 381–391.

Rockwell, F.V. (1956) 'Psychotherapy in the older individual', in *Mental disorders in later life*, (Ed. O.J. Kaplan) 2nd ed., California, Stanford University Press, Ch. 16, pp. 423–445.

Roth, M. (1955) 'The natural history of mental disorder in old age', *J. Ment. Sci.*, **101**, 281–301.

Roth, M., and Kay, D.W.K. (1956) 'Affective disorders arising in the senium. Part II: Physical disability as an aetiological factor', *J. Ment. Sci.*, **102**, 141–150.

Savage, R.D. (1973) 'Old age', in *Handbook of abnormal psychology*, (Ed. H.J. Eysenck) 2nd ed., London, Pitman Medical, Ch. 8, pp. 645–688.

Schapira, K., Roth, M., Kerr, T.A., and Gurney, C. (1972) 'The prognosis of affective disorders: the differentiation of anxiety states from depressive illnesses', *Br. J. Psychiat.*, **121**, 175–181.

Schilder, P. (1940) 'Psychiatric aspects of old age and aging', *Am. J. Orthopsychiat.*, **10**, 62–72.

Sealey, A.P.E.L. (1965) 'Age trends in adult personality as measured by the 16PF test', *Bull. Br. Psychol. Soc.*, **18**, 19.

Seligman, M.E.P. (1975) *Helplessness—on depression, development and death*, San Francisco, W. H. Freeman.

Shepherd, M., Cooper, B., Brown, A.C., and Kalton, G.W. (1966) *Psychiatric illness in general practice*, London, Oxford University Press.

Shepherd, M., and Gruenberg, E.M. (1957) 'The age for neuroses', *Milbank Memorial Fund Quart.*, **35**, 258–265.

Simon, A. (1968) 'Mental health of community-resident versus hospitalized aged', in *Aging in modern society*, (Ed. A. Simon and L.J. Epstein), Washington, American Psychiatric Association, Ch. 11, pp. 161–169.

Slater, E., and Shields, J. (1969) 'Genetical aspects of anxiety', *Br. J. Psychiat.*, Spec. Pub. 3, pp. 62–71.

Social trends (1975) No. 6. (Ed. M. Nissel), Central Statistical Office, London, H.M.S.O.

Straker, M. (1963) 'Prognosis for psychiatric illness in the aged', *Am. J. Psychiat.*, **119**, 1069–1075.

Susser, M.W., and Watson, W. (1971) 'Community: status, roles, networks, mobility', in *Sociology in medicine*, 2nd ed., London, Oxford University Press, pp. 177–206.

Swenson, W.M. (1961) 'Structured personality testing in the aged: an MMPI study of the gerontic population', *J. Clin. Psychol.*, **17**, 302–304.

Townsend, P. (1957) *The family of old people*, London, Routledge and Kegan Paul.

Tunstall, J. (1966) *Old and alone—a sociological study of old people*, London, Routledge and Kegan Paul.

Vispo, R.H. (1962) 'Pre-morbid personality in the functional psychoses of the senium: a comparison of ex-patients with healthy controls', *J. Ment. Sci.*, **108**, 790–800.

Watts, C.A.H., and Watts, B.M. (1952) *Psychiatry in general practice*, London, Churchill.

Williamson, J., Stokoe, I.H., Gray, S., Fisher, M., Smith, A., McGhee, A., and Stephenson, E. (1964) 'Old people at home—their unreported needs', *Lancet*, **i**, 1117–1120.

Wilmot, P., and Young, M. (1960) *Family and class in a London suburb*, London, Routledge and Kegan Paul.

Wollf, H.H. (1973) 'The place of psychotherapy in the district psychiatric services', in *Policy for action*, (Ed. R. Cawley and G. McLashlan), Nuffield Provincial Hospitals Trust, London, Oxford University Press, pp. 117–128.

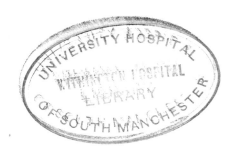

4

THE FUNCTIONAL PSYCHOSES

F. Post

Introduction

In this chapter the term 'functional psychosis' will be used over-inclusively. Conditions will be described in which patients are by no means always and necessarily, grossly deluded or hallucinated. As we shall see, mental disorders without physically based cerebral failure or damage almost always occur in elderly persons with longstanding neurotic problems or character deviations, which had however, only rarely been seriously disabling. For this reason neurotic admixtures such as obsessional, phobic, and especially hypochondriacal symptoms are almost always present in, and often overshadow, the classical features of melancholia, mania, or schizophrenia in the elderly and aged.

We shall not consider here, except in passing, patients growing old after suffering for many years from chronic or recurrent psychoses. The life course of schizophrenics has recently been documented by Bleuler (1972), who demonstrated that these patients often made fair adjustments, rarely deteriorated after the first few years of illness (which in any case often pursued a remitting course), and were able to spend long periods outside institutions. By contrast, depressive, manic, and bipolar affective psychoses recurring from an earlier age do not become less severe and disruptive as patients become older. Attacks tend to become increasingly frequent; sometimes attacks become increasingly similar. Less well documented is the frequency with which earlier episodes had been labelled, with good reason, as neurotic reactions (Post, 1972).

Functional psychoses first appearing during the fifth and sixth decades of life are still regarded by some as separate illnesses, and the debate continues as to whether paraphrenics and paranoid schizophrenics are 'real' schizophrenics. On the other hand, in the case of involutional melancholia, Stenstedt (1959) conclusively failed to demonstrate any genetic differences between involutional and earlier onset manic depressive patients. As we shall see, similarities rather than differences between early and late life psychoses have been stressed in recent work, and any differences in clinical phenomenology have been attributed to age changes in personality structure.

Manic illnesses, for instance, are said to show the effect of ageing in being often characterized with advancing age by less overt and infectious elation and much more by a surly, disgruntled affect, and persecutory content. Flight of ideas may be less conspicuous than over production of speech with a circumstantial, discursive, and anecdotal pattern. Possibly more important may be the observation that depressive admixtures are much more frequently encountered than in younger manics, and to note the frequent occurrences of mixed manic depressive illnesses in the elderly. Similarly, mixtures between depressive and schizophrenic symptoms may become increasingly more common with advancing age, and schizo-affective conditions may become established, which will be briefly discussed in the final section of this chapter, and which are probably not related to the cycloid psychoses of Leonhard found to be confined to younger persons by Perris (1974).

Manic, melancholic, and schizophrenic phenomena singly, or possibly more often in various combinations, may colour or for a time overshadow acute or subacute cerebral failure (confusional states, organic brain syndromes). Early differential diagnosis may be impossible. Slowly progressive cerebral failure as in the dementias of late life (chronic brain syndromes) is also often associated with more persistent states of euphoria and overactivity, with depression, or with paranoid-schizophrenic symptomatology. Differentiation is usually much easier as there is no complicating somatic illness and examination of the cognitive state is more readily carried out. As a rule intellectual decline precedes any psychotic symptoms by many months in dementing illnesses.

From an immediate practical point of view these diagnostic difficulties should not be overstressed. With few exceptions, there are in psychiatry no disease entities, but only individual patients exhibiting mental symptoms, sometimes of one kind only, but especially in late life more often of several kinds. There is no causal therapy, but only a variety of agents which abolish or suppress symptoms. Somatic diseases and deficiencies are treated *secundum artem* when they are discovered. Depressive, manic, and schizophrenic symptoms need to be recognized and distinguished, because specific symptomatic remedies are now available.

Though every patient presents in a highly personal way, and requires an individualized therapeutic approach, most of them, when observed over a period of time, and by stressing similarities rather than differences, can be thought of as suffering from one kind of 'illness' rather than from another.

Affective conditions

Epidemiology

Prevalence figures for several functional psychoses vary between four and one per cent of elderly community samples (Kay *et al.*, 1964). However, the frequency of depression among selected groups tends to be a good deal higher, especially when neurotic depressions are included. Harwin (1973) reported a prevalence of some 30 per cent in elderly invalids visited by a domiciliary nursing service. It is not always recognized that severe depressions are essentially disorders of late life. Those requiring hospital admission occur for the first time most frequently between the ages of 50 and 65; first depressions become a rarity only after the age of 80 (for details see Post, 1968). In the elderly, suicidal acts are almost always associated with well established depressive states, even though 'cry for help' psychodynamics are frequently present as well. Accordingly, many investigators (e.g. Sainsbury, 1968; Ross and Kreitman, 1975) have discovered that the rates for attempted and completed suicide increase steadily into the highest age ranges. Figures for manic illnesses in the elderly have not been discovered by the writer, but it is well known that these are far rarer than depressions, with which in later life they are almost always closely associated.

Psychopathology

Classical senile melancholics suffering for many years from nihilistic and enormity delusions in a setting of severe agitation or near stupor are rarely seen nowadays. To what extent this is attributable to modern and early treatment, or to the possibility that in the past textbook writers had based themselves too exclusively on patients under their care in mental institutions, is far from clear. Having considered, and found wanting, a quite complex classificatory system (Post, 1965), the author (Post, 1972) has come to suggest a far simpler framework.

Ninety-two consecutively admitted depressives over the age of 60 were personally assessed and followed through for three years after discharge from inpatient treatment. Some 37 per cent were very severely ill in terms of retardation, agitation, and perplexity. Their severe emotional disturbance was clearly communicated to the observer as a mood of sadness and fear, alone or in combination. In three-quarters of these patients, thoughts, beliefs, and experiences were easily elicited which were characteristic of severe melancholic states. There were firmly held ideas of being dirty and poor, of having no clothes, of being shunned and talked about by others. They felt themselves targets of obscene remarks. More frequent perhaps were ideas of bowel blockage or of the presence of cancer. A very few patients exhibited a classical Cotard's syndrome with delusions concerning emptiness of head or abdomen, hollowness of bones, thinning of blood, etc. Having committed the unpardonable sin or having sinned against the Holy Ghost were delusions voiced only once or twice by patients, who had, after all, spent the greatest parts of their lives during the twentieth century! However, in this materialistic age, ideas of guilt and self-reproach concerning more mundane matters, especially past dishonesties, were frequently voiced. In about one-quarter of these severely psychotic depressives little thought content of any kind was communicated.

Twenty-four per cent of the sample seemed less severely depressed, and were far less incapacitated in their conduct on the ward, causing less concern on account of restlessness, self neglect, or food refusal. In one-third of their number, no or little depression was communicated, sometimes only seemingly empty agitation. Like other patients in this group of intermediate psychotic depressives they voiced delusional beliefs of physical disease, guilt, and victimization frequently associated with auditory experiences. Initial doubts concerning a possible diagnosis of senile paraphrenia were entertained most frequently in these patients.

Finally, there were some 39 per cent of patients who were dubbed descriptively as neurotic depressives. They communicated little or no sadness of affect, but much more anxiety with, however, little agitation. They had lost interest, showed some sleep disturbance and poor appetite. They complained about unpleasant sensations in abdomen, pelvis, or head with hypochondriacal fears rather than convictions. They tended to blame others rather than themselves. Some patients were phobic of going out on their own or of staying alone; a few had obsessional ruminations or compulsions. All of them had required admission, either because outpatient treatment had failed or because they had become increasingly distressed or distressing in their home surroundings. These conditions were probably equivalent to masked depressions described in younger patients.

Anxiety was felt to be present in 75 per cent of the clinical states of the neurotic depressives, a little less frequently in the intermediate group, and significantly less often, but even so in as many as 47 per cent of severely psychotic patients, documenting the importance of anxiety in elderly depressives. By contrast, attention seeking, histrionic, almost hysterical behaviour was exhibited by only one severely psychotic depressive, but by half the neurotic depressives, while patients in the intermediate psychotic group also occupied, in this respect, an intermediate position.

In spite of all these striking and easily associated differences in symptomatology, all attempts at making them the basis of a classification in terms of aetiology, response to different types of treatment, and of long term course failed.

Aetiology

Common sense would regard the increasing incidence of first depressions, and their tendency to recur even more frequently with rising age, as in no way surprising. Older people do experience life events of a depressing sort much more often than younger persons. We noted that depressions in the very old become increasingly rare, and this may be thought to be due to their decreasing contact with the outside world (disengagement). As summarized elsewhere (Post, 1968), death of a spouse, severe illness of a spouse, moving away of children, retirement, move from the old home, and, most importantly, acutely threatening physical illness have been reported as preceding depression by a few days or weeks in the great majority of affective illness of people over 60. Events of this kind as well as some less clear cut sources of emotional turmoil were deemed to have triggered off the illness in some 78 per cent of the 92 patients described in the previous section. However, using a far more sophisticated method for evaluating the aetiological importance of life events or major difficulties, Brown and his associates (1975) found such to have occurred in between 75 and 86 per cent of female depressives aged 18–65; the incidence of these events over the same period in matched controls had been only 31 per cent. Thus, the idea that traumatic experiences and stresses of various sorts might be of special importance in precipitating the depressions of elderly persons, and thus explain the increasing frequency of these disorders with rising age, does not seem to hold water.

It might still be thought that precipitating events would be more frequently recorded in patients exhibiting neurotic rather than psychotic ('endogenous') clinical pictures. Against expectation, this was found the case only to a statistically insignificant degree. In fact the most easily identified and timed life events (losses or threatened losses of beloved persons) occurred in 41 per cent of severely psychotic, in 32 per cent of intermediate, and in only 29 per cent of neurotic depressives. Retirement, removal from home, physical illness, and other less well defined events were only to an insignificant extent most often associated with neurotic affective states.

Almost half of the recently investigated sample of elderly depressives had been handicapped during their past life by sexual maladjustment, by abnormalities of habitual mood, and by a variety of neurotic propensities. Longstanding interpersonal difficulties had overshadowed the past lives of 75 per cent of neurotic depressives as against those of 50 per cent of the psychotics, but the only statistically significant differences concerned the striking preponderance in neurotic depressives of past phobic and obsessional traits or symptoms. On a global measure of personality deviation (compounded of a number of variables), the three clinical groups could be differentiated at a highly significant level, with greatest past deviation being characteristic of the neurotic group and most stable personalities being recorded for severely psychotic depressives.

Turning to family factors, loss of parents in childhood occurred more frequently in elderly depressives than in the general population, (confirming similar findings by McDonald, 1969), but was not related to type of symptomatology. Typical affective illnesses had occurred in the first degree relatives of 44 per cent of severely psychotic patients, but only insignificantly less often in those of neurotic depressives (31 per cent). Atypical disorders, especially alcoholism, were insignificantly most often ascertained in the relatives of the intermediate, and in many ways most atypical depressives.

Manic states occurred spontaneously or in relation to treatment in 17 of 92 depressives, and interestingly all but two of them had exhibited psychotic depressive symptomatology. This was the only piece of evidence in favour of the traditional view of psychotic depressions of manic depressive type being basically separate illnesses contrasting them with neurotic depressions. Otherwise, experience with elderly depressives would appear to favour the continuum hypothesis of affective illnesses (most recently expounded by Kendell, 1969), in that each depressive state is best conceptualized as a highly individual affair. Regardless of the type of clinical picture shown by the patient, there is often evidence of affective heredity and almost always reactive precipitation. The place where individual patients fall along the continuum between psychotic and neurotic depressions seems to depend much more on the patient's lifelong personality adjustment, and perhaps especially on any previously established neurotic patterns or their absence. Clinical type in no way related to age at first depression, to number of previous attacks, or to longterm outcome. (For a detailed discussion, see Post, 1972.)

Returning to the question as to why depressive illnesses should occur with increasing frequency towards late life, we will briefly note that several investigations have shown that late onset depressives have significantly less family history of affective illness than early onset depressives (Kay, 1959; Hopkinson, 1964; Chesser, 1965; Post, 1972) and that late life depression is not a separate hereditary entity.

Apart from less genetic loading, in some ways late life depressives have been found to be characterized by rather more stable prepsychotic personalities (Roth, 1955). To a statistically significant extent late onset depressives showed less often than early onset patients personality problems such as moodiness, lack of sociability, sexual difficulties, and anxious-hypochondriacal traits (Chesser, 1965).

We saw earlier in this section that the increasing frequency of depressions in late life could not be attributed to greater life stress, which may however play a role in one or two specific circumstances. Roth and Kay (1956) reported physical illness to be an unduly frequent precipitating factor of first depressions in old men, and Chesser (1965) suggested that the loss of a spouse may be a more potent precipitant of late life depression.

In the end, we seem to be forced back to a position traditionally occupied by earlier psychiatrists, to the effect that depressions occurring for the first time late in life were forerunners of the dementias of old age. In fact, the follow-up of elderly depressives carried out at different centres (Kay et al., 1955; Kay, 1962; Post, 1962, 1972) has shown that many of them do develop multi-infarct or senile (Alzheimer pathology) dementias, but that this did not occur more frequently than might be expected in age-matched samples of the general population.

At the height of their illness, a considerable proportion of elderly patients with affective disorders exhibit some cognitive impairment, and in nearly one-fifth of patients this impairment could be objectified by the use of certain tests of new learning of verbal material and of psychomotor speed (Kendrick et al., 1965). However, neither this almost always reversible defect ('pseudodementia', Post, 1975), nor isolated or doubtful neurological signs were found to predict the subsequent occurrence of dementia (Post, 1962). In a later investigation (Cawley et al., 1973) it was shown that a transitory lowering of psychological test performance could be demonstrated a good deal more frequently than clinically obvious pseudodementia, especially in the more severe and psychotic types of depression of the elderly. Equally reversible reductions of physiological measures of brain functioning were shown to be more marked in late onset as against in early onset depressives. The transitory cognitive impairment was demonstrated to be different from that occurring in dementia (Whitehead, 1973), and these findings (which require confirmation) suggested that physiological rather than pathological processes of ageing may facilitate the occurrence of depression.

Prognosis

The further outlook in affective illnesses of late life will be discussed before their treatment, because in a number of ways the management of the individual attack is influenced by what has been learnt about the further life histories of elderly depressives.

There is a strong impression, which is difficult to prove conclusively in retrospect, that before the introduction of electroplexy for elderly subjects in the 1940s, many patients tended to pursue a course lasting a number of years, or died of intercurrent illnesses in mental institutions. In the presence of reasonably good physical health, it is now possible to terminate or vastly improve depression or mania of the elderly in all but some 15 per cent of cases. On the other hand, it has emerged that long lasting remissions are rare, in that recurrent attacks with and without some form of mental invalidism tend to be the rule. Like most geriatric conditions, affective illnesses of the elderly and aged acquire chronicity and increasing incapacity.

In following two consecutive samples of patients admitted to the same unit (Post, 1962, 1972), it was discovered that only one-third of patients maintained a permanently recovered status over the next few years; a further third suffered more depressions and had remissions of varying quality; the majority of the remaining third continued to suffer from a form of invalidism characterized by moodiness, anxiety, poor sleep, and somatic preoccupations, often punctuated by further depressive attacks. Finally, between 11 and 17 per cent of the two samples remained mentally ill, though not necessarily hospitalized, throughout the observation periods. The first sample were treated in the years 1950–51, and in the absence at that time of any effective treatment other than electroconvulsive therapies, very few had received ambulant treatment before admission. Thymoleptic drugs had been introduced by the time the second sample was treated in the years 1965–66, and 61 per cent of patients had received unsuccessful drug therapy before admission (Post, 1972). Accordingly, the more recently treated series almost certainly contained a higher proportion of patients presenting greater therapeutic problems, and the finding that there were no significant differences in long term outcome between the earlier and later series does not necessarily mean that there had not been any improvement in our therapeutic techniques.

The analysis of follow-up findings of the 1950–51 series produced only a few prognostic indicators. Using group comparisons, patients did better long term when they had been below the age of 70, had been continuously ill for less than two years before admission, had remained free of all disabling and progressive physical illness, had an extraverted social adjustment, and had shown a clinical picture approaching the manic depressive stereotype. The usefulness of these prognostic indicators, which in any case would not help much in forecasting the future of individual patients, was only weakly confirmed for the 1965–66 series. There was a strong impression that social adjustment depended on clinical progress, rather than the other way round. The appearance of serious extracerebral disease, which was more likely to occur in persons over the age of 75, influenced prognosis for life and mental health even more adversely than the presence or new development of atherosclerotic or senile dementia. In fact, a few patients where depression was associated with recent strokes (and they tended to have a strong family history of typical depressions) responded well to treatment, at any rate initially.

Treatment

The management of elderly patients with affective disorders should be planned on the assumption that one will have to work with the patient and his family not just during the present attack, but for many years to come. Dynamic psychopathology often lies very close to the surface in elderly psychotics, and especially in depressions after bereavements processes of identification and introjection of the ambivalently loved lost object are temptingly obvious. In the writer's experience, interpretations and 'working through' always lead to withdrawal of the patient from verbal communication or worsening of the psychosis. It seems better to build up a caring relationship with the patient and his family, in order to promote their continued co-operation during the illness and its aftermath. Failure to take medication, which is usually a sign of distrust of the doctor, is an important reason for which elderly depressives may require admission, and this is usually imperative when the patient has little supervision at home, shows severe agitation, food refusal, hypochondriacal, importuning, and suicidal behaviour. Recent and sudden worsening of the affective state almost always indicates that this downward course is likely to continue rapidly, and that it will lead to an emergency situation before treatment has had a chance of effect.

In choosing the appropriate method of treatment, many psychiatrists are led by the belief that symptoms should be removed as quickly as possible by immediately using all available treatments concurrently: minor or major tranquillizers, thymoleptic preparations, plus in severe cases electroplexy. Apart from the risk of producing toxic confusional states and extrapyramidal symptoms, such blunderbuss therapy will make it impossible to know which of the agents used had been responsible for any beneficial change in the clinical picture. As the large majority of patients will require further treatment for some years to come, it is clearly important to know which remedy had been effective. Also, if at all possible each method of treatment should be given an adequate trial before changing, or before resorting to any combination of therapies.

In the older age groups, electroconvulsive therapies remove depressive–retarded and depressive–anxious–agitated symptoms in the great majority of patients: four to twelve treatments may be required, but rarely more than eight. However, the immediate relapse rate is high. As a first therapeutic approach, ECT is therefore limited to patients in whose case the psychosis is life threatening (refusal of food, exhausting agitation). In these circumstances, or where patients are not fit for ECT under anaesthesia and a muscle relaxant, intravenous infusions of tricyclic antidepressants (such as clomipramine) are indicated, possibly more acceptable to the patient's relatives, but in the writer's experience much less effective.

In the outpatient clinic and in the case of many inpatients, treatment with oral tricyclic and similar antidepressant preparations will be one's first choice. Paradoxically, they are in the elderly less 'safe' than properly administered ECT. Apart from the usual side effects, these drugs may produce confusion, visual hallucinations, and more seriously and more frequently, falls and fractures. With an ever changing market, no specific drugs can be recommended: possibly amitriptyline is specially suited to the agitated elderly (single dose at night for outpatients), and iprindole to those with a tendency to cardiac arrhythmias. A very low initial dosage is slowly increased. Remission may only occur after four weeks, and in a few patients tolerance may be astonishingly high; a little lady of 70 repeatedly failed to respond until 275 mg of amitriptyline daily was reached. Most preparations can be given in a syrup, where tablet swallowing presents a problem. A partial remission on tricyclics, should lead to additional use of ECT. Where this is refused, a monoamine oxidase inhibitor may be tried, (with the usual precautions quite safely), and a few of the writer's patients appear to remain symptom free only on the even more feared combination of tricyclic and MAO inhibiting preparations.

Unfortunately the type of presenting symptomatology does not help in the choice of the treatment most likely to produce remission. ECT had been the first choice in 59 per cent of severely psychotic depressives as against in 24 per cent of those with a mainly neurotic symptomatology (Post, 1972). Nearly half the patients had drugs as well as ECT in succession. The treatment given immediately preceding discharge, and thus presumably the most effective one, was ECT rather than drug therapy in 53 per cent of the severe psychotics, in 36 per cent of the intermediate depressives, and surprisingly in 41 per cent of neurotic depressives, in spite of the presence in them of features which according to the textbooks would contraindicate the use of electroconvulsive therapy; anxious rather than depressed, manipulative, blaming others rather than themselves!

Some 15 per cent of older persons with affective illnesses fail to respond to any of the treatments so far discussed, initially and following repeated courses. In the recent past, psychosurgery was considered after elderly patients had been continuously ill for more than 18 months. Modified open leucotomies were in fact particularly successful in persistently agitated depressions of late life (Post et al., 1968). In recent years, however, the writer has referred hardly any elderly patients for psychosurgery, because depressives failing to respond to current therapies singly or in combination usually suffer from slowly progressive senile dementia, or much more frequently from a progressive and incurable physical illness. Patients of either kind may be operable, but tend to die within a few weeks or months of a brain operation.

As was indicated earlier, cognitive impairment even where associated with undoubted and progressive cerebral pathology does not present any contraindication to the treatment of affective symptoms. Cautious drug therapy only is usually indicated, but a few ECT may be life saving. Probably far too many distressing states of depression are allowed to go on untreated on account of suspected or confirmed dementing conditions.

The most difficult therapeutic problems continue to be presented by old people with serious physical disease and depression. Depressively coloured confusional states tend to clear up following the successful treatment of the underlying physical condition, but persistent depressive illnesses are hardly ever improved after cardiac failure, a urinary infection, myxoedema, and many other conditions have been dealt with. Failure to help depressives who had been successfully treated in previous attacks is usually due to the development of a persistent physical disorder.

Maintenance treatment

In the recently studied series, only seven per cent of patients followed for three years after discharge received no further psychiatric treatment, and in only 18 per cent had it been possible to discontinue antidepressant medication permanently soon after return to the community. The remainder, i.e. some 75 per cent, relapsed or threatened to relapse when dosages were lowered after a few months, or after follow-up supervision had broken down. Some 38 per cent of patients continued to need tricyclic drugs intermittently or continuously. Some 20 per cent also required further ECT and some 18 per cent received other forms of treatment, among them lithium salts, which on present and preliminary impression may have an important place in the prophylaxis of affective conditions without manic components. Social workers can be very helpful in making follow-up arrangements effective. Resocialization through attendance at clubs and day centres seems useful in some cases, but is resisted by many patients. Psychosocial attempts at prophylaxis are rarely feasible as patients cannot be protected from traumatic life events. There is a small group of depressives who break down again and again with initially neurotic, but soon increasingly psychotic features, after return to their lonely home surroundings. They remain well only after they have been persuaded to go into a community home for the elderly.

Manic states

Manic states, whether of recent or of more remote origin, always prove to be recurrent in the elderly, and are almost always associated with depressive admixtures or depressive phases. Treatment does not vary much from that of manic states of younger persons. Major tranquillizers are especially perhaps haloperidol (cautious increase of dosage!) where it is imperative to achieve rapid control and lithium salts where there is less urgency. All these patients will require maintenance therapy, which is facilitated by preparations of lithium given once a day only. Changes in physical state may make patients more sensitive, to the point of producing mild canfusion. Regular monitoring of serum levels, which should be kept at the lower end of the effective range, is required, the frequency depending on the clinical state. So, these patients need to be seen by the psychiatrist at least every two months. As in younger patients, checks of thyroid functions must also be carried out regularly. Further research will be needed to assess the efficacy of lithium prophylaxis as well as its optimal duration.

Persecutory states

Introductory remarks

Paranoid, and occasionally classical schizophrenic symptoms may occur in the setting of an acute brain syndrome, and they almost always prove to be of a transitory nature. Persistent persecutory states are also found in association with any of the dementing disorders of late life, but usually only while cognitive impairment is still relatively mild. Schizophrenia-like conditions arising for the first time late in life and not apparently related to gross brain changes have only been studied since Kleist suggested that perhaps some of his cases of involutional paranoia were identical with Kraepelin's paraphrenics, and since Bleuler's (1943) monograph concerning late (i.e.

after the age of 40) onset schizophrenia. The literature has been reviewed elsewhere (Post, 1966) and is largely of historical interest. Most later writers have concerned themselves with patients over 60, whose symptoms had first appeared after the age of 50, and with the really meaningless question as to whether these patients were schizophrenics or paraphrenics, as well as with the special clinical features presented by these patients.

Probably only some ten per cent of persons admitted to psychiatric hospitals after the age of 60 suffer from paraphrenic conditions (Roth and Morrissey, 1952), and these have been discovered in only one or two per cent of elderly community residents (Parsons, 1964; Williamson *et al.*, 1964). Probably, many milder cases escape ascertainment during surveys.

Symptomatology

The present writer (Post, 1966) was impressed with three different forms which symptomatology took in a consecutive series of hospital patients. Further experience has shown that these three separate types continue to be recognized, and that patients do not pass from one to the other.

Firstly, and perhaps most commonly in the community, there are paranoid states often with a largely auditory hallucinosis. Typically, an old woman who lives alone develops the conviction that people interfere with her property; there is an intruder who secretly displaces objects in the patient's home and sometimes steals them. People want her to get out of her home; she overhears remarks from next door or upstairs. Many of these old people, who continue to look after themselves quite adequately, become regular recipients of reassurance at their local police station. A few become so disturbing in their neighbourhood that they are finally referred to psychiatrists.

Less frequent, but usually more overtly disturbed are patients with more widespread paranoid experiences and with a belief in a more extensive conspiracy. Persons in the street behave strangely and significantly. Obscene remarks are overheard. Accusatory voices are heard, perhaps produced by a tape recorder. The home is bugged; some optical appliance is built into the ceiling; the patient is observed in embarrassing situations. Cars circle the house, lights are shone at night. Occasionally there are delusions of marital irregularities being committed by the spouse. In this group, there are thus no truly schizophrenic, but only schizophrenic-like or schizophreniform clinical phenomena.

Finally, there is a group of patients in whose case most psychiatrists would agree on a schizophrenic label. Voices talk about the patient in the third person singular; they comment on his or her activities; they repeat or even anticipate his thoughts. Sensations are produced in the patient's body by telepathic means. The content of the abnormal beliefs and experiences is frequently and, considering the patient's age, incongruously, erotic, e.g. the phantom lover may be felt to have sexual relations with the patient from a considerable distance. Symptoms are largely of a paranoid-schizophrenic kind, and catatonic features and disruption of formal thought are rarely seen in late onset schizophrenics.

These three clinical types do not differ from one another in terms of aetiological factors or response to treatment, except that paranoid-hallucinatory states and schizophreniform disorders quite often clear up, at least for a time, when patients are moved from their homes to more sheltered surroundings, while it has never been possible to abolish or ameliorate truly schizophrenic symptoms by social measures.

Aetiology

In late schizophrenics a family history of schizophrenia is far less often obtained than in the case of young schizophrenics, but still significantly more frequently than in control populations (Kay, 1963). The presence of genetic aetiological factors is also suggested by a generally reported striking excess of female over male patients (4:1). While elderly paraphrenic tend to be physically healthier than elderly depressives, long standing social deafness is strongly associated with late schizophrenia (for details see Cooper *et al.*, 1974). An association of persistent schizophrenic symptoms with dementing conditions of late life was confirmed over the course of a three year observation period in 15 per cent of a consecutive series of inpatients. In a further 18 per cent the development of senile dementia could not be ruled out with certainty, because in these patients evaluation continues to be difficult on account of their frequent deafness and poor accessibility. No type of paraphrenic symptomatology was found unduly frequently in association with organic cerebral disease or with deafness. Whether occurring in the setting of dementia or in cerebrally intact persons, paranoid-hallucinatory, schizophreniform, and schizophrenic syndromes almost always arose in relation to well defined personality characteristics.

In contrast with younger schizophrenics, elderly paraphrenics have usually had quite a good work record, and have tended not to show any social decline. However, they had usually been socially somewhat withdrawn, this leading in some cases to an isolated existence as senile recluses. Membership of esoteric cults was not uncommon. The greatest deficiency in the personality of late schizophrenics arose from failure in more intimate relationships. Marriage rate was found to be strikingly low; marriage when it did occur took place relatively late in life, and sometimes not even following the birth of illegitimate children. It is most unusual to obtain a convincing account of satisfactory sexual adjustment. Identical observations on pre-illness personality have been made in as widely differing settings as rural Southern England, London, Stockholm, and Moscow (Kay and Roth, 1961; Post, 1966; Kay, 1963; Sternberg, 1972). These findings have led the British workers to suggest that the patients' abnormal personalities might be evidence of a longstanding latent schizophrenic disorder, which is finally brought into the open by the further social deprivations of late life, by deafness, by some cerebral aspects of the ageing process (unbalancing of arousal systems?), or in a few patients by more definite cerebral pathological events. Sternberg, however, claims that in about half of the late life schizophrenics attending a Moscow dispensary there had been early attacks without psychiatric referral. These had often taken the guise of atypical anxiety states, depressive, or obsessional episodes. In the present writer's experience, however, it is unusual to obtain accounts of previous overt psychiatric breakdowns of any sort in late schizophrenics; this is very much in contrast to what one finds in elderly depressives.

Treatment

As was mentioned earlier, except in the presence of truly schizophrenic symptoms, social measures directed at diminishing the patient's loneliness and social isolation are sometimes successful. But, as with all forms of treatment of paranoid illnesses, the main obstacle arises from the patient's negative attitude towards therapy, because, obviously they do not think they are ill; they only want their grievances to be dealt with. However, many young and older schizophrenics can be treated informally in hospital or in the outpatient clinic because of the schizophrenic's attitude of ambivalence. While saying they are not ill and in need of treatment, many patients will in fact co-operate with medication, especially if a head-on collision with arguments is avoided, a good relationship can be built up, and medication made acceptable as designed to protect the patient from his unpleasant experiences. This sort of approach succeeds more frequently, and especially with older patients, than might be expected. With some, admission by a compulsory method may be necessary, and this should not be avoided as so many of these patients can be brought under therapeutic control, and once an improvement has been produced may become quite co-operative.

The results of treatment of late life schizophrenics with phenothiazine preparations have been fully described elsewhere (Post, 1966) and concerned 73 consecutive in- and outpatients. Only two of the last mentioned initially defaulted from treatment. Complete failure of therapy occurred in only six of the remaining 71 patients, possibly because they had really been schizophrenic for much longer than their histories had suggested. Abnormal experiences continued to be reported by 22 patients, whose general adjustment might be best described as one of social recovery. Complete remissions could be claimed for 43 patients, though only 14 of them were able to describe in retrospect their past experiences as having been due to confusion or mental breakdown. In the case of the majority the disappearance of symptoms was attributed to changes in the environment without any real or at best dubious realization of recent mental illness. During an average follow-up period of three years, progress was very clearly and closely correlated to success or failure of drug therapy maintenance. Thirty-three of the 43 patients making complete remission remained well throughout, but it was possible to stop drugs lastingly in only seven (and a number of these are known to have relapsed after the study was completed). One-third of patients had occasional periods of symptoms usually responding to treatment, and a final third turned out to have remained psychotic though usually not as severely disabled as before treatment. Social factors seemed to influence long term outcome only as far as they contributed to success in maintenance therapy: e.g. patients maintaining reasonably good relationships with their spouse did better than the rest. Paranoid, schizophreniform, and schizophrenic patients continued to be equally responsive to drug therapy, confirming perhaps that basically these three clinical subtypes are all manifestations with different degrees of penetration of the same pathological deviation. Where schizophrenic ways of thinking and experiencing coloured organic cerebral disorders, functional symptoms seemed to yield more quickly and to lower dosages or major tranquillizers, but quite apart from any worsening of their cerebral state these patients appeared to do less well in the long term.

There is no need to stress that older people are especially sensitive to major tranquillizers, and those active in small dosages (and thus more likely to produce neurological side effects such as parkinsonism and not always reversible dyskinesias) should not be one's first choice. The writer has found thioridazine or chlorpromazine most satisfactory in the great majority of patients, most of whom show a response on 150–200 mg daily. In only a few instances has there been any need to resort to more neuroleptic preparations such as trifluoperazine or haloperidol. With all these drugs stepwise increases of dosage are advisable, if at all possible allowing at least ten days to pass before increasing the amount prescribed. This gives the preparation a chance to produce its effects, and lessens the risk of giving unnecessarily big doses. The need to give antiparkinsonian preparations can thus usually be avoided, and should not be prescribed as a routine. Few older patients fail to learn that stopping their tablets leads to trouble, and intramuscular depot injections, whose ill effects take time to reverse, are only needed in an occasional case. No doubt there are settings where a fortnightly injection may be the only way of maintaining treatment, but in Western urban practice this should rarely be necessary in this age group because, unlike as with so many younger patients, the removal of psychotic symptoms often leaves behind a responsible person who will co-operate in reasonable arrangements.

The correct maintenance dose is usually about a quarter of that needed to suppress the symptoms. Efforts should be made every six months or so to lower and finally stop medication. As we saw above this is rarely successful; usually the patient soon begins to feel tense and uncomfortable, and fleeting delusional ideas may be reported.

In the recent past, paraphrenic states of the elderly were regarded as incurable. Those patients who required admission only rarely left hospital again, but survived there for long periods (Roth and Morrissey, 1952; Gabriel, 1974). Now, almost all patients respond with improvement or complete control of the disorder. Hospital admission is often unnecessary. Recognition of persecutory symptoms in the elderly is particularly important at family doctor level. Their sudden appearance may signify a toxic or metabolic delirious reaction requiring treatment of the causative condition; gradual onset and persistence of paranoid beliefs and experience is more likely to be part and parcel of a late schizophrenic illness amenable to simple drug therapy, which in these cases may be more smoothly initiated by the trusted family doctor.

Schizo-affective illnesses

When severely disturbed old people are first seen, and physical causes for the mental disorder have as far as possible been excluded, the symptoms displayed may suggest a mixture of affective and schizophrenic phenomena. In one of the previously referred to series of depressives (Post, 1961), 38 per cent exhibited paranoid symptoms, and in some of them they were by no means clearly related to the depressive affect (e.g. guilt-laden), but schizophrenic in form and content. On the other hand, in 58 per cent of late schizophrenics referred to in the preceding section depressive mood changes were at one time or other prominent, and some delusions and hallucinations had a decidedly depressive colouring.

Over a period of six years, all elderly inpatients in whom serious doubts as regards the differential diagnosis between an affective and a schizophrenic disorder had arisen were earmarked and followed over a number of years (Post, 1971). Only six per cent of all functional patients gave rise to this kind of diagnostic doubt, and this could not be speedily resolved in half of them. So, in the end there were only 29 patients who continued to exhibit both depressive and schizophrenic phenomena either simultaneously or in succession. They were compared with both late schizophrenics and elderly depressives on a number of characteristics which had distinguished these two groups. Paraphrenics had shown less family history of affective illness, were characterized by a considerable excess of women, poorer sexual adjustment, lower marriage rates, and lower socioeconomic status. They had hardly ever exhibited overt psychiatric conditions before the age of 50, and there was (in striking contrast to the sequence of events in depressives) no evidence for external precipitation of the illness, which had developed gradually out of the previous personality. On all these biological and psychosocial variables schizoaffective patients occupied an intermediate position. Abnormal personality traits, which in a recent study (Kay et al., 1976), have been shown once again to differentiate elderly depressives from schizophrenics, were even more frequently reported for schizo-affectives. These were also characterized by a far higher loading with psychiatric family histories of all kinds (in 86 per cent of the 29 patients), and burdened significantly more frequently with various kinds of cerebral pathology. In only a few instances, schizo-affective illnesses seemed to run in the family, but elderly schizo-affectives should not be confounded with Leonhard's cycloid psychotics characterized by genetic homogeneity (Perris, 1974).

The concept schizo-affective has had a chequered career, which has been evaluated elsewhere (Post, 1971), but whatever logical and theoretical objections may have been raised, there is a small group of elderly patients who suffer from both types of symptoms, and who have been shown to benefit at different times from either thymoleptic or tranquillizing therapies; a few seemed to show a response only when both types of treatment were used in combination and simultaneously. As might be predicted from severe loading of these schizo-affective patients with psychiatric heredity of all kinds, with longstanding personality defects, and with cerebral pathology, their long term prognosis was found to be strikingly worse than that of elderly depressives or of late paraphrenics co-operating with treatment; nearly one-half as against one-third of other functional psychotics tend to remain disabled.

Some concluding thoughts

In the writer's opinion, the affective and schizophrenic disturbances of late life are for the time being best seen within a framework which also applies to these disorders in earlier life. To enter states of anxiety, sadness, elation, or dissocation together with the accompanying deviations of thinking and experiencing is in different strengths and proportions characteristic of all humans. In dreaming, during artistic creation, under emotional stress, and with metabolic cerebral disturbance, these deviations may singly or in combination come to dominate awareness and conduct for short periods. Whenever this domination and deviation becomes protracted, we begin to speak of mental illnesses, whose form and content derives from the patients' temperamental endowments.

Though some psychological and physical precipitating factors almost always determine the actual onset of the disorder, strong hereditary tendencies towards a similar type of psychosis are usually demonstrable in younger subjects, whose further personality development tends to be unfavourably influenced by the persistence or recurrence of the mental illness. Where there is less genetic predisposition to psychotic breakdown, some temperamental deviations may increasingly colour personality and life pattern, becoming seriously disabling only under exceptional stresses in the course of adult existence. Shifts in personality structure due to ageing or cerebral disease, as well as in consequence of increasing lack of emotional support, may be among the factors responsible for affective and schizophrenic illnesses occurring for the first time only late in the life of persons with little family history of psychosis, and with temperamental deviations which had not led to earlier breakdowns.

Until we can influence personality development, we are limited to diminishing or suppressing mental symptoms, and when these are at all severe the only remedies available at this time are physical agents. Progress made in this endeavour during the last 30 years, and especially in the case of the elderly, should not be undervalued.

References

Bleuler, M. (1943) 'Die spätschizophrenen Krankheitsbilder', *Fortschritte der Neurologie und Psychiatrie*, **15**, 259.

Bleuler, M. (1972) *Die Schizophrenen Geistesstörungen*, Stuttgart, Georg Thieme.

Brown, G.W., Bhrolchain, M.N., and Harris, T. (1975) 'Social class and psychiatric disturbance among women in an urban population', *Sociology*, **9**, 225–254.

Cawley, R.H., Post, F., and Whitehead, A. (1973) 'Barbiturate tolerance and psychological functioning in elderly depressed patients', *Psychological Medicine*, **3**, 39–52.

Chesser, E.S. (1965) *A study of some aetiological factors in the affective disorders of old age*, unpublished dissertation, Institute of Psychiatry, University of London.

Cooper, A.F., Kay, D.W.K., Curry, A.R., Garside, R.F., and Roth, M. (1974) 'Hearing loss in paranoid and affective psychoses of the elderly', *Lancet*, **ii,** 851–61.

Gabriel, E. (1974) 'Der langfristige Verlauf Schizophrener Späterkrankungen', *Psychiatrica Clinica*, **7**, 172–80.

Harwin, B. (1973) 'Psychiatric morbidity among the physically impaired elderly in the community', in *Roots of evaluation—the epidemiological basis for planning psychiatric services*, (Ed. J.K. Wing and H. Häfner) London, Oxford University Press.

Hopkinson, F.J. (1964) 'A genetic study of affective illness in patients over 50', *British Journal of Psychiatry*, **110**, 244–54.

Kay, D.W.K. (1959) 'Observations on the natural history and genetics of old age psychoses', *Proceedings of the Royal Society of Medicine*, **52**, 791–7.

Kay, D.W.K. (1962) 'Outcome and cause of death in mental disorders of old age: a long-term follow-up of functional and organic psychoses', *Acta Psychiatrica Scandinavica*, **38**, 249–276.

Kay, D.W.K. (1963) 'Late paraphrenia and its bearing on the aetiology of schizophrenia', *Acta Psychiatrica Scandinavica*, **39**, 159–69.

Kay, D.W.K., Beamish, P., and Roth, M. (1964) 'Old age mental disorders in Newcastle upon Tyne. Part I: A study of prevalence', *British Journal of Psychiatry*, **110**, 146–158.

Kay, D.W.K., Cooper, A.F., Garside, R.F., and Roth, M. (1976) 'The differentiation of paranoid from affective psychoses by patients' premorbid characteristics', *British Journal of Psychiatry*, **129**, 207–15.

Kay, D.W.K., and Roth, M. (1961) 'Environmental and hereditary factors in the schizophrenias of old age ("late paraphrenia") and their bearing on the general problem of causation in schizophrenia', *Journal of Mental Science*, **107**, 649–86.

Kay, D.W.K., Roth, M., and Hopkins, B. (1955) 'Affective disorders in the senium: I. Their association with organic cerebral degeneration', *Journal of Mental Science*, **101**, 302–318.

Kendell, R.E. (1969) 'The continuum model of depressive illness', *Proceedings of the Royal Society of Medicine*, **62**, 335–9.

Kendrick, D.C., Parboosingh, R.C., and Post, F. (1965) 'A synonym learning test for use with elderly psychiatric subjects: A validation study', *British Journal of Social and Clinical Psychology*, **4**, 63–71.

Parsons, P.L. (1964) 'Mental health of Swansea's old folk', *British Journal of Preventive and Social Medicine*, **19**, 43–47.

McDonald, C. (1969) 'Parental deprivation and psychiatric illness in old age', *Australian and New Zealand Journal of Psychiatry*, **3**, 401–3.

Perris, C. (1974) 'A study of cycloid psychoses', *Acta Psychiatrica Scandinavica*, supp. 253.

Post, F. (1962) *The significance of affective symptoms in old age*, London, Oxford University Press.

Post, F. (1965) *The clinical psychiatry of late life*, Oxford, Pergamon Press.

Post, F. (1966) *Persistent persecutory states of the elderly*, Oxford, Pergamon Press.

Post, F. (1968) 'The factor of ageing in affective illness', in *Recent developments of affective disorders*, (Ed. A. Oppen and A. Walk) *British Journal of Psychiatry*, Special Publication No. 2.

Post, F. (1971) 'Schizo-affective symptomatology in late life', *British Journal of Psychiatry*, **118**, 437–45.

Post, F. (1972) 'The management and nature of depressive illnesses in late life: a follow-through study', *British Journal of Psychiatry*, **121**, 393–404.

Post, F. (1975) 'Dementia, depression and pseudo-dementia', in *Psychiatric aspects of neurologic disease*, (Ed. D.F. Benson and D. Blumer) New York, Grune and Stratton.

Post, F., Rees, W.L., and Schurr, P. (1968) 'An evaluation of bi-medial leucotomy', *British Journal of Psychiatry*, **114**, 1223–46.

Ross, O. and Kreitman, N. (1975) 'A further investigation of differences in the suicide rates of England and Wales and of Scotland', *British Journal of Psychiatry*, **127**, 575–82.

Roth, M. (1955) 'The natural history of mental disorders in old age', *Journal of Mental Science*, **101**, 281–301.

Roth, M., and Kay, D.W.K. (1956) 'Affective disorders arising in the senium: II. Physical disabilities as aetiological factors', *Journal of Mental Science*, **102**, 141–52.

Roth, M., and Morrissey, J.D. (1952) 'Problems of diagnosis and classification of mental disorders in old age', *Journal of Mental Science*, **98**, 66–80.

Sainsbury, P. (1968) 'Suicide and depression', in *Recent developments in affective disorders*, (Ed. A. Coppen and A. Walk) *British Journal of Psychiatry*, Special Publication No. 2.

Stenstedt, A. (1959) *Involutional Melancholia*, *Acta Psychiatrica Neurologica Scandinavica*, supp. 127.

Sternberg, E. (1972) 'Neuere Forschungsergebnisse bei spätschizophrenen Psychosen', *Fortschritte der Neurologie und Psychiatrie*, **40**, 631–64.

Whitehead, A. (1973) 'Verbal learning and memory in elderly depressives', *British Journal of Psychiatry*, **123,** 203–8.

Williamson, J., Stokoe, I.H., Gray, S., Fisher, I.M. and Smith, A. (1964) 'Old people at home: their unreported needs', *Lancet*, **i,** 1117–1120.

5

THE DIAGNOSIS OF DEMENTIA

C.D. Marsden

Introduction

Dementia in the elderly is common and costly. Geriatric medicine, as it is currently organized in the United Kingdom, necessarily involves the institutional care of many elderly, demented patients, and a much greater number are cared for in the community by relatives, or in homes provided by the social services or private enterprise. Up to about ten per cent of those over the age of 65 years are likely to show evidence of dementia (see Chapter 9) of which some 25 per cent will be in institutional care and 75 per cent will be in the community. Crude estimates indicate that by 1980 the population of Great Britain will be about 60 million, of which about seven million will be over the age of 65 years. By then there will be some 700 000 demented elderly patients of which close to 200 000 will require institutional care.

In contrast to the frequency of dementia in the elderly, dementia with onset under the age of 65 years is comparatively uncommon. However, such 'pre-senile' demented patients are more intensively investigated. As a result, the neurologist obtains a view of the problem of dementia that is distorted by concentration of diagnostic skills on the younger patients. The reasons for such a pattern of referrals are partly social and partly medical. The appearance of dementia in the elderly is frequently accepted as the inevitable consequence of ageing, and is not considered to justify intensive investigation. In any case, the yield of such time consuming and expensive studies is small, and the risks of some of the investigations required are prohibitive in the very elderly. The neurologist therefore, sees predominantly those patients whose dementia appears before the age of 65 or 70. More elderly patients are referred to geriatric services, both medical and social.

The neurologist's attitude to the clinical problem of dementia as he sees it in younger patients is simple. Although the majority will have untreatable primary cerebral degenerations, a significant minority will be discovered to have treatable conditions. Extensive, and even uncomfortable, or potentially harmful investigations, are fully justifiable to discover the few who can be treated. How far this attitude can be applied to the elderly demented depends on a balanced judgment of the likely yield of investigation weighed against the risks and cost-effectiveness of such studies. Many have taken the view that unless there are clinical clues to suggest a treatable cause, there is little point in extensively investigating the elderly dement (Arie, 1973). Indeed, a large proportion of such patients are handled directly by the social services.

While this practical attitude may be sensible, in terms of use of available resources, it has resulted in a relative academic ignorance of the true incidence and character of the various conditions that may cause dementia in the elderly. Such an admittedly realistic approach to this large problem has been based on the undoubted risks of some investigations, such as cerebral arteriography and air encephalography, in elderly patients. However, with the advent of safe non-invasive techniques, such as computerized axial tomographic scanning (CAT scan or EMI scan), it is now possible to visualize intracranial anatomy without risk to the patient. Further advances in non-invasive techniques for measurement of regional cerebral blood flow, in biochemical investigation of CSF constitutents of cerebral metabolism, and electrophysiological methods of study of cerebral physiology may well provide simple and safe means of accurate diagnosis of dementia in even the very elderly patient. In view of the increasing size of the problem, the application of such an approach to selected samples is required at least to establish facts. Whether such knowledge would alter practical management remains to be discovered. If it did, the financial implications would pose another problem in an age of decision-making based on community—rather than patient cost-effectiveness.

Against this background, I propose to review the diagnosis of dementia initially from the standpoint of the neurologist's concern primarily with those under the age of 65 to 70 years. I will then attempt to relate such information to the problem of dementia in the elderly.

Definition

The term dementia is used in different ways by neurologists, psychiatrists, and geriatricians. Many psychiatrists employ the term to describe only those patients with progressive and irreversible diffuse structural brain damage. Used in this sense dementia is synonymous with untreatable progressive disintegration of the brain, with the consequence that the application of the label precludes any hope of a treatable cause or therapy. Yet, in practice, the label of dementia is applied to describe a syndrome of generalized, global loss of higher mental function, irrespective of its cause. The syndrome is identified at clinical interview, or by formal psychological testing, when deficits in many or all mental spheres are apparent. Such a patient is said to be demented, no matter what the cause, which is often not apparent at this stage of the assessment.

For the purpose of this chapter, *dementia* is defined as the syndrome of global disturbance of higher mental functions in an alert patient. Dementia may be static, as after cerebral anoxia or head injury, or progressive; it may be irreversible, as in Alzheimer's disease, or reversible, as in some forms of hydrocephalus.

Dementia is distinguished from *delirium*, which is defined as the syndrome of global disturbance of higher mental function occurring in a patient with clouded consciousness, usually as an acute or subacute illness, often associated with hallucinations, usually visual, and motor restlessness.

TABLE 5.1. Symptoms indicating a disorder of higher mental function

Intellect	Personality	Memory	Speech and cognitive function	
Loss of power of abstract thought	Loss of interest and initiative	Forgetfulness	Loss of fluency	
Deficits in reasoning, judgment and planning	Emotional blunting or disinhibition	Inability to learn	Loss of comprehension	
Loss of concentration	Social misconduct	Disorientation in time and space	Topographical disorientation	
	Personal neglect		Visual and spatial disorientation	
May be due to:				
Psychosis	Focal neurological syndrome	Focal neurological syndrome	Global neurological syndrome	
			Delirium	Dementia
Severe depression or elation	Fits		Halucinations	
Retardation or agitation	Focal signs		Motor restlessness	
Delusions	Raised intracranial pressure			
Gradual onset	Acute or chronic onset		Acute or subacute onset	Usually gradual onset
Clear consciousness	Alert or drowsy		Clouded consciousness	Clear consciousness

Delirium may occur on top of dementia, as when the patient with Alzheimer's disease develops bronchopneumonia.

The critical distinction between dementia and delirium is the patient's level of consciousness. The simplest bedside test is the capacity to repeat 7 ± 2 digits. An alert patient, even with a dense amnesic syndrome, is quite capable of this, but the drowsy or inattentive delirious patient cannot.

Delirium must be distinguished from the drowsiness associated with raised intracranial pressure, by the associated hallucinations and motor restlessness.

Synonyms for dementia (chronic brain failure, chronic brain syndrome) and delirium (toxic confusional state, acute brain failure, acute brain syndrome) will be avoided.

The diagnosis of the syndrome of dementia

In the patient presenting with symptoms indicating a disorder of higher mental function (Table 5.1) it is first necessary to establish whether these are due to:

(1) A psychotic illness
(2) A focal neurological syndrome
(3) A global neurological syndrome, which may be:
   (a) Delirium
   (b) Dementia.

A practical distinction is between patients who present with acute or subacute symptoms, and those with chronic symptoms.

Acute or *subacute symptoms* may be due to delirium (Table 5.2), a focal neurological deficit, or, more rarely, a psychotic illness, and will not be discussed further.

TABLE 5.2. Causes of delirium

Overwhelming infection	Renal failure
Anaemia	Hepatic failure
Carcinomatosis	Drug intoxication
Stroke	Electrolyte disturbance
Epilepsy	Endocrine disturbance
Cardiac failure	Vitamin deficiency
Respiratory failure	Hypothermia

Chronic symptoms may be due to psychiatric illness, focal neurological deficit, or dementia.

Differentiation from psychiatric illness

A number of psychiatric conditions may masquerade as an apparent dementia (Kiloh, 1961; Post, 1975). Depression is the commonest and most important. The loss of interest, failure at work, and memory difficulty may be the prime cause of referral, but the mood disorder, frequent paranoia and delusional state are usually quite apparent. Difficulty arises because depression is not uncommon in patients with dementia; many retain insight into their inadequate intellectual performance for some time, and react to their waning intellectual powers by becoming depressed. The differentiation of depression from dementia may require careful assessment of intellectual, memory, and cognitive function to detect the clues to organic brain damage.

TABLE 5.3. Psychiatric illness that may mimic dementia

| Depressive psychosis |
| Schizophreniform psychosis |
| Hysteria |
| Malingering |

Depression and other psychiatric illnesses which may mimic dementia (Table 5.3) are discussed in detail in Chapter 4. Their distinction from dementia by psychological testing is described in Chapter 8. Suffice to say here that it is wise to consider the possibility of such psychiatric illness, which may be eminently treatable, in every patient presenting with an apparent dementia.

Differentiation from focal neurological syndromes

Focal lesions of the frontal, temporal, or parietal lobes of the brain may produce restricted deficits in higher mental functions that may be confused with dementia (Table 5.4). The intellectual abnormalities produced by focal brain lesions are not as consistent as the more obvious motor, sensory, visual, or speech deficits. However, lesions in specific brain areas do tend to produce particular types of mental abnormality.

Frontal lobe lesions cause a disintegration of personality, leading to apathy, indifference, and lack of initiative. There may be neglect of personal cleanliness in dress, toilet, and manners, as well as insensitivity and lack of normal inhibitions in social behaviour and morality. Indifference to urinary or faecal incontinence is characteristic, and lack of insight is common. Rarely, there may be euphoria, facetiousness, and grandiose delusions. In contrast to dementia, focal frontal lobe lesions often do not affect measured IQ or memory. Other evidence of a frontal lobe lesion may be a Broca's aphasia, a grasp reflex, or adversive focal seizures.

Focal temporal lobe lesions affecting the dominant hemisphere produce a Wernicke's aphasia, which may be mistaken for dementia. The gross abnormalities of the fluent spoken and written speech, and the severe inability to comprehend speech combine to produce an apparent chaos of thought which may be

TABLE 5.4. Focal deficits in higher mental function

Type	Nature of deficits	Other signs	Functions often preserved
Frontal lobe syndrome	Social disintergration Emotional disinhibition Personal neglect Loss of judgment	Incontinence Adversive seizures Anosmia Grasp reflex Word finding difficulty Broca's aphasia	IQ Memory Cognitive function
Amnesic syndrome	Loss of recent memory Inability to learn new material Confabulation	Hemianopia Temporal lobe seizures Wernicke's aphasia	IQ Personality Cognitive function
Parietal lobe syndromes	Loss of visuo-spatial recognition Topographical disorganisation Agnosia for space and self	Cortical sensory loss Hemianopia	IQ Personality Memory

misinterpreted unless the dysphasia is recognized. Although the temporal lobes are concerned with the processes of memory, unilateral temporal lobe lesions do not usually produce severe memory deficit. However, left temporal lobe lesions affect verbal memory and learning when tested formally (and, hence, are associated with a selective reduction in verbal scores on IQ testing); while, right temporal lesions affect visual memory and learning (and are associated with a selective reduction in performance scores on IQ testing). The single most important sign indicating a temporal lobe lesion is the contralateral upper quadrantic hemianopia. The wide variety of focal seizures due to temporal lobe lesions is well known.

The so called amnesic syndrome deserves special mention. A selective loss of memory and learning ability, with preservation of intellect and personality, occurs in a number of conditions, all of which affect the regions of the hippocampus–fornix–mammilary body system bilaterally. Memory loss is associated with disorientation, and often confabulation, but the preservation of intellectual faculties and of personality distinguishes the amnesic syndrome from dementia. The amnesic syndrome may be due to ischaemia in the distribution of both posterior cerebral arteries (as in vertebra-basilar disease), trauma, alcohol, and vitamin B deficiency (Korsakoff's psychosis), encephalitis, and, rarely, tumours of the diencephalon or third ventricle. An interesting, but unexplained, amnesic syndrome may occur episodically in otherwise normal people (so called transient global amnesia) (Fisher and Adam, 1964). Transient global amnesia may represent focal bilateral transient ischaemia in posterior cerebral artery distribution affecting the medial temporal regions.

Focal parietal lobe lesions may produce florid and bizarre mental deficits. Typical are visuospatial disorganization causing difficulty in tasks involving appreciation of three-dimensional spatial relations; for example, difficulty with car driving, using machinery, dressing, laying a table, drawing or other constructional tasks, and loss of topographic organization. Neglect of the opposite side of the body and of space is seen more commonly with right than with left parietal lesions. Inability to recognize or name body parts (for example, finger agnosia), associated with disorientation for right and left, are components of the so called Gerstmann syndrome, often associated with left parietal lesions (the other features of the Gerstmann syndrome are dysgraphia and dyscalculia). Lesions of the dominant parietal lobe produce conduction or anomic aphasia, and apraxia. Anterior parietal lesions encroach on the primary sensory cortex, causing contralateral cortical sensory loss, which is marked by the ability to recognize the basic sensory stimuli of pain, temperature, touch, or vibration, but a loss of the capacity to interpret these sensations. As a result, there is loss of recognition of joint position or movement, inability to judge size, shape, weight or texture of objects held in the hand, and defective tactile localization or discrimination between two or more stimuli. Parietal lobe lesions also encroach on the visual pathways to cause a contralateral lower quadrantic hemianopia, or, if posteriorly placed, they may cause a visual agnosia. Anterior parietal lesions produce focal sensory seizures, while posterior lesions may lead to unformed visual seizures.

Differentiation from the effects of raised intracranial pressure

One further practical problem requires emphasis. As stated earlier, consciousness is always preserved in all but the very advanced cases of dementia, so confusion of dementia with the apathy, slowness, and obtundation of patients with raised intracranial pressure should not prove too difficult. However, mistakes are made, particularly in patients with considerably raised intracranial pressure with few, if any, localizing neurological signs, as with subdural haematomata, space-occupying lesions in silent areas (N.B. right frontal or temporal lobe tumours) and hydrocephalus of any cause. Papilloedema is usually present in such patients, but may not be. The essential clue to the raised intracranial pressure is the loss of alertness, sleepiness, and difficulty in rousing such patients. When stimulated, they may converse and respond to command, only to lapse back into sleep when left alone. Such patients are sleepy because of severe brainstem distortion due to

TABLE 5.5. The causes of progressive dementia

Primary cerebral degenerations
    Alzheimer's disease and senile dementia
    Multi-infarct dementia
    Pick's disease
    Huntington's chorea
    Jakob–Creutzfeldt disease
    Disseminated sclerosis
    Spinocerebellar degenerations
    Wilson's disease
    Parkinsonism and its variants
    Punch-drunk syndrome
Cerebral infections and inflammations
    Neurosyphilis
    Cranial arteritis
    Disseminated lupus erythmatosus
    Limbic encephalitis
    Multi-focal leucoencephalopathy
Intracranial mass lesions
    Tumour
    Subdural haematomas
Hydrocephalus
    Obstructive
    Communicating
Secondary to systemic disease
    Hypothyroidism
    Hypocalcaemia
    Hypoglycaemia
    Porphyria
    Vitamin B_{12} deficiency
    Hepatic encephalopathy
    Renal dialysis
    Malabsorption syndrome
    Dementia in alcoholics

transtentorial herniation, and require urgent neurological investigation and treatment.

The presentation of dementia

Every textbook lists a large number of conditions that may cause dementia (Table 5.5). In practice, however, dementia appears in three guises:

(1) The patient with an obvious and established neurological or other illness develops dementia as an additional symptom of brain damage. This situation obtains in most patients with, for example, disseminated sclerosis or a spinocerebellar degeneration, who dement. On rare occasions dementia may be the presenting symptom of such diseases.
(2) The patient presents with the symptoms and signs of dementia. In this situation, the diagnostic possibilities become much fewer.
(3) The patient presents with a psychiatric illness, based on an underlying dementia. The common situations are the presentation of dementia with an episode of delirium due to intercurrent illness, such as infection or heart failure, or with a psychotic illness.

We are concerned here primarily with those diseases in which dementia is the common presenting symptom, or those that may be discovered by investigation of the patients presenting with dementia. The classical clinical features of Alzheimer's diseases and other primary cerebral degenerations causing dementia are described extensively elsewhere and need not be reiterated. Rather, I will concentrate on certain areas of controversy or uncertainty in relation to illnesses presenting with dementia.

'Arteriosclerotic dementia'—an overused misnomer

Cerebral arteriosclerosis is blamed as the cause of dementia in perhaps 50 per cent of cases. In fact, cerebral arteriosclerosis by itself does not produce dementia, and cerebrovascular disease is an uncommon cause of dementia.

The concept that atherosclerosis of cerebral blood vessels leads to dementia by a general reduction in blood supply to the brain is incorrect, (Hachinski *et al.*, 1974). The human cerebral circulation has a remarkable capacity to adjust blood flow in the face of wide fluctuations in perfusion pressure. Such autoregulation of cerebral blood flow is usually preserved in the face of atherosclerosis, except in malignant hypertension. As a result, even severe reductions in the size of the lumen of major blood vessels supplying the brain, and large drops in systemic blood pressure, do not compromise flow. A reduction of 95 per cent or more in the lumen of the carotid artery is required to reduce flow. A drop of mean arterial blood pressure to below about 50 or 60 mm Hg is required before cerebral blood flow is affected. This latter point is well illustrated by the fact that during sleep blood pressure commonly falls to about 80 mm Hg in normal subjects for long periods. For atherosclerosis to cause dementia by reducing cerebral blood flow, it would be necessary for most or all of the major cerebral blood vessels to be almost totally obstructed.

The commonest mechanism whereby atheroma causes brain damage is by embolization. Cholesterol, fibrin, or platelet emboli from atheromatous plaques in carotid or vertebrobasilar arteries is now recognized as the major cause of cerebrovascular disease. Such emboli cause abrupt neurological deficits, in the form of the familiar transient ischaemic attack or completed stroke. Repeated emboli from atheroma of the major extracranial blood vessels usually affect the same vascular territory. To produce dementia, emboli must be widespread to infarct numerous sites throughout the brain which is unusual. The patient then presents with multiple strokes, the dementia being the end product of such a series of catastrophies.

Multiple cerebral infarction and softening most commonly occurs in association with hypertension. Multiple cavities are found in the brain at *post mortem*, particularly in the region of basal ganglia, internal capsulae and thalamus (*état lacunaire*). Such multiple lacunes are now believed to result from infarction and microscopic haemorrhage occuring in the distribution of the deep perforating arteries that supply these regions of the brain, in association with the micro-aneurysms described by Charcot and Bouchard which affect these blood vessels, and which are so frequent in those with hypertensive vascular disease (Russell, 1963).

In summary, cerebrovascular disease may cause dementia only by multiple widespread emboli from major cerebral blood vessels, or as a result of the multiple lacunes that occur in hypertension. Multi-infarct dementia correctly emphasizes the true pathological basis of such cases.

In fact, multi-infarct dementia is uncommon, probably accounting for 20 per cent or less of all patients with dementia (Blessed *et al.*, 1968; Sourander and Sjögren, 1970). It is characterized by abrupt episodes of weakness, sensory change and speech disturbance (strokes) culminating in a reasonably distinct clinical picture of dementia, pseudobulbar palsy (with dysarthria, dysphagia, and emotional incontinence), small-stepped gait, and bilateral pyramidal signs, usually in association with hypertension. Insidiously progressive dementia without definite episodes of stroke is most unlikely to be due to cerebrovascular disease, particularly if the patient is normotensive.

Brain tumour and dementia

Brain tumours characteristically cause progressive focal neurological deficit with evidence of raised intracranial pressure. However, slowly growing tumour, notably meningiomas in clinically silent areas of the brain, sometimes present with global deficits of higher mental function in a more or less alert patient. Such global deficits are a consequence of the local damage caused by the tumour, plus remote effects due to distortion of intracranial structures and hydrocephalus (see below). Certain tumours are well known for occasionally presenting in this fashion (Sachs, 1950; Avery, 1971) (Table 5.6), and include not only neoplasms, but also other mass lesions such as aneurysms (Bull, 1969) and subdural haematoma (Selecki, 1965). Symptoms of raised intracranial pressure may be absent, and the optic discs may be normal. Such tumours may only be detected by further investigation of the demented patient.

Hydrocephalus is one of the mechanisms whereby such tumours lead to dementia, but hydrocephalus may be due to other causes and requires further consideration.

TABLE 5.6. Tumours that may present with dementia

Frontal lobe tumours	Convexity meningiomas
Non-dominant temporal lobe tumours	Olfactory groove meningiomas
	Sphenoidal ridge meningiomas
	Gliomas
Parapituitary tumours	Pituitary adenomas
	Craniopharyngiomas
	Hypothalmic tumours
	Aneurysms
Intraventricular tumours	Colloid cyst of third ventricle
	Intraventricular meningioma
Pineal tumours	Pinealoma
	Dermoids
Corpus callosal glioma	
Secondary deposits	
Subdural haematomas	

Hydrocephalus and dementia

Obstruction to CSF flow, at whatever site, causes ventricular dilatation, which may lead to widespread damage to the cerebral cortex.

Hydrocephalus due to tumour

Hydrocephalus is usually due to tumour disturbing CSF pathways, particularly tumours in the posterior fossa which cause early obstruction of the cerebral aqueduct. Such tumours usually present with symptoms and signs due to the local damage they cause, such as cerebellar ataxia, accompanied or followed by the symptoms and signs of raised intracranial pressure. However, such tumours may give rise to so little local symptomatology that they present with the results of hydrocephalus. If CSF obstruction occurs relatively rapidly, these are those of intracranial pressure, but if the tumour is benign and slow growing, the presenting picture may be one of dementia. Notorious in this regard are intraventricular tumours (such as colloid cysts of the third ventricle, or intracranial meningiomas) (Riddoch, 1936), pineal masses, and parapituitary tumours (White and Cobb, 1955; Tiberin et al., 1958). Intraventricular tumours cause no local signs. Pineal masses, by compression of the posterior aspect of the midbrain cause the syndrome of Parinaud, but this may produce few symptoms. Parapituitary tumours cause typical visual and hormonal deficits, but these may be ignored by the patient, and may be very difficult to detect in the dement. On rare occasions, even a massive cerebellar vermis tumour may cause little or no local symptomatology if it grows only very slowly. In all these situations, dementia may be the presenting symptom, local signs may be absent or undetected, and the responsible lesion is only discovered on investigation.

Aqueduct stenosis and other non-communicating hydrocephalus

Obstruction to CSF flow out of the ventricular system (non-communicating hydrocephalus) may be due to congenital or inflammatory obliteration of the cerebral aqueduct or outflow foramina in the roof of the fourth ventricle. Aqueduct stenosis, in particular, may not become apparent until adult life, even though the pathology responsible occurs congenitally or in childhood. A balance is struck between CSF formation and CSF absorption, which occurs at least in part via the enlarged ventricular surface. This compensation may break down at any age to cause progressive symptoms. Initially, these are those of dementia, with the early appearance of difficulty in walking (a gait dyspraxia) and incontinence, both of which may be due to frontal lobe damage. There is often no evidence of raised intracranial pressure in such cases and the correct diagnosis can only be established by investigation.

Communicating hydrocephalus

Hydrocephalus may also be caused by obstruction to the flow of CSF in the subarachnoid space, in which case the cerebral ventricular system freely communicates with the basal cisterns in the posterior fossa (hence the term communicating hydrocephalus). CSF normally flows from the basal cisterns up to the supratentorial subarachnoid space to be absorbed into the venous channels in the arachnoid villi adjacent to the saggital sinus. The narrowest and most vulnerable section of this pathway is at the tentorial opening, which may easily become obstructed by the fibrous reaction to blood or pus, or even tumour. The result is back pressure and dilatation of basal cisterns, and of the whole ventricular system, particularly of the lateral ventricles.

Such a situation is not uncommon in the weeks after a subarachnoid haemorrhage (Kibler *et al.*, 1961), a severe head injury causing intracranial bleeding, or meningitis. Following initial improvement after the acute illness, such patients develop progressive drowsiness, delirium, incontinence, and raised intracranial pressure. Some may require ventricular drainage to relieve the communicating hydrocephalus, but spontaneous remission occurs in many others. Clearly such patients do not present *de novo* with dementia.

Adams and colleagues (1965) drew attention to patients, in whom communicating hydrocephalus occurred many years after subarachnoid haemorrhage, head injury, or meningitis, who presented with a progressive dementia, in the absence of evidence of raised intracranial pressure. Air encephalography demonstrated massive ventricular dilatation with failure of air to pass into the cerebral cortical subarachnoid space, indicating tentorial block, and CSF pressure was normal. The concept of 'normal pressure hydrocephalus' was introduced, and physical laws were invoked to explain ventricular dilatation in the absence of raised pressure. Furthermore, cases of such normal pressure communicating hydrocephalus were identified, with dramatic response to ventriculo-atrial shunting operations, in whom there was no antecedent history of subarachnoid haemorrhage, head injury or meningitis.

The concept of normal pressure communicating hydrocephalus immediately attracted considerable attention, for a new treatable cause of dementia had been identified. Hitherto, many such patients, who might be in their sxties or seventies, would have been dismissed as cases of cerebral atrophy, probably due to Alzheimer's disease. Problems arose because of difficulty in establishing the diagnosis. The air encephalogram, and the more recent EMI–CAT scan, only give static anatomical information, so techniques were devised to study the dynamics of CSF flow. Of these, the intrathecal injection of a radionucleotide, such as radio-iodinated human serum albumin (RIHSA), has been most widely employed to visualize the flow of CSF in the head. The technical details of these and other such investigative techniques are beyond the scope of this chapter (see Benson, 1975) Sufficient to say that none are entirely satisfactory in establishing the diagnosis of communicating hydrocephalus or in predicting a successful outcome to surgical treatment (Wood *et al.*, 1974). Experience has indicated that those in whom air encephalography and RIHSA scanning unequivocally indicate the diagnosis will respond to ventriculo-atrial shunting, while, in general, those in whom these investigations are suggestive, but not diagnostic, will not benefit from treatment. However, unexpected success occurs and this remains a field in which improvements in diagnostic techniques are required.

Hydrocephalus as a cause of dementia

The various forms of hydrocephalus are not common causes of dementia, but their importance lies in the fact that they are treatable. Unfortunately, there are few clinical clues to indicate the diagnosis. The most valuable are: (1) the history of a previous subarachnoid haemorrhage, head injury, or meningitis, and (2) the early appearance of incontinence and gait disturbance. Difficulty in walking and incontinence are common in advanced dementia of whatever cause, but when they appear early in the illness at a time when the dementia is not advanced, they should always raise the suspicion of hydrocephalus.

That hydrocephalus and unsuspected brain tumours may present with dementia is the reason why air encephalography, despite its risks, has been undertaken as part of the full investigation of any patient with dementia under the age of 65 or 70 years. The safe EMI–CAT scan may replace air encephalography, and could well be applied without risk to the elderly dement.

Dementia and cancer

In a few patients, dementia can be attributed to the effects of a primary neoplasm outside the head, causing either metastatic involvement of the brain, or one of the non-metastatic cerebral syndromes.

Secondary cerebral deposits are usually multiple, but grow fast and provoke intense cerebral oedema. Global loss of higher mental function in such cases is nearly always accompanied by clouding of consciousness, so the patient is not strictly demented. However, on occasion tumour may infiltrate the brain and/or meninges to cause true dementia. Multiple cranial nerve palsies usually occur, and detection of malignant cells in the CSF provides the definitive diagnosis.

The non-metastatic cerebral complications of remote neoplasms may cause a dementing illness in an alert patient, at least in the initial stages.

The cerebellar cortical degeneration associated with carcinoma (Brain *et al.*, 1951) is frequently accompanied by dementia, in addition to the florid cerebellar syndrome. The illness may antedate or follow discovery of the underlying neoplasm, usually a carcinoma of bronchus, by up to three years. Symptoms are usually rapidly progressive and are not influenced by treatment of the neoplasm. The CSF characteristically exhibits a pleocytosis, raised protein and paretic Lange curve.

Progressive multifocal leucoencephalopathy (Astrom *et al.*, 1958) may present as a subacute dementing illness, usually accompanied by focal neurological deficits and normal CSF. This rare disorder is most frequently associated with lymphomas and leukaemias, occasionally carcinomas or sarcoidosis. It appears to result from opportunist viral invasion of the brain in an immunodeficient host.

Limbic encephalitis (Corsellis *et al.*, 1968) in which the medial temporal lobe structures exhibit a combination of degenerative and inflammatory change, usually presents as a subacute amnesic syndrome, but can manifest as a global dementia. Carcinoma of the bronchus is the commonest cause, the course is subacute, and the CSF usually contains excess lymphocytes, a raised protein, and paretic Lange curve.

Finally, the non-metastic endocrine syndromes associated with remote neoplasia, such as inappropriate secretion of an antidiuretic hormone, may cause a metabolic encephalopaphy. Such conditions usually present as delirium rather than dementia.

Metabolic and nutritional causes of dementia

It is well-known that patients with a variety of metabolic or nutritional disorders may exhibit a global loss of higher mental function as part of more widespread symptomatology. For example, it has become apparent that a proportion of those on chronic renal dialysis may, in time, dement. Interestingly, this has been attributed to aluminium toxicity resulting from the use of aluminium hydroxide for the control of hyperphosphataemia (Alfrey *et al.*, 1976). Aluminium toxicity has been implicated in Alzheimer's disease because it can cause neurofibrillary tangles in experimental animals, and because there is a suggestion that brain aluminium content is raised in such patients (Crapper *et al.*, 1973). In this situation, the dementia occurs in an obvious clinical setting, and although of great interest, is of no relevance to the problem of the patient who presents with dementia. The same is true for dementia occurring in those with malabsorption syndromes, or chronic liver disease, and is also true of the majority of those with vitamin B_{12} deficiency, hypothyroidism or hypocalcaemia. However, on rare occasions patients with the last three diseases may present with dementia as the outstanding feature of the illness.

Vitamin B_{12} deficiency

Patients with pernicious anaemia, or other causes of malabsorption of vitamin B_{12}, nearly always present with peripheral paraesthesiae and difficulty in walking, due to the combination of a peripheral neuropathy and subacute combined degeneration of the spinal cord. Many will be found to have changes in personality and intellectual performance, if carefully examined (Holmes, 1956; Roos, 1974). Such abnormalities of higher mental function are nowadays rarely florid enough or widespread enough to justify the diagnosis of dementia, and, even if they are, the other symptoms and signs usually clearly point to the correct cause. Whether vitamin B_{12} deficiency can ever present with progressive dementia in the absence of such clues is questionable. Smith (1960), and Strachen and Henderson (1965) have reported cases in which mental disorders were the predominant feature of B_{12} deficiency, but none of the patients described appear to have presented with alert dementia. Surveys of elderly patients, including many with dementia, have unearthed low vitamin B_{12} levels in a proportion of cases (Schulman, 1967), but the associated dementia did not respond to B_{12} therapy. Nevertheless, on these tenuous grounds, B_{12} deficiency has entered the lists of potentially treatable causes of dementia.

Personally, I have not encountered a case of dementia without other diagnostic symptoms and signs, in which B_{12} deficiency has been demonstrated to be the cause. However, in view of the potential success of treatment, all cases of dementia in younger patients warrant investigation for B_{12} deficiency. Since the haematological changes may not be apparent in those with neurological symptoms, measurement of blood levels of vitamin B_{12} are required.

Folic acid and dementia

Strachen and Henderson (1967) attributed dementia to folic acid deficiency in two patients who improved after treatment with folate. Folate deficiency is common amongst those with dementia, but is due to defective nutrition. That folate deficiency causes dementia has not been established, and folate therapy does not affect the course of the illness. At present, the relation of folate deficiency to neurological disorder is uncertain (see Reynolds et al., 1973).

Hypothyroidism

A large proportion of those with myxoedema undergo a change in personality and drive, which, if severe, may produce a syndrome reminiscent of frontal lobe damage. Such changes may be florid, and have led to the concept of 'myxoedema madness' (Olivarius and Röder, 1970). True dementia, with global loss of higher mental function is very uncommon (Bahemuka and Hodkinson, 1975). Careful testing of such patients normally indicates that intellectual and cognitive function is preserved. However, the initial impression may be that of dementia and the clinical features of myxoedema may be inconspicuous. For these reasons, routine thyroid function tests on rare occasions may detect hypothyroidism in the patient presenting with apparent dementia.

Hypocalcaemia

Idiopathic hypoparathyroidism may rarely present as dementia (Robinson et al.,

1954). Hypoparathyroidism is a rare condition, and as a cause of dementia it must be almost unknown in most physicians' experience. In any event, the associated fits, tetany, skin changes, and cataract are likely to indicate the correct diagnosis. However, measurement of serum calcium level is simple.

'Subcortical' dementias

Most diseases cause dementia by damage to the cerebral cortex, but there are some conditions in which dementia occurs with lesions more or less confined to subcortical structures. One of the earliest reports of such a situation is that by Stern (1939) in which severe dementia was associated with bilateral symmetrical degeneration of the thalamus.

Recently, Albert *et al.* (1974) have reviewed the nature of the so-called dementia that occurs in progressive supranuclear palsy, a condition in which pathological changes affect diencephalic and brainstem structures. Such patients, who are usually middle-aged or elderly, present with a progressive akinetic-rigid syndrome and a characteristic supranuclear gaze palsy. Many have been reported to show 'mild dementia', but careful analysis has revealed that this takes the form of alteration of personality, usually apathy, and slowness of thought processes and memory. Although complaining of being forgetful, given time, memory can be shown to be preserved. Aphasia, apraxia, and agnosia are notably absent, in striking contrast to the situation in Alzheimer's disease and other cortical pathologies (Table 5.7). Albert and colleagues drew attention to the similarity of the mental changes in progressive supranuclear palsy to those of frontal lobe disease. The implication is that such mental changes are the result of loss of input from subcortical 'activating centres' to

TABLE 5.7.

Cortical dementia	Subcortical dementia
Features	
Personality change	Personality change
Intellectual decline	Slowness of thought and memory
Memory loss	
Speech and cognitive deficits	
Pathophysiology	
Cerebral cortical damage	Subcortical damage with preserved cerebral cortex
Aetiology	
Alzheimer's disease	Thalamic damage
Multi-infarct dementia	Progressive supranuclear palsy
Pick's disease	Parkinson's disease
	Olivo–ponto–cerebellar degeneration
	Progressive pallidal degeneration

intact frontal lobe cortical neurones; in the absence of such input, the affected cortical areas no longer function. This raises the therapeutic possibility that the intact cortex could be made to work by drugs affecting these alerting systems.

The concept of subcortical dementia may have more widespread application, in particular to the longstanding debate on whether dementia occurs in Parkinson's disease. This issue has been clouded by misinterpretation. Greatest of these has been the misuse of the term 'arteriosclerotic parkinsonism'. Any disease causing widespread brain damage will affect, amongst other regions, the extrapyramidal system, which will lead to an akinetic-rigid syndrome as part of the clinical picture. A large proportion of those with Alzheimer's disease or multi-nfarct dementia will exhibit akinesia, rigidity, and postural flexion (Pearce, 1974). Critchley (1931) observed that such signs resemble those of Parkinson's disease. However, such patients have Alzheimer's disease or multi-infarct dementia, with pathological changes in the basal ganglia, as well as the rest of the brain. These patients do not have Parkinson's disease, which is well defined pathologically as due to degeneration of brainstem neurones, containing melanin, especially those of the substantia nigra. In fact, cerebrovascular disease does not cause bilateral infarction or haemorrhage into the substantia nigra, and is not a cause of Parkinson's disease.

When patients with Alzheimer's disease or multi-infarct dementia with prominent akinesia and rigidity are misdiagnosed as suffering from Parkinson's disease, the apparent incidence of dementia in the latter condition will be high. However, even if such errors are avoided, and it must be admitted that such a distinction can be difficult, the question remains whether patients with true Parkinson's disease dement. Undoubtedly this occurs, but patients with Parkinson's disease are of an age when concurrent Alzheimer's disease and multi-infarct dementia are common. Whether patients with Parkinson's disease dement more frequently than a similar aged-matched control population has never been answered satisfactorily. Also there are the complicating factors of other diseases in which dementia occurs and which may mimic Parkinson's disease almost exactly, such as strionigral degeneration, and the difficulties introduced by drug therapy. At present it seems wisest to conclude that true dementia when it occurs in a patient with Parkinson's disease is likely to be due to another pathology.

However, a significant proportion of those with Parkinson's disease do exhibit mental changes of greater or lesser degree. Typically they are those of lack of drive and initiative with slowness of thought process and memory. In other words, they are the symptoms of 'subcortical dementia'. Again it may be that these changes in mental function, which are not truly those of a dementia, are due to the brainstem lesions of Parkinson's disease.

It will be apparent in this brief discussion of 'subcortical dementia' that the term is being misapplied. Such patients exhibit not the global decline in all higher mental function that is diagnostic of dementia, but a more restricted deficit reminiscent of focal frontal lobe pathology. Perhaps the term should be replaced by 'subcortical frontal lobe syndrome'.

The investigation of dementia

Against the background of the known causes of the syndrome of dementia, it is apparent which investigations are required to establish the cause (Table 5.8). In general, the patient under the age of 70 requires all these tests before it can be assumed that no treatable condition exists.

TABLE 5.8. The investigation of dementia

Blood count and film
ESR
WR and serology
Thyroid function tests
Electrolytes and urea, and liver function tests
Plasma calcium
Vitamin B_{12}
Chest X-ray
Skull X-ray
EEG
Radioisotope brain scan
EMI–CAT scan (or air encephalography)
CSF examination

Few of these investigations merit comment, but the interpretation of radiologically demonstrated cerebral atrophy warrants further consideration.

Cerebral atrophy

The demonstration of atrophy of the brain in demented patients used to require air encephalography, but can now be shown safely and without discomfort to the patient by the EMI–CAT scan. The demonstration of cerebral atrophy is, however, neither diagnostic of dementia, nor does it necessarily imply a progressive deterioration. Furthermore, cerebral atrophy may not be visible in some undoubtedly demented patients. The studies of Gosling (1955) and Mann (1973) have highlighted these important practical points.

Gosling examined the air encephalogram of 68 cases of dementia occurring after the age of 45 without evident cause. Eighty-five per cent had evidence of cerebral atrophy, but 15 per cent did not. At the same time, some eleven per cent of air encephalograms undertaken for reasons other than dementia revealed evidence of cerebral atrophy. Mann examined 54 patients with radiological evidence of cerebral atrophy, of which 49 were followed up five to ten years later. Thirty-three of them were considered to be demented at the time of the radiological investigation; the remainder were thought to have a primary psychiatric disorder (eight), epilepsy (eight), or other neurological condition (five). At the follow-up, 33 were dead, and none of the 16 living patients were demented. Thus about one-third of those with radiological evidence of cerebral atrophy were alive and not demented five to ten years later; most had been treated for depression. This study highlights the risks of equating radiological evidence of cerebral atrophy with progressive dementia and a hopeless prognosis. While the use of the EMI–CAT scan, particularly the feasibility for repeated examinations, may strengthen the diagnostic and prognostic value of demonstrating cerebral atrophy in life, at present such tests are primarily concerned with excluding other treatable causes of dementia.

The yield of investigation

Some indication of the yield of extensive investigation in a population of patients with dementia referred for neurological assessment of dementia, most of whom were under the age of 70, is given in lable 5.9 (Marsden and Harrison, 1972).

TABLE 5.9. Outcome of investigation of dementia in relation to age at the time of the investigation

| | Age in years | | | | |
	50	50–59	60–69	70 +	Total
No. of patients	8	40	43	15	106
Not demented	5	10	5	2	22
Demented					
Intracranial space occupying mass	—	2	5	1	8
Multi-infarct dementia	—	1	5	2	8
Dementia in alcoholics	—	4	2	—	6
Possible normal pressure hydrocephalus	—	1	3	1	5
Creutzfeldt-Jakob disease	—	1	1	1	3
Huntington's chorea	2	1	—	—	3
Post-traumatic cerebral atrophy	—	1	—	—	1
Post-subarachnoid haemorrhage	1	—	—	—	1
Limbic encephalitis	—	—	1	—	1
Cerebral atrophy of unknown cause	—	19	21	8	48

The significant observations are that no less than 22 of the 106 patients, although initially considered to be demented, were found to have primary psychiatric illnesses, usually depression. Of the demented patients, ten per cent were discovered by investigation to harbour an unsuspected cerebral tumour. Over all, about 15 per cent of the whole series had a potentially remediable cause. Similar figures have been obtained on a comparable series of patients by Pearce (personal communication).

By far the majority of demented patients were finally considered to have 'cerebral atrophy of unknown cause'. Most of these would have been cases of Alzheimer's disease, but there are no means of making this diagnosis with certainty in life (other than cerebral biopsy which was not undertaken in the series).

Inspection of Table 5.9 does not suggest that the causes of dementia are materially different at various ages, but the data is limited and further studies to investigate this point have not been undertaken.

Nosological problems of dementia in the elderly

There was a tendency in the past to attribute all mental illness in the elderly to organic brain disease, and to consider the latter under the single diagnosis of senile dementia. Careful psychiatric analysis of the mental disorders of old age has shown that the affective and schizophreniform psychoses of late life can be differentiated from dementia in most cases (see Roth, 1971, and Post, 1975). Dementia in the elderly can be diagnosed most reliably on the basis of (1) a history of progressive decline in higher mental functions over a matter of some months or years prior to the onset of the psychotic illness, or delirious state, that brings the patient to medical attention, and (2) assessment of the mental state over a number of weeks, which allows time for resolution of psychotic behaviour or delirium, and for accurate estimation of residual higher mental function.

If a confident diagnosis of dementia is established in the elderly, there is a tendency to consider the syndrome as due to 'senile dementia'. The latter is thus incorrectly raised to the status of disease.

Difficulty has arisen because senile dementia has been equated with the pathological changes of senile plaques and neurofibrillary tangles that are found in the brains of many such patients. Such pathological changes are referred to as those of senile dementia, whereas they represent one of the causes of that syndrome. The matter has been complicated further by the fact that many undemented old people have a number of senile plaques, and a few have neurofibrillary tangles, in the brain. These pathological changes have therefore been equated with senility, irrespective of the presence or absence of dementia.

Confusion can be avoided if the term senile dementia is restricted to describe the syndrome of dementia in the elderly, whatever its cause, and if the pathological change of plaques and tangles is referred to as Alzheimer's change. Alzheimer's change occurs in most normal old people, but if extensive enough causes senile dementia, and is, of course, the pathological change responsible for Alzheimer's disease when it occurs in the younger patient. Three questions are posed by the ubiquitous Alzheimer's change: (1) Is Alzheimer's disease in the younger patient different from senile dementia due to Alzheimer's change, except in age of onset? (2) Is senile dementia due to Alzheimer's change different from the milder Alzheimer's change seen in most normal old people, except in degree? (3) If the answer to (1) and (2) is no, then is Alzheimer's disease no more than an early and exaggerated form of the milder Alzheimer's change found in normal old people, i.e. is Alzheimer's disease in the young due to a premature ageing of the brain?

These questions are dealt with in detail in Chapter 6. Suffice it to say here that pathologically it has not yet proved possible to distinguish between the changes of Alzheimer's disease in the young patient and those of senile dementia due to Alzheimer's change, nor between the Alzheimer's change in elderly demented patients and normal old people, except in degree. Nor have genetic studies clearly separated these entities as distinct diseases.

A second problem arises in attributing dementia in the elderly to cerebrovascular disease. A diagnosis of 'arteriosclerotic dementia' is misapplied all too frequently on the tenuous grounds of minor changes in retinal blood vessels, evidence of ischaemia affecting the heart or leg blood vessels, minor hypertension, or doubtful evidence of prior stroke, such as previous episodes of 'confusion' (which were probably due to fever, etc.) or an extensor plantar response (which might well be due to cervical spondylosis). As argued earlier, arteriosclerosis *per se* does not cause dementia, and the dementia due to cerebrovascular disease—multi-infarct dementia—is uncommon. It can only be diagnosed with confidence when there is a clear history of multiple strokes, evidence of the typical clinical features of a pseudobulbar palsy and gait disturbance, and significant hypertension. Obviously all of these criteria are not present in every case of multi-infarct dementia, but even if rigorously employed, one will probably not greatly underestimate the incidence of the disease.

In conclusion, senile dementia can reasonably be defined as the syndrome of dementia in the elderly, irrespective of its cause. The two commonest causes are Alzheimer's change and multiple infarcts. The next problem is to what extent do these two pathologies account for all dementia in the elderly?

Causes of dementia in the elderly

The extensive studies of Corsellis, and Roth and his colleagues (see Corsellis, 1962; Roth, 1971; Smith, 1970) have clarified the relative contribution of Alzheimer's change and multiple infarcts to senile dementia. These two pathologies account for about 85 per cent or more of the elderly who die demented. Some 50 per cent of such patients show marked Alzheimer's change; about 15 per cent show predominant multi-infarct changes; a further 20 per cent show both.

Thus, 15 per cent or less of elderly dements are found to have pathology other than Alzheimer's change or multiple infarcts. Many of these patients have other uncommon, and untreatable, degenerative diseases. Such studies suggest, at first sight, that treatable causes of dementia in the elderly are very rare, with the implication that extensive investigation is unnecessary.

However, these studies were carried out on patients who died in chronic hospitals. Treatable causes of dementia should have been sorted out from such a population and would not achieve their true incidence amongst *post mortem* material. What is required is the relative incidence of different causes of the dementia syndrome in the elderly, as established during life. However, data similar to that presented in Table 5.9 is not available for such a population. Hitherto it has not been reasonable to subject all elderly dements to air encephalography in order to exclude tumour or hydrocephalus. The risks of the investigation far outweighed the potential yield in the age group. However, with the advent of the safe EMI–CAT scan, such a survey can be undertaken, and, in conjunction with the other simple tests indicated in Table 5.8, it will be possible to obtain reliable data on the incidence of the various diseases that may cause dementia in the elderly.

In practice, the neurologist encounters occasional examples of most of the conditions listed in Table 5.5 in elderly dements. However, the geriatrician, with extensive experience of large numbers of such patients only rarely discovers treatable causes for the syndrome. Such as do occur are usually indicated by clinical clues (Arie, 1973). It is against this background that one must consider the problem of investigation of dementia in the elderly.

Investigation of dementia in the elderly

The practical approach to investigation of dementia in the elderly must be guided by a number of considerations. The risks and discomfort, time and expertise involved, and cost must be weighed against the yield of results that may influence management. The latter is likely to be very small, but in an ideal situation it would be reasonable to undertake skull X-rays, chest X-rays, blood serology, thyroid function tests, biochemical studies, including calcium, blood count, and serum B_{12}, in all such cases. None of these investigations will harm the patient, and all are capable of detecting other diseases in a population renowned for multiple pathology. Further investigation is probably unwarranted in this age group unless other clinical clues indicate the need, although, were it not for cost, a case would be made for undertaking an EMI–CAT scan to achieve the greatest degree of diagnostic accuracy. Even the battery of simple tests may be deemed unnecessary as a routine, but neurologists, aware of clinical fallibility, have opted for such an approach in the younger dement in order to pick up the odd treatable case that might otherwise have been missed. There seems no reason why a similar approach should not be followed in the elderly, even if the useful result is to discover a single unexpected case of myxoedema over a period of years. If such an argument is persuasive, and sufficient money is available to allow such a course of action, the earlier such assessment is carried out in elderly dementing patients, the greater the chance of successful treatment of any treatable conditions.

References

Adams, R.D., Fisher, C.M., Hakim, S., Ojemann, R., and Sweet, W.H. (1965) 'Symptomatic occult hydrocephalus with "normal" cerebrospinal fluid pressure. A treatable syndrome', *New England Journal of Medicine*, **273**, 117–126.

Albert, M.L., Feldman, R.G., and Willis, A.L. (1974) 'The "subcortical dementia" of progressive supranuclear palsy', *Journal of Neurology, Neurosurgery, and Psychiatry*, **37**, 121–130.

Alfrey, A.C., LeGendre, G.R., and Kaehny, W.D. (1976) 'The dialysis-encephalopathy syndrome: possible aluminium intoxication', *New England Journal of Medicine*, **294**, 184–188.

Arie, T. (1973) 'Dementia in the elderly: diagnosis and assessment', *British Medical Journal*, **iv**, 540–543.

Astrom, K.E., Mancall, E.L., and Richardson, E.P. (1958) 'Progressive multifocal leuco-encephalopathy: a hitherto unrecognized complication of chronic lymphatic leukaemia and Hodgkin's disease', *Brain*, **81**, 93–111.

Avery, T.L. (1971) 'Seven cases of frontal tumour with psychiatric presentation', *British Journal of Psychiatry*, **119**, 19–23.

Bahemuka, M., and Hodkinson, H.M. (1975) 'Screening for hypothydroidism in elderly inpatients', *British Medical Journal*, **ii**, 601–603.

Benson, D.F. (1975) 'The hydrocephalic dementias', in *Psychiatric aspects of neurological diseases*, (Ed. D.F. Benson and D. Blumer) New York, Grune and Stratton, pp. 83–97.

Blessed, G., Tomlinson, B.E., and Roth, M. (1968) 'The association between quantitative measures of dementia and of senile change in the cerebral gray matter of elderly subjects', *British Journal of Psychiatry*, **114**, 797–811.

Brian, W.R., Daniel, P.M. and Greenfield, J.G. (1951) 'Subacute cortical cerebellar degeneration and its relation to carcinoma', *Journal of Neurology, Neurosurgery, and Psychiatry*, **14**, 59–75.

Bull, J. (1969) 'Massive aneurysms at the base of the brain', *Brain*, **92**, 535–570.

Crapper, D.R., Krishnan, S.S., and Dalton, A.J. (1973) 'Brain aluminium distribution in Alzheimer's disease and experimental neurofibrillary degeneration', *Science*, **180**, 511–513.

Corsellis, J.A.N., Goldberg, G.J., and Norton, A.R. (1968) 'Limbic encephalitis and its association with carcinoma', *Brain*, **91**, 481–496.

Corsellis, J.A.N. (1962) *Mental illness and the ageing brain*, London, Oxford University Press.

Critchley, M. (1931) 'The neurology of old age', *Lancet*, **i**, 1119–1127; 1221–1230.

Dayan, A.D. (1971) 'Comparative neuropathology of ageing. Studies on the brains of 47 species of vertebrates', *Brain*, **94**, 31–42.

Fisher, C.M., and Adams, R.D. (1964) 'Transient global amnesia', *Acta neurologica Scandinavica*, **40**, suppl. 9.

Gosling, R.H. (1955) 'The association of dementia with radiologically demonstrated cerebral atrophy', *Journal of Neurology, Neurosurgery, and Psychiatry*, **18**, 129–133.

Hachinski, V.C., Lassen, N.A., and Marshall, J. (1974) 'Multi-infarct dementia. A cause of mental deterioration in the elderly', *Lancet*, **ii**, 207–210.

Holmes, J.M. (1956) 'Cerebral manifestations of vitamin B_{12} deficiency', *British Medical Journal*, **ii**, 1394–1398.

Kibler, R.F., Couch, R.S.C., and Crompton, M.R. (1961) 'Hydrocephalus in the adult following spontaneous subarachnoid haemorrhage', *Brain*, **84**, 45–61.

Kiloh, L.G. (1961) 'Pseudo-dementia', *Acta Psychiatrica Scandinavica*, **37**, 336–351.

Mann, A.H. (1973) 'Cortical atrophy and air encephalography: a clinical and radiological study', *Psychological Medicine*, **3**, 374–378.

MacDonald, C. (1969) 'Clinical heterogenecity in senile dementia', *British Journal of Psychiatry*, **115**, 267–271.

Marsden, C.D., and Harrison, M.J.G. (1972) 'Outcome of investigation of patients with presenile dementia', *British Medical Journal*, **i**, 249–252.

Olivarius, B.F., and Röder, E. (1970) 'Reversible psychosis and dementia in myxoedema', *Acta Psychiatrica Scandinavica*, **46**, 1–13.

Pearce, J. (1974) 'The extrapyramidal disorder of Alzheimer's disease', *European Neurology*, **12**, 94–103.

Post, F. (1975) 'Dementia, depression and pseudodementia', in *Psychiatric aspects of neurologic disease*, (Ed. D.F. Benson and D. Blumer) New York, Grune and Stratton, pp. 99–120.

Reynolds, E.H., Rothfeld, P., and Pincus, J.H. (1973) 'Neurological disease associated with folate deficiency', *British Medical Journal*, **ii**, 398–400.

Riddoch, G. (1936) 'Progressive dementia, without headache or changes in the optic discs, due to tumour of the third ventricle', *Brain*, **59**, 225–233.

Robinson, K.C., Kallberg, M.H., and Crowley, M.F. (1954) 'Idiopathic hypoparathyroidism presenting as dementia', *British Medical Journal*, **ii**, 1203–1206.

Roos, D. (1974) 'Neurological symptoms and signs in a selected group of partially gastrectomized patients with particular reference to B_{12} deficiency', *Acta Neurologica Scandinavica*, **50**, 719–752.

Roth, M. (1971) 'Classification and aetiology in mental disorders of old age. Some recent developments', in *Recent developments in psychogeriatrics*, (Ed. D.W.K. Kay and A. Walk) *British Journal of Psychiatry*, Special Publication, No. 6, pp. 1–18.

Russell, R.W.R. (1963) 'Observations on intracranial aneurysms', *Brain*, **86**, 425–442.

Sachs, S. (1950) 'Meningioma with dementia as the first and presenting feature', *Journal of Mental Science*, **96**, 998–1007.

Schulman, R. (1967) 'Vitamin B_{12} deficiency and psychiatric illness', *British Journal of Psychiatry*, **113**, 252–256.

118

Selecki, B.R. (1965) 'Intracranial space-occupying lesions amongst patients admitted to mental hospitals', *Medical Journal of Australia*, **1**, 383–390.

Smith, A.D.M. (1960) 'Megaloblastic madness', *British Medical Journal*, **ii**,1840–1845.

Smith, W.T. (1970) 'The pathology of the organic dementias', *Modern Trends in Neurology*, **5**, 96–126.

Stern, K. (1939) 'Severe dementia associated with bilateral symmetrical degeneration of the thalamus', *Brain*, **62**,157–171.

Strachan, R.W., and Henderson, J.G. (1965) 'Psychiatric syndromes due to avitaminosis B_{12} with normal blood and marrow', *Quarterly Journal of Medicine*, **34**, 303–317.

Strachan, R.W., and Henderson, J.G. (1967) 'Dementia and folate deficiency', *Quarterly Journal of Medicine*, **36**,189.

Sourander, P., and Sjögren, H. (1970) 'The concept of Alzheimer's disease and its clinical implications', in *Alzheimer's disease and related conditions*, (Ed. G.E.W. Wolsterholme and M. O'Connor) London, Churchill, pp. 11–36.

Tiberin, P., Goldberg, G.M., and Schwartz, A. (1958) 'Craniopharyngiomas in the aged', *Neurology, Minneapolis*, **8**, 51–54.

Tomlinson, B.E., Blessed, G., and Roth, M. (1968) 'Observations on the brains of non-demented old people', *Journal of the Neurological Sciences*, **7**, 331–356.

White, J.C., and Cobb, S. (1955) 'Psychological changes associated with giant pituitary neoplasms', *Archives of Neurology and Psychiatry*, **74**, 383–396.

Wood, J.H., Bartlett, D., James, A.E., and Udverhelyi, G.B. (1974) 'Normal-pressure hydrocephalus: diagnosis and patient selection for shunt surgery', *Neurology, Minneapolis*, **24**, 517–526.

6

DEMENTIAS WITH SENILE PLAQUES AND NEUROFIBRILLARY CHANGES

J. Constantinidis, J.Richard, and J. de Ajuriaguerra

Introduction

It is now accepted that from the nosological point of view the clinico-anatomical diseases previously described under the names of presbyophrenia, simple senile dementia, 'Alzheimerized' senile dementia, and Alzheimer's presenile dementia, or Alzheimer's disease, are variants of the same degenerative disorder of the central nervous system, the common histological characteristic of which is the existence in the brain of two essential types of lesion that are quantitatively significant: senile plaques (SP) and neurofibrillary changes (NFC). It is for this reason that we have made them the common subject of the present study.

We shall present here the clinical symptoms which form the main stages of disintegration in higher nervous functions, particularly from the psychological, neuropsychological, and neurological points of view. We shall emphasize the clinical concept of the homogeneity of general disintegration in certain of the functions studied.

We shall not enter into histological descriptions (by optic and electronic microscopy) of the cerebral lesions found in these dementias. Readers interested in their morphology, topography, and pathogenesis (SP, degenerative dysphoric, and congophilic angiopathies, granulovacuolar neural degeneration and neurofibrillary changes, GVD and NFC) should turn to specialized works on these subjects.

We shall deal with the specificity of SP and NFC, and with their occurrence in cases which show no clinical signs of a dementing state.

Finally we shall present some statistical data concerning histoclinical correlations, in particular between the density of NFC, memory disorders and the age of their onset, instrumental disorders, and the rate of clinical progress of the disease.

Historical summary

The history of dementias with SP and NFC does not really begin until the end of the nineteenth century. For some time before then, and particularly from Esquirol onwards (1816), the general concept of a dementing state had been developing. Dementia was distinguished from congenital mental deficiency or idiocy and from certain acute states, traumatic or transitory, such as Georget's state and stupidity (1820), which first having become Delasiauve's state of stupor was later integrated by Chaslin into the huge clinical area of mental confusion. Bayle's study of general paralysis (1922) demonstrated the organic nature of certain states of dementia. It offered the hope, not immediately recognized, of possible therapeutic action in these diseases. In 1853 Marcé drew attention to atheromatous lesions of the cerebral vessels and in the same year Kjelburg affirmed the syphilitic origin of general paralysis. Baillarger (1889) discussed the relationship between dementia and premature ageing. The idea of a presenile pathology of dementia was introduced by Binswanger and developed by Kraepelin. The isolation of arteriopathic dementia began with Klippel (1891). In 1894 Binswanger drew a distinction between this dementia, which he called arterioschlerotic, and general paralysis, and he described a special form of dementia of subcortical localization. In 1895 Magnan recognized the diffuse or localized nature of organic lesions in dementia. The history of dementia with SP and NFC began when Charcot and then Kraepelin (1896) tried to differentiate arteriosclerotic processes from those of senile dementia, emphasizing that they were very often combined. In 1898 Alzheimer showed that certain lesions which were observed in senile dementia could not be attributed to arteriosclerosis.

In 1905 Klippel and Lhermitte put forward a new clinico-anatomical entity, that of pure senile dementia, which was not of vascular aetiology and which they considered akin to presbyophrenia, isolated in 1890 by Wernicke.

The concept of presbyophrenia was to be the subject of much discussion, particularly at the beginning of this century. In 1900 Wernicke restricted use of the term to cover disorientation in time and place, amnesia for recent events, false recognition, and confabulation: he hoped thereby to give it a proper nosological place, alongside senility but distinct from senile dementia.

He related presbyophrenia to Korsakoff's psychosis, but with this Kraepelin disagreed. Fischer (1910), under the name of 'spherotrichia cerebri multiplex', described disseminated cerebral lesions, considering them as presbyophrenia's histological substratum and affirming that they did not exist in senile dementia. The autonomy of presbyophrenia was defended in France by Marchand and Nouët (1912), while Dupré and Charpentier (1909) refused to recognize it and insisted that latent signs of polyneuritis were very frequently present. These two authors considered presbyophrenia to be a chronic form of Korsakoff's syndrome which forms part of the picture of mental confusion. This concept was to be revived by Bessière (1948) who suggested retaining an entity which he called the Wernicke–Korsakoff syndrome, although dementia is not found in Korsakoff's psychoses, although the alcoholic aetiology of that psychosis cannot be invoked in presbyophrenia, and although the frequency of polyneuritis associated with presbyophrenia may be contested, as well as the assimilation of presbyophrenia into the state of mental confusion.

It was Kraepelin who, in 1910, assigned originality to the disorder by conferring on it the name of *Alzheimer's disease*, an early presenile form of dementia with SP and NFC. This was made possible by a series of studies, of which we will recall only the principal stages. First Block and Marinesco (1892) discovered senile plaques in the brain. In 1907 Alzheimer found these senile plaques in the brain of a woman of 51 who suffered from dementia, and he described, in addition, particular neurofibrillary changes. Benfiglio (1908) and Perusini (1909), on the basis of other clinical-anatomical observations, finally described a demential disorder that could be distinguished from senile dementias by its early development and its focal symptomatology. The studies carried out by Alzheimer, Perusini, and Simchowicz between 1910 and 1914 advanced our knowledge of senile plaques, neurofibrillary and granulovacuolar changes viewed as histological accompaniments of pure senile dementia.

The parallel studies of Pick (1892–1904) on focal cerebral atrophies, and Alzheimer's histological studies, in particular his description in 1911 of two cases of atrophic dementia with no SP or NFC, but with an abundance of neuronal swellings and argyrophilic inclusions, pointed to the existence of another type of dementia which was at first considered to be presenile and to which in 1926 Onari and Spatz gave the name of Pick's disease. After this original clinico-anatomical synthesis, it was not until Escourolle's publication in 1956 that the major differential criteria were recognized for Pick's disease and Alzheimer's disease, thus bringing to an end the diagnostic uncertainties that had existed between these two disorders (see also Constantinidis et al., 1974; Tissot et al., 1975).

Study of the so called presenile dementia thus gradually eroded the category of senile dementia. But while the distinction between senile dementia and Pick's disease became easy, the distinction between senile dementia and Alzheimer's disease remained a much more delicate matter and as a result of further studies was to be subjected to renewed investigations later. From 1924 onwards, such studies included a series of histological investigations which tried to define more precisely the morphology (Van Braunmuhl, 1931, 1932, 1939; Jacob, 1939, 1952), the topography (Grünthal, 1926–1952; Simma, 1949, 1959), the histochemistry (Alexander and Looney, 1938; Divry, 1927–1952; Morel and Wildi, 1952) and the pathogenesis (Simchowicz, 1924; Lowenberg, 1925; Ferraro, 1931; Divry, 1939) of so called senile lesions. Attention was drawn to the irregular occurrence of SP. The concept of dysphoric angiopathy emerged from the observations of Schölz (1938), Divry (1941–1942), and Morel and Wildi (1943–1955). In 1954 Pantelakis described congophilic angiopathy. Interest was shown also in the relationship between senile dementia and senescence and in mixed senile dementias (degenerative and vascular) and the frequency of their occurrence (Uyematsu, 1923; Rothschild, 1941).

While genetic studies were being developed (Sjögren et al., 1952) and after Marchand (1937, 1938) had tried to obtain acceptance of the term 'encephaloses' to cover a regrouping of Pick's and Alzheimer's diseases and dementia without cerebral arethoma, all to be regarded as different modalities of the same degenerative process, Mutrux (1947, 1958), Newton (1949), and later Arab (1960) and Albert (1964) took up once more the problem of the relationship between Alzheimer's disease and senile dementia. They thus paved the way for a unitary theory of these two entities, which was definitely accepted from 1968 (Lauter and Meyer) and according to which the two disorders are early and late forms of the same degenerative dementia, as distinct from Pick's disease.

From 1964 onwards de Ajuriaguerra and Tissot have directed a structural clinical analysis of these forms of dementia and to this end they have adapted the methods of genetic psychology and applied them to the problems of old age. Their work has led to the concept of a homogeneous multiple disintegration of higher nervous functioning, a concept which has proved useful in the differential diagnosis of dementias with SP and NFC (Alzheimer's disease and senile dementia) on the one hand and dementias of other aetiology, in particular vascular, on the other. Subsequent studies have clarified other aspects of dementia with SP and NFC, namely, neurological (Paulson and Gottlieb, 1968; Seitelberger, 1969; Fot et al., 1970; Vernea, 1973), neuropsychological (Savage and Bolton, 1968; Irving et al., 1970; Miller, 1971), psychiatric (Jonsson et al., 1972; Ferm, 1974) and social (Luke, 1973; Wang, 1975).

During the last few years pathological anatomy has been enriched by the findings of electromicroscopy (Kidd, 1963, 1964; Terry, 1963; Schlote, 1965; Hirano et al., 1968; Hirano, 1970; Gonatas and Gambetti, 1970; Lampert, 1971; Nikaido et al., 1971, 1972; Wisniewski and Terry, 1973; Miyakawa et al., 1974). The morphology and pathogenesis of SP, NFC, GVD, and dysphoric angiopathy have thus become more clear. Biochemical studies (Shelanski and Taylor, 1970; Crapper, 1973), enzyme studies (Suzuki and Terry, 1967; Rotin, 1972), serum and hormone investigations (Constantinidis, 1960, 1962a, 1962b) and immunological researches (Duheille et al., 1973) have also been pursued. There has been a series of genetic publications (Nielsen, 1968; Pratt, 1970; Mark and Brun, 1973; Constantinidis et al., 1965a, 1965b, 1969, 1972). The neurophysiological approach has become better defined (Dejaiffe et al., 1964; Constantinidis et al., 1969; Levy et al., 1970, 1971; Crapper, 1973). There have likewise been studies concerned with cerebral circulation (Obrist, 1970; Collard, 1972; Gustafson and Risberg, 1974).

Finally there have been publications on methods of inpatient and outpatient care and on ways of making these patients mobile: ergotherapy, sociotherapy, and physiotherapy (Richard and de Bus, 1973; Arie, 1973; Bhasker, 1974).

Clinical aspects

In order to provide a better understanding of the problems which face the clinician dealing with states of dementia, particularly those with SP and NFC, it seems to us that the following are necessary.

(1) To try to describe some of the progressive stages of dementia with SP and NFC, starting with an analysis which may be called structural, in other words to study first certain modalities of individual and multiple disintegration in higher nervous functioning that are found in these dementias.
(2) To indicate the essential characteristics of the main clinical forms of dementia, i.e. simple senile dementia, 'Alzheimerized' senile dementia, and Alzheimer's disease.

Our attitude towards elderly patients has changed considerably in the last few years and there have also been developments in the methods of care given them. The clinico-anatomical pictures have, however, not been subjected to adequate clinical study and have still not been made relevant to the real problems which these patients pose. As they are presented today they are of no real help with the rehabilitation and social integration of the elderly dementing patients, which is one of the immediate concerns of the doctor and his auxiliary team.

Acccurate assessment of the symptoms which are of real diagnostic value is always hampered by the possibility of misidentifying underestimating, overestimating or mistaking the origins of the symptoms. Symptom misidentification occurs much more easily in elderly than in other patients and to avoid it we must usually carry out an active investigation. The same symptom may mean many different things and failure to investigate its mechanism may lead us to underestimate its importance. The reaction of the elderly patient to his illness and to its consequences can also give rise to additional symptoms which can and must be controlled if we are not to hamper certain clinical, anatomical, biological, or therapeutic investigations, or cause them to give misleading results.

In cases of dementia the clinician is still too often apt to forget how necessary it is to describe the symptoms in plain language, with as little medical terminology as possible, and to employ a vague terminology, so that there is a risk of paying too little attention to the clinical evolution of the disease and of passing too quickly to a stage of interpreting ill defined symptoms. Finally, it is more important in clinical practice to understand the semiology presented, to try to grasp the structure of the patient's reasoning or action, than to assess the consequences.

One last general remark concerns the clinician's difficulty in drawing up positive rather than negative balance sheets. It is essential to remember that the doctor must assess accurately what assets the patient still possesses, which may assist in his social rehabilitation even if only briefly, and use them in relation to any physical and mental handicaps. This means that the clinician cannot limit his activity to observing the patient across the desk in his consulting room, but must study his behaviour in his ordinary environment, in contact with his family and his colleagues and, if he is an inpatient, in his relationship with other patients and with the nursing staff.

The principal stages of disintegration in higher nervous functioning (The structural analysis of these states of dementia)

Leaving aside purely neurological problems, we shall consider here only certain essential aspects of cognitive functioning in the course of disintegration in dementias accompanied by SP and NFC.

The isolated or multiple disorganization which we shall study here covers operationality, memory, language, praxias, gnosias, and motor-behaviour; in dementias with SP and NFC disorganization occurs according to a predictable progression which supports the clinical concept of homogeneity in dementia (de Ajuriaguerra and Tissot, 1968; Richard, 1964, 1971; Richard and de Bus, 1973).

Individual disintegration of certain functions

This will now be reviewed semiologically from the psychological, neuropsychological and neurological points of view.

Psychological: intelligence and operationality (de Ajuriaguerra *et al.*, 1960, 1964, 1967a, 1969, 1970a, 1970b; Müller, 1961; de Ajuriaguerra and Tissot, 1966; Tissot, 1973; Tissot *et al.*, 1972; Richard, 1974; Richard and Tissot, 1974; Burnand *et al.*, 1972).

For reasons which we cannot go into here, it has become common in geriatric practice to substitute qualitative for quantitative appreciation in the assessment of intelligence. From this point of view it therefore seems more important to know how an elderly patient achieves a performance, and why he does not achieve it or no longer achieves, than to determine whether he did achieve it, did not achieve it, or no longer achieves it. Genetic psychology tests, especially those devised by Piaget to which we shall refer, have thus proved best for our purpose. They represent in fact genetic scales in the full sense of the word. They do not give us more or less immediate or arbitrary levels such as the mental ages provided by classical psychometric tests, but point rather to stages of cognitive activity.

By using them we can show that elderly patients with dementia accompanied by SP and NFC pass through stages which are characteristic of the ontogenesis of cognitive functions. Their operational performance has now been established in most of the main areas of cognitive activity, namely those concerned with physical quantities, space, time, elementary logic, and chance.

We know that patients suffering from these dementias show a levelling of performance at the point of transition to preformal reasoning. All their behaviour tends then to reach the same level though there is a partial loss of efficiency in certain tests. The levelling off occurs precisely at the performance level of those functions which we call concrete. Quasi-instrumental factors are later superimposed on this phenomenon at the pre-operational level.

It is interesting to note, particularly in the areas of space and time, that the level of performance falls below that found in a child with the same functional level so far as conservation of physical quantities is concerned.

The specific attitude of patients in operational tests may account for the falling off observed in certain tests in which performance is clearly below the average level of functioning. These attitudes, the incidence of which varies according to the stage of disintegration reached, are as follows:

Forgetting the starting and finishing instructions of the problem;
Difficulty in manipulating or apprehending many elements of the test, or pieces of information;
Distractability;
Fluctuation in performance;
Imprecise use of former automatic concepts, when the operations which normally underly them and which were a necessary part of their acquisition, have already been lost;
Lack of representational anticipation.

Some means of facilitating the task in question are used spontaneously by the patient. Others have to be supplied. Although they constitute an obvious handicap in the difficulties encountered at a higher level, they may enable us to understand better the nature of the deficits which they are intended to relieve. From this point of view the forms of behaviour frequently resorted to or accepted by patients are:

Successive approaches which are all the more effective when a clue is left open to view;

Decrease in the number of elements to be manipulated, which in the more deteriorated patients seems to compensate for the narrowing of the perceptive field and difficulties of perceptive decentering. In less deteriorated patients it seems to eliminate the difficulty of passing from one concept to another;

Verbalization of the real or virtual action in progress, which may be suggested by an inadequate or not quite adequate exploration on the part of the examiner;

Use of concrete facts;

Changes effected by the examiner himself;

Manipulation, when it narrows contact with the problem, and permits the patient to proceed by trial and error.

The fall in level which we have mentioned seems also to be connected with a lack of representational anticipation, which is one of the first processes to be affected by dementia with SP and NFC. In dementing patients everything takes place as if the operational schemes were still effective when applied to problems that do not call for preliminary organization of successively apprehended facts. Actions are in this case regulated internally and do not have to be confronted with external reality. But the operational capacity in question becoming inoperative when it has to select its own regulations for observing external events. In this situation the individual has continually to submit to the hypothesis that results from applying an operational scheme to a confrontation with observed events. He has to maintain his intention, as well as the systematic decentering that leads to a comparison of supposed and real events. The operation must therefore anticipate a configuration of events, in order to compare it with what is observed. It is here that we come up against difficulties of inductive reasoning.

There is thus a clear distinction between the dementing patient and a child or adult of the same operational capacity. It is easy for the dement to reason deductively by using logical structures that are pre-adapted to events. It is very difficult for him to reason inductively by grouping successive data in order to confront them with a hypothesis.

Complementary tests of transitivity and of causality have enabled us to confirm that conservation of physical quantities, like logical structures pre-adapted to events, depends on an operational mechanism and not just on simple automatisms or preservation of structures that have already disappeared, although sometimes conservation of weight without transitivity presupposes an operational structure akin to that which underlies the invariance of matter. In effect the level of operational structurism underlying tests of causality and tests of conservation of physical quantities is one and the same.

The differences in operational level thus do not conflict with the hypothesis of a relatively homogeneous disorder of operational capacity in dementing patients. But if the stage of equilibrium of organization and of operational involution are the same, they do not seem to be sustained by identical mechanisms.

Let us recall that in the first stage of demential disintegration ocular exploration is also a good criterion of cognitive activity. The amount of oculomotor activity that takes place when an individual voluntarily looks at something corresponds almost to the total amount of information that he deems it necessary to gather. Where his eye rests represents a selection made from all the potential information that the stimulus offers. Moreover, the localization of visual inspection represents an outline of the strategy chosen in gathering information. Therefore a random distribution of glances represents an absence of hypotheses, of anticipation, of strategy in the search for information. So long as the patient's sensorimotor system remains strictly speaking intact so far as his oculomotor apparatus is concerned, his visual exploration is regular, methodical, more extensive and of longer duration, although it leads to difficulties in visual recognition, in particular pictures of objects. Relating past information to present information in order to anticipate the future is one of the functions of visual exploration. Other observations permit us to say also that in visual exploration the dementing patient experiences difficulties in ridding himself of certain notions acquired by experience (in other words, he shows a lack of intellectual 'plasticity', a decrease or loss of dynamic cognition). He also can no longer resist the attempt to obtain greater precision of forms, which tends to lead to errors in visual recognition.

The limited active visual exploration of the dement might also be explained, at least partially, in terms of a lack of pragmatism. But although the methods the dement employs to facilitate his task show that he is not making full use of his actual oculomotor potentialities; nevertheless these begin to modify his ways of relating to the external world. Cognitive variables in behaviour are intimately bound up with affective variables in his motivation and in the interest with which he approaches anything novel or unusual. To infer a law implies a strategy. It implies, too, the maintenance of a constant intention throughout a complex series of proceedings.

It should also be noted that the operational level of the patients in whom we are interested does not depend directly on memory impairment, since this may be present in initial stages of demential disintegration without any accompanying operational disturbances. But after the initial phase, when operational levels decline, the converse is by no means true. It seems, on the contrary that there is a very good correlation between operational and instrumental levels of disintegration.

Neuropsychological

(1) Memory: Sufficient consideration has not been given to the possible conservation of memory as compared with the obvious conservation of operational schemes. Such consideration might, without excluding the existence of specific mechanisms based on equally specific functional anatomical systems (the circuit of Papez, for example, for successive forgetting), perhaps have kept us in mind of the fact that the integrity of memory processes is inconceivable without functional integrity in the brain as a whole.

In fact mnesic impairment, as measured by the degree of orientation in space and time, power of registration and recall, and other clinical signs such as ecmnesia, iterations, confabulation, false recognition and misidentification, and as defined within the framework of memory in the strict Piagetian sense of the term, does not run parallel with impairment of operational and instrumental capacities (i.e. language disorder, praxias, and gnosias), although the two aggravate each other as histological lesions become more extensive. It is thus common to find that in the less advanced stages of dementia a patient is disoriented in time and space and shows clear amnesia of registration and recall, although no operational and instrumental deficits have yet appeared.

In dementing patients with SP and NFC, however, we find that mastery of physical and chronological time, without which memories cannot be organized, is closely correlated with operational capacity. As such it is independent both of registration amnesia and of the capacity to relate past events to the present.

At the higher level of concrete operations, the reproduction of rhythm is not much affected in these patients. When spatial symbols have to be translated into rhythmic figures, reproduction is at first carried out on the same spot, then spatialization later begins to appear. Isochronicity of successive periods is rarely conserved. With practice subjects become able to equalize synchronous periods, but they are not able to generalize from one situation to another. When there is cinematic interference the duration of perceived events is conserved, though not without an initial tendency to dissociate space–action–time. Some subjects overestimate the action itself. One subject out of two estimates the duration of the action on the basis of the task accomplished and not on speed (more work or effort equals more time, rather than higher speed equals less time).

There are few, if any, difficulties in placing regularly events within the conventional chronological system. The first difficulties emerge when putting action pictures into serial order, but after some groping this can still be successfully achieved. Disorientation in time is clearcut. The year, month, and date are no longer known.

At the middle level of concrete operations, failures are markedly more frequent in reproducing rhythmic structures. When the patient is asked to space rhythmic reproductions on the basis of spatial symbols, he regularly does this on a horizontal line. So far as physical time is concerned, space time and task time are only partly differentiated, or not at all. The only constant achievement is the estimation of the duration of events where there is no cinematic interference. So far as action time itself is concerned, the duration of action is overestimated in most cases. Its estimation is based on the task accomplished. In chronological time, difficulties regularly arise in placing less regularly occurring events which have no fixed place on the temporal axis.

Serialization of action pictures is clearly hampered by the impossibilty of keeping hold of one central person who is shown in changing situations. If the series is complicated, fragmentation becomes complete. Disorientation in time may be superimposed on that of the preceding group.

At the lower level of concrete operations and at the pre-occupational level failures to reproduce rhythmic structures are not much more frequent than in the group just described.

Short structures (five elements or under, lasting not less than 2·5 s—Fraisse's unit of the perceived present) are on the whole successfully achieved. When the subject tries to translate rhythms starting from spatial images, there is at first some spatialization, but later neither rhythm nor spatialization can be observed.

So far as physical time is concerned, space and time are not differentiated which, *a fortiori*, means no differentiation between speed and work accomplished.

So far as action itself is concerned, the duration of the action is overestimated, but no reason is given.

So far as chronological time is concerned, the patient is still able to place correctly on the chronological axis those temporal landmarks which are habitual and fixed. Serial ordering of action pictures is no longer possible or is achieved only with difficulties and when the changes do not involve more than one element in the pictures and do not number more than two or three. Temporal disorientation is complete for both long and short durations of time.

While it is true that some disorders concerned with social and historical time seem to be connected with memory deficit in the strict sense, and while in certain cases a relative conservation of this memory seems to play a corrective role, the relative integrity of this particular memory is not sufficient to maintain the integrity of temporal operations, nor is amnesia in the strict sense sufficient to abolish them.

In the disintegration of chronological time there may exist, alongside operational disorders, a loss or relative conservation of automation in regard to learned facts, together with some element of amnesic disorders in the strict sense, and of praxic or gnosic disorders peculiar to the demential disorganization.

But the semiology of dementias with SP and NFC shows—more clearly than in the case of focal lesions—that knowledge, recognition, and recall of concepts and signs are inseparable from the functioning of the sensorimotor and operational schemes which give rise to them.

In dements with SP and NFC the ability to integrate the past and the present in order to anticipate the future—an integration which helps organize the past temporally—does not explain either the mastery of physical and chronological time or amnesia in its strict sense. But when it is affected, it contributes to the disturbance of memory in the strict sense.

Mastery of the past is in itself bound up with short term and long term registration of the present. While it admittedly calls for integrity in the circuit of Papez, lesions of this anatomical apparatus cannot alone account for disorders of memory in the strict sense as observed in dementing patients. For short term retention the important factor here is the absence of any interference between obtaining the information and its recall. The dement is able to acquire not a memory but a scheme of action which embodies those perceptual signs which are necessary if successful conditioning is to take place. One is led to believe that by means of this conditioning one can pass from the domain of memory in the strict sense to memory as a broad concept. We rediscover here the intrinsic capacity to conserve schemas whether they are of habit, of action or operational, as opposed to the fragility of 'memory images' as seen in memory in the strict sense. This is why in the practical area of re-education it is necessary to bring into play the potentialities of 'schematism' in the Piagetian sense, in order to compensate for deficits of memory in the strict sense.

(2) Language: When language disintegration occurs in dements with SP and NFC it seems possible to distinguish the following.

(a) Disturbances of language which seem to be related to defects in operational functioning.

Language in degenerative dements rapidly becomes elliptic and pleonastic. Prepositions are left hanging without the nouns or phrases which should follow them, terms which are essential to the situation are omitted. Predicates are multiplied. Language seems to be used in its practical form as an auxiliary of action and no longer as a vehicle of explicit thought. The superfluity of words may be explained by the need to qualify. Lack of the right word, which becomes apparent, seems to be momentarily remedied by the use of common paraphrases. The expression of asymmetrical relationships is difficult. Classifications are no longer extensive but intensive.

Disorganization of the semantic fields becomes concrete with the appearance of semantic paraphasias or of primary articulation. When the patient is asked to name objects his replies thus move from the adequate word to the one that has no apparent semantic connection with the object, with intermediate semantic deviations of every kind. Some of these clearly suggest a cognitive disturbance or even a loss of differentiation which is akin to the lack of differentiation found in the semantic fields of children. Other phenomena are more difficult to interpret— the way in which the patient appeals to a generic class, or slips semantically towards a neighbouring term of the same class, or passes to a related subfield.

Language disturbances along the syntactical axis of the language are less in evidence than those on the lexical or paradigmatic axes. The arguments used by dements, for example to justify their responses when faced with comprehending a series of events or actions whose order can be expressed only by morphosyntax (tense of verbs and order of words), correlates well with their operational level. Where the morphosyntactic linguistic values seem, in a purely linguistic context comparable to those of classical syllogisms, to share the fate of concepts based on intellectual operations, they are preserved for a very long time within the framework of more or less automatic verbal utterances.

(b) Disturbances of language that are semiologically akin to those of secondary aphasis found in cases with circumscribed lesions.

It is difficult to determine the point at which the semantic paraphasias, or those of primary articulation already mentioned, take on the character of frank aphasis.

Paraphasias of secondary articulation, which occur less frequently in the course of demential disintegration and appear later than the semantic paraphasias, do not seem to show any semiological characteristics which would distinguish them from the phonemic paraphasias of Wernicke's aphasia.

Phonemic interchanges (commutations) are very rarely found in spontaneous and repetitive language until an advanced stage of dementia has been reached.

They abound, however, in the iteration of logatomes by patients who are not yet severely affected. As in the syndrome of phonetic disintegration in anarthria or Broca's aphasia, described by T. Alajouanine, A. Ombredanne, and M. Durand, vowels are better retained than consonants. There are also numerous elisions, metathesis, interconsonantal assimilations and displacements of consonants under the influence of neighbouring vowels. While the most frequent phenomenon observed is the oralization of nasal vowels, nasalization of oral vowels is not uncommon. The elements more frequently affected are the constrictives, which interact by exchanging the point of articulation while keeping the same degree of mouth, according to contextual influences, the relevant serial characteristics— voicelessness, sonority, nasalization—are generally preserved. The transition from one series to another is not always in the same direction. Sonorization is more frequent than voicelessness, though this does occur. While oralization predominates, nasalization is not rare. From this it is natural to wonder whether these commutations are not more akin to phonemic than to phonetic disturbances, and whether they might not be interpreted, as regards both apprehension and utterance, as a loss of the distinctive characteristics of phonemes.

(c) Disturbances of language occurring within a framework of motor disintegration.

What we shall consider here are phonemic iterations in the strict sense rather than the substitutive perseverations of verbal confusions which seem by their form and by the context in which they develop to be identical with those aphasias that occur in patients with circumscribed lesions. Phonemic repetitions or logoclonias, more frequently syllabic than verbal, can occur in the middle of a linguistic utterance which is still relatively well structured. They may also occur spontaneously, or they may accompany any intentional tightening of the buccophonatory organs. They exist simultaneously with graphic and other motor iterations such as spontaneous unvocalized oral activity, kneading the bedclothes, tramping the feet, crossing and uncrossing the legs, to which we shall return later. They also occur in conjunction with a disturbance of muscular tonus and with the reappearance of primitive forms of behaviour and primitive reflexes. They generally manifest themselves at a stage when language is severely disorganized. But this disorganization does not seem to be a necessary or sufficient cause.

Language disintegration in dements with SP and NFC is therefore the result of different kinds of disturbance. Initial impoverishment of vocabulary, failure to find the right word, disorders of syntax, semantic and phonemic paraphasias, logoclonias which appear as dementia progresses—these cannot be reduced to a common denominator. Such defects cannot be attributed to a decline in global intellectual capacity, nor to purely instrumental disturbances.

(3) Apraxias (de Ajuriaguerra and Kluser, 1965; de Ajuriaguerra et al., 1967b; Gainotti, 1970).

The first defects to appear are constructional apraxias. In the study of graphic constructional praxias, which are the usual baseline studies, cubic perspectives are at first spontaneously reproduced but disappear progressively when copied, several forms of flattening being shown. First, the reproduction shows only two surfaces of the cube, then only one, while in Bender's test in which the patient has to copy a bicycle or a double hexagon, it becomes difficult to join the different elements together. Finally topological relationships are lost and the parts of the model are jumbled together.

Difficulties begin to appear in copying hand movements from the Bergès–Lezine test for children, particularly reverse movements such as putting the index and little fingers of one hand against the little and index fingers of the other. These are followed by difficulties in executing spontaneous or imitated conventional symbolic ideomotor gestures (putting one's finger to one's nose, a military salute, making the sign of the cross, etc.).

Symbolic praxic difficulties appear when there is frank ideomotor apraxia. It becomes impossible to indicate the gestures which accompany the use of an object, and later to manipulate an object with or without preliminary demonstration. It should be recalled here that Piaget's loss of object permanence follows symbolic apraxia.

Praxic difficulties in dressing appear first in putting clothes on, and then taking them off. Certain attitudes before dressing, for example lack of spontaneity or of pragmatism, discontinuity in action, may be found in other forms of behaviour without being of particular semiological significance. But they may also herald the first specific disturbances in dressing. Other symptoms occupy an intermediate position between disturbances in affective an and in cognitive behaviour. Confabulatory digressions, which could not occur without memory disturbance, also represent a means of eluding and masking failures to accomplish the task to be done. More specific disturbances are those that affect the order in which clothes are put on or taken off, the sequence of actions required for putting on and taking off a particular garment, mistakes in positioning the garment—holding it either wrongly in itself or wrongly in relation to the body. In the end such disturbances may affect the relationship between one part of a garment and another, or between one garment and another, or may affect recognition of an article of clothing and its utilization.

Buccofacial apraxias, if any, appear at a very late stage. Certain disorder of deglutition seem to have an air of aphagopraxia.

(4) Agnosias (Tissot *et al.*, 1972; Guilleminault, 1968; Gaillard, 1970; Cornu, 1974; Richard, 1974, 1975).

In the visual field, the difficulties which occur at a very early stage are concerned essentially with recognition of the mixed images of objects and figures in Poppelreuter's test. Object recognition remains unimpaired for a very long time. The patient is still able to classify colours, even at an advanced stage of his disorder.

We have already drawn attention to the importance of the exploratory ocular activity which leads to recognition. We shall see later how this recognition is influenced by conjunct oculomotor disturbance in the strict sense. We have never confirmed the presence of true auditory agnosia.

All the tests used to study hylognosia (heat conductivity, resistance, rugosity, weight, hydrometry) can still be excellently performed by dementing patients with SP and NFC, provided one uses, if necessary, the method of multiple choice with a minimum of three elements.

From the morphognostic point of view:

(a) Ordinary objects require a much shorter period of exploration than geometric shapes and no mistakes are made.

(b) Three-dimensional shapes are always recognized when there are only four possibilities to choose from and when these possibilities are all different. When three choices are offered that are similar and non-spherical in shape but of different sizes, mistakes are made at the pre-occupational stage, either macro- or micro-agnosia, neither predominating over the other. Large shapes are always recognized, but medium sized and small shapes are confused in a third of the cases. Spheres of different sizes are, on the other hand, always differentiated.

(c) When the shapes to be identified are two-dimensional, open and closed shapes are well differentiated and round shapes are clearly preferred to those with angles.

When the transition is made to pre-formal operations, mistakes are made between lozenge shapes and irregular quadrilateral shapes. At the level of concrete operations, only round shapes are recognized, as well as rounded shapes with notches, though mistakes do occur in the size of the notch. Patients at this level do not recognize shapes which have both curved and straight lines, nor do they distinguish between a cross and a feathered cross, nor between a round plaque with a hole in the middle and one with a hole that is not in the middle. Angles that point outwards and angles that point inwards are often confused.

At the pre-operational stage, the square is confused with the circle, the feathered cross with the star. Angles that point outwards are regularly confused with angles that point inwards, and the circle which has a quarter of its area removed is likewise confused with the lozenge or the square.

There are no instances of patients being able to identify shapes concerned with Euclidean relationships, nor do they discriminate at this stage between shapes that are topologically different.

The results fluctuate and there is overlapping between the different degrees of the over-all scale. Thus a patient who can still discriminate between shapes whose identification depends on Euclidean relationships, may already have difficulty in picking out shapes whose identification depends on topological relationships.

The confusion between shapes which have an angle in common (a circle which has a quarter of its area removed confused with a square, a circle with a segment removed confused with a lozenge) is peculiar to the dementing patient and has not been found in children.

The dement thus shows a contrast between conservation of identity, down to the lowest level, so far as familiar objects and polyhedra are concerned, and premature difficulties in recognizing two-dimensional shapes.

The time spent by the dement on exploration before he comes to the pre-operational stage is proportional to the difficulty which that exploration presents. Familiar objects are recognized with a few quick touches. Geometric shapes require a distinctly longer exploratory period.

At the pre-operational stage, when exploration calls for some stimulation of the patient, he feels the object with a kind of 'gliding' touch. The object is held against the palm of his hand and all four fingers together glide over its surface. No one finger is used separately, and only exceptionally does he use his thumb.

At the lower level of concrete operations the index finger brushes over the object, and one may also detect some palpation in the fingertips.

At the level of concrete operations touch becomes systematic. A distinctive feature is sought, which can form the starting point of an analysis. Next comes a synthesizing study of the object, in which the thumb and the index finger play an important part.

In dements there is a considerable discordancy between their operational capacity so far as conservation of physical quantities is concerned and their ability to get the feel of a two-dimensional shape.

Finger agnosia appears at an early stage, in the form of bilateral digital autotopoagnosia. In its final form it shows in right–left mistakes in the Piaget–Head test. Body autotopoagnosia is next to appear. It would seem that the ways of reacting to pain, which finally appear, cannot be interpreted as the equivalent of the asymbolia for pain found in focal cortical lesions. In fact at the most advanced stage of dementia pain is no longer related to a precise body schema. It is no longer localized but is expressed as a diffuse feeling of suffering and disagreeableness, while the patient is unable to organize movements which would permit him to avoid it.

Neurological (de Ajuriaguerra *et al.*, 1963a, 1963b; de Ajuriaguerra and Gauthier, 1964; Gainotti, 1970; Fot *et al.*, 1970; Tissot *et al.*, 1972; Richard, 1974).

At the first stage neurological examination shows practically no abnormality, apart from slight trembling and some synkinetic mimicry. But vertical extinction of sensation is a frequent phenomenon. It seems at first to be evinced when a stimulus is applied simultaneously to one foot and one hand, perception of the foot stimulus being effaced. Then, when a stimulus is applied both to the hand and the cheek, only the facial stimulus is perceived. Extinction thus occurs first at foot level and then at hand level. There may also at this stage be some motor habits which assume the character of an invariable fixation.

At the second stage the face may be expressionless but quickly livens up in the course of conversation. When standing spontaneously, the patient is a little rigid and his trunk is bent slightly forward. His head is motionless. He looks at the ground and his arms are usually hanging flat at his side. He does not move. When he is asked to move, his gait seems to have lost its suppleness, although he does not yet take short steps. Automatic arm movements are restricted, but the forearm is not bent as in parkinsonism. It seems difficult for him to start walking and this takes some time. Very occasionally the start may be accelerated. Stopping is not always easy and is preceded by some wavering. It is difficult to make a half-turn. When seated, the patient's posture (attitude) remains rigid. He sits stiffly and does not lean against the back of his chair. His hands are placed on his knees and it is not long before they begin an incessant movement to which we shall return later. Any attempt to relax the upper and lower limbs ends either in his conserving his posture or, if he is lying down, in his limbs being forcibly positioned on the bed. The concentration required to carry out the request disturbs progress of the action that has to be performed. The resistance encountered in restoring part of the limb in question to its original position disappears when the patient's attention is distracted. There is a marked, symmetrical, and constant decrease in swinging of the limbs. When the limbs are passively moved, there is progressive resistant hypertonia, which seems most marked in the lower limbs. This may be accompanied by motor anticipation when the patient anticipates the passive movement imposed by the examiner, and by motor iteration. The patient then continues the imposed movement after the examiner has stopped moving the limb in question. The motor anticipation may disappear after several flexion–extension movements. Conservation of posture is common, especially in the upper limbs. A certain amount of tonic preseveration may be observed when the patient is shaking hands. His ability to make a quick, suitable gesture, such as is required in order to catch a ball and throw it to the examiner, sometimes shows that, if he catches the ball successfully, he cannot let it go to throw it until it is just at the level of the examiner's hand. When this happens his fingers often do not open properly.

At this stage too the upper limbs once more show a forced tactile or proprioceptive grasping reflex or both at the same time. This reflex is more easily and more constantly released if the examiner gets the patient to speak and so distracts his attention. It is not always symmetrical. Palmomental and pellicomental reflexes are fairly common. Appearance of the oral visual reflex is preceded by the cephalobuccal reflex and usually followed by the oral tactile reflex. These reflexes are produced in response to long pointed objects but not to round flat objects. The most simple response to visual and tactile stimuli is a round or rectangular opening of the mouth. Other responses to tactile stimulus are a fish-like opening of the mouth, licking the lips, sucking the object with the mouth half open. This sucking, which is at this stage only short and strong with quick opening and closing of the mouth, is accompanied by frowning.

Synkinesis is frequent, bilateral, and varies from one moment to the next according to the attention paid by the examiner or the patient to the motionless limb. It is almost always tonicokinetic, very rarely tonic, pure, or median.

Stereotypes occur in the form of the isolated kneading movement described, when the patient is in bed, plucking his bedclothes. It may be triggered at first by emotion, then by stimulation of the cavus conchae of the external ear, or by putting paper or tissue in the patient's hand. Stereotypes appear immediately after the occurrence of the grasping reflexes.

Ocular motility is equally affected. The first symptoms to attract attention are difficulties in ocular fixation. Vertical optokinetic nystagmus is inhibited (OKN). When the patient is asked to look at a central spot, these difficulties show in slipping movements or slight ocular displacement, which may be vertical or horizontal, while in the pendulum test he loses sight of the oscillations.

These difficulties go curiously hand in hand with a fixation of gaze. When the patient is asked to describe a picture of large dimensions his eyes first wander and then become riveted on what is actually only a part of the picture. This fixation is maintained for a considerable time and the patient can pass to other elements in the picture only if one insists energetically on his doing so. Fixation of this kind does not usually occur with pictures of smaller dimensions—it happens in fact when he is trying to achieve OKN. Chronologically, wandering, and fixation appear later than the forced grasping reflex observed at hand level.

Changes in ocular pursuit are also expressed in difficulties in ocular 'braking', in which we find his eyes overshooting the mark, then returning, with ocular pauses and jumps. There is also a tendency for eye movements to be accompanied by movements of the head.

There is a third stage at which the phenomena just described become more acute. So far as walking is concerned, it is not unusual for the patient to mark time when he is starting to walk, when he stops, and when he is close to obstacles. The forced grasping reflex observed in the upper limbs now reaches a climax, with the hand being drawn magnetically towards any object that approaches it. In the lower limbs we find a plantar support reaction, a Pötzl phenomenon (paradoxical contraction of the quadricept in Lasègue's manoeuvre), a forced grasping plantar reflex, and conservation of postures.

Oral activity may occur spontaneously or may be evoked. Opening the mouth and putting out the tongue, opening the mouth and trying to catch an object, on the one hand, sucking everything that lightly touches the mouth on the other—these are additional responses to visual and tactile stimuli respectively and emphasize the existence of the cardinal points of André Thomas (for tongue mouth and head) where there is simultaneous response to the two types of stimulus. These oral forms of behaviour are triggered by any object whatsoever. Spontaneous oral activity is represented by buccofacial stereotypes.. They consist in opening the mouth roundly or in a rectangle, sucking and licking with the tip of the tongue, masticating and rumination, sucking the fingers and massaging the gums, sucking, and licking. Sometimes anything that comes into contact with the hand is spontaneously put into the mouth.

Other stereotypes may be noted: marking time with the feet, accompanied by smoothing, tapping with the hands, rubbing of the hands alone or accompanied by foot stamping, smoothing and tapping, rubbing between the thumb and index finger, rubbing the hands on the thighs and knees, polymorphic movements of the lower limbs which occur in many patients who have difficulty in walking and which consist of bending and stretching one or both legs, crossing the feet, moving the whole body. All this corresponds to a global motor disturbance, the various activities occurring and mingling in no strict order. In many cases the model extends to graphic and gestural activities.

At this last stage spontaneous oculomotor activity is reduced. It is further hampered by aggravation of the fixed gaze phenomenon and by the simultaneous existence of marked wavering eye movements.

The anarchic ocular movements observed when the gaze is centrally fixed thus seem to be independent of any effort at fixation, being produced rather 'in a vacuum'. When the patient tries to read, his eyes jump from one line to another, if they do not become fixed. These symptoms seem to correspond to a more or less degraded form of Balint's syndrome.

It seems justifiable to ask whether some clinical aspects of the fixed stare or wavering eyes might be connected with the conservation of posture observed in the limbs and whether other aspects might be related to the difficulties of grasp noted in advanced dementia, when the patient has to be asked over and over again to accept an object, while once he has taken hold of it, with or without help, his grasp is retained to an exaggerated degree.

Oculomotor activity continues to be hampered by synchronized movements of the eyes and head.

This synchronization is such that the carriage of the head may inhibit the patient's eye movements. If he is given test instructions in the normal manner, as if he understood what was expected of him, traces of ocular exploration may persist, some normal and brief, others reminiscent of an earlier stage, for example, when the test is one of concentrating the gaze on a peripheral spot and reading a text, or when the patient is examining pictures.

As these dementias develop, oculomotor activity, both automatic and voluntary, deteriorates progressively in the following ways:

Attempts to initiate OKN;
Realization of ocular convergence;
Ocular pursuit of an object which the examiner holds and moves;
Ocular pursuit of a pendulum with large or average oscillations;
Ocular pursuit, especially unguided pursuit, of the perimeter of a square;
Enumeration of scattered points or of counters that have been scattered or arranged;
During exploration aimed at estimating the relative lengths of two sides of an 'L', of two fixed sides of a rectangle, and of two straight lines of unequal length, either parallel or not parallel;
During exploration aimed at estimating the relative lengths of two sides of an 'L' and two sides of a rectangle, when one remains constant and the other is increased in length;
When assessing the depth of two objects in a dynamic situation.

This decline in conjunct oculomotor performance, both automatic and voluntary, may occur in very different modalities:

Appearance and aggravation of a single symptom in a given test, for example, fixation of gaze;
Appearance in the same test of a series of symptoms which further hamper ocular motility, for example, OKN, with difficulties occurring first in the vertical and then in the horizontal plane;
A defect which is common to different experimental situations, as when ocular convergence in the course of demential disintegration starts by being obtainable on request, later can be achieved only with the help of an external point of fixation (an object held by the examiner, the examiner's finger), later still can be achieved only with the help of a point of fixation that is connected with proprioceptive afferent nerves (an object held by the subject, his finger, which is brought near to his nose), and finally cannot be achieved at all.

Simultaneous disintegration of operational, mnesic, instrumental and motor functions. The concept of homogeneity in general demential disintegration in patients with SP and NFC

This general disintegration of evoked functions is a homogenous phenomenon in dements with SP and NFC. General homogenous disintegration implies that when a sign of disintegration appears in one function, another known sign of disintegration will be found at the same moment in another function.

We could draw up clinical tables of general homogenous disintegration in three areas—operational, instrumental, and motor. But the most useful clinical table of general disintegration at the present stage of our knowledge seems to be one which describes concurrent defects of language, praxias, and gnosias and which is limited therefore to the instrumental field.

The main points of reference which enable us to establish clinical stages are the following:

(1) Inability to find the right word, onset of constructual graphic apraxia in the form of impaired ability to reproduce perspective, difficulties in recognizing pictures of objects—at first if they are incomplete, blurred or superimposed, and digital autotopoagnosia (when the examiner touches the finger of one hand the patient locates this in the other hand).
(2) Paraphasias, loss of perspective in graphic praxic constructural reproduction, difficulties in copying complicated hand gestures, constant digital autotopognosia.
(3) Substitution of words, drawing cubes in two-dimensions, then in one-dimension, errors of articulation in constructual graphic reproductions, ideomotor praxic difficulties in copying conventional symbolic gestures, and bilateral stereognosias.
(4) Mistakes made in forming individual words, jumbling of parts of the model in drawing, ideomotor apraxia, praxic difficulties in ideation, body autotopoagnosia, and loss of normal reactions to pain.

This description may, in spite of its precision, seem arbitrary. It is of real importance for positive clinical diagnosis of dementia with SP and NFC. It indicates that the introduction of a syndrome of aphasia–apraxia–agnosia follows relatively precise rules when the aetiology of the disease is degenerative.

Clinical forms of dementia with SP and NFC
(Richard and Constantinidis, 1970, 1975)

Simple senile dementia

In this the clinical onset of the disorder is usually progressive and insidious. Disorders of memory are usually the first to appear. They are accompanied by intellectual fatigability and sometimes by depressive dysthymia often associated with some awareness (nosognosia) of failing intellectual faculties, or by contrast a state of affective indifference. Ill-structured delusional ideas of prejudice or persecution centred on those immediately around, most frequently based on memory (forgetting) or interpretation (false construction) are not infrequent, nor are behaviour disorders such as diurnal and nocturnal agitation, tendencies to wander, aggressiveness. The patient neglects bodily hygiene, his dress, his food. Acute onset is less frequent.

As memory disturbances grow worse, there is increasing disorientation in time and space, which becomes more and more complete and affects long and short periods of time, large and small areas of space; we also find faulty registration and loss of recall, at first for recent, later for earlier events, confabulation, false recognitions, misidentifications and babbling. The patient becomes anosognosic, irritable, incontinent, insomniac. He shows disorders of attention. His activity is disorganized and incoherent. Disorders of intellectual functioning can easily be demonstrated by using Piaget's genetic tests.

At this stage we get impoverishment of language, the patient cannot find the right word, there is constructual apraxia, but no other signs of aphasis–apraxia–agnosia. Apart from slight hypertonia in the limbs, slight or inconstant forced grasping reflexes in the hands and some vertical extinction of sensation, neurological examination is normal.

The course of the disorder is slowly progressive, and in general lasts three to eight years. Disorientation in time and space becomes total, and mnesic and operational abilities disappear, though instrumental functions are not seriously impaired. The patient gradually enters his dotage, he becomes bedridden and cachechtic. Sometimes there is contraction of joints. Death usually occurs in the course of an intercurrent disease, often a cardiac or infection illness.

While there are early and late forms of simple dementia, presbyophrenia, which could be merely one stage in the evolution of simple senile dementia, is another and frequent clinical form. It cannot at present be judged clinically as very different from Korsakoff's syndrome. It resembles that disorder in the prominence and the quality of its memory disturbance and in the absence of operational, instrumental and motor disorder.

'Alzheimerized' senile dementia

This is an evolutionary form of simple senile dementia. It is characterized by the more or less progressive intrusion into the clinical picture above of simple senile dementia of a syndrome of increasingly complete aphasia–apraxia–agnosia, which follows the decline in operational capacity and which is accompanied by increasingly overt symptoms of so called prefrontal origin (forced tactile and proprioceptive grasp reflex of the hands, forced plantar reflexes, oral visual and tactile reflexes with cardinal points, Pötzl's phenomenon, support reaction, conservation of attitudes, etc.), with increasingly marked resistance hypertonia, stereotypes and signs of conjunct oculomotor disturbance reminiscent of a degraded form of Balint's syndrome. Combined disturbance of language, praxias, and gnosias occur fairly regularly and in the predetermined order which we have already indicated.

As the illness progresses, the degree of dependency increases. Verbal iterations appear (echolalia, palilalia, logoclonia). The patient no longer recognizes himself in a mirror and no longer uses the mirror image. (When objects are held over his shoulder while he is looking in the mirror, he tries to catch them in or behind the mirror.) There are no pyramidal and no cerebellar labyrinthic symptoms. There may be generalized epileptic seizures. Death occurs in circumstances similar to those described for simple senile dementia.

Alzheimer's presenile dementia

This comes on usually before the age of 65. The clinico-anatomical picture is comparable to that of the 'Alzheimerized' senile dementia described above, for which it has served as a model for study, since although it is less frequent its description came earlier. The syndrome of aphasia–apraxia–agnosia seems, however, to be more rapid in onset and less regular in its chronological evolution than 'Alzheimerized' senile dementia.

Neuropathology

The anatomical and histological substratum of these degenerative dementias consists of cerebral atrophy with SP and NFC. Almost every case also shows granulovacuolar degeneration in the neurones of the hippocampal allocortex. In a proportion of cases there is also dysphoric angiopathy, particularly in the occipital cortex, as well as congophilic angiopathy.

We will not deal here with the morphology or pathogenesis of these cerebral changes. We shall limit our discussion to SP and NFC, their specificity, and the correlation between the density of these lesions and the degree of dementia.

This is an area worth studying, for we find SP and NFC in the brains of elderly patients who have shown no signs of dementia. According to Gellerstedt (1933), SP were found in the non-dementing aged brain in 84 per cent of cases and NFC in 64 per cent. Matsuyama *et al.* (1965) studied the brains of 680 patients, none of whom had senile dementia or Alzheimer's disease; they found that the number of cases with SP and NFC increased in linear proportion to age. Dayan (1970a and b) and Dusheiko (1972) reached similar conclusions.

How specific are these lesions for degenerative dementias, and what are the histoclinical correlations?

These problems have been studied in different ways, of which we shall give a few examples as follows.

Comparison of the incidence of SP and NFC in aged dements and non-dements

Malamud's study (1965) covered 411 patients between 60 and 84 years. He found the incidence of SP and NFC to be as follows:

220 cases with a chronic cerebral organic syndrome	153 cases =	69·5%
116 cases of functional psychosis	21 cases =	18·1%
75 old persons with no signs of dementia	3 cases =	4%

Studies carried out by Wildi *et al.* (1964, 1967, 1968) and Dago-Akribi (1969) covered three series of patients:

Series 1: 606 brains of patients who died in the psychiatric clinic, including dementias and other forms of psychiatric disorder but excluding schizophrenia.

Series 2: 75 brains of patients with schizophrenia who died in the psychiatric clinic.

Series 3: 303 brains of patients who died in the general hospital from a variety of diseases.

The following findings emerged:

(1) Frequency of cases with SP
  (a) Comparison between series 1 and 2
    Series 1: over-all frequency 71 per cent
    Series 2: over-all frequency 44 per cent
  (b) Comparison between series 1 and 3
    Series 1: group aged between 80 and 91 years, 86 per cent
    Series 3: group aged between 80 and 91 years, 60·6 per cent
(2) Frequency of cases with NFC
  (a) Comparison between series 1 and 2 (Table 6.1)

TABLE 6.1. Frequency of cases with NFC, series 1 and 2

	Series 1	Series 2
Hippocampal allocortex	59%	29%
Hippocampal isocortex	57%	20%
Frontal neocortex	24%	5%
Occipital neocortex	8%	1%

  (b) Comparison between series 1 and 3
    Series 1: presence of NFC in neocortex of group aged between 80 and 91 years, 30 per cent
    Series 3: presence of NFC in neocortex of group aged between 80 and 91 years, two per cent

These findings show that in series 1, which included many dements, SP and NFC occurred far more frequently at the same age than in schizophrenics (series 2) or in patients who died in the general hospital (series 3). If we take only neocortical NFC, they were present in 30 per cent of series 1, and five per cent of series 2 and two per cent of series 3.

Comparison between the density of SP and NFC in the brains of aged dements and non-dements

Blessed *et al.* (1968) counted the SP found in different cerebral fields in 60 patients with an average age of more than 70. Their results are given in Table 6.2. Small quantities of SP were found in non-dements, but they were present in large quantities in patients with senile dementia.

TABLE 6.2.

	Average no. of SP per field
Senile dementia	20·85
Depression	1·14
Paraphrenia	5·00
Confusional states	2·75
Delusional states	2·64
Physical illnesses	5·13

Tomlinson *et al.* (1968, 1970) carried out a quantitative study of SP and NFC in dements and non-dements. Table 6.3 summarizes their findings.

TABLE 6.3.

	Dements	Non-dements
No. of cases	50	28
Average age	76·4	75·4
Average no. of SP per field	14·7	3·3
NFC in the hypocumpus:	28%	44%
	(+)16%	24%
	+ 18%	32%
	+ + 38%	0%
NFC in the neocortex	62%	11%

(+) low density; + average 40. density; + + high density

These results show that qualitatively the same lesions are found in dements and in non-dements, but that quantitatively they are far less numerous in the latter:

four times fewer SP (3·3 as compared with 14·7 per cent)
six times fewer NFC in the neocortex (eleven as compared with 62 per cent)

NFC are found in the hippocampus of slightly more than half of the non-dements, but they are present only in small or moderate quantities, whereas in dements they are more frequently found (four-fifths of the cases) and are present in large quantities. These findings show that SP and NFC may be observed in non-dementing elderly subjects but in far smaller quantities than in the case in the brains of patients with degenerative dementia. Moreover these changes may be absent, even up to an extremely advanced age. It is therefore the quantity of lesions which is specific for these dementias. There are, however, still some questions to be asked. Are these changes (SP and NFC), when present in small quantities, a normal or inevitable phenomenon of the ageing brain? It is difficult to answer this question. Some people have reached the age of 100 without showing any of these lesions: but perhaps they would have shown them if they had lived even longer! Some elderly patients have small quantities of SP and NFC without having shown any signs of dementia. If these patients had lived longer, would the lesions have become more numerous and would the patients have shown signs of dementia?

It is again difficult to answer. In the present state of our knowledge we may say that SP and NFC are present in the brains of a large number of elderly persons, and that the incidence of these changes increases with age. There is probably a greater or lesser tendency to senility in everyone, and individual resistance to these changes varies in accordance with constitutional and acquired factors, such resistance generally decreasing with age. These changes must take place in a certain quantity before clinical signs of dementia appear.

Study of the correlations between density of SP and NFC, degree of dementia, age of onset of clinical signs, and rate at which the disorder develops

We have seen that SP and NFC must be present in certain quantities before demential disorders appear. Gellerstedt (1933) considered that the presence of SP did not necessarily have any clinical significance. Neumann and Cohn (1953), found a correlation between profusion of SP and NFC and the degree of dementia characterized by memory and instrumental disorders, and insisted that the presence of SP in itself was of no clinical significance. Roth *et al.* (1966) found a correlation between density of SP and degree of dementia. Sim *et al.* (1966), who carried out frontal and temporal biopsies in elderly subjects, found a very clear correlation between clinical symptomatology and the presence of NFC. In our own study we have tried to measure the correlations between SP and NFC on the one hand and demential disturbances on the other, using cases from the psychiatric clinic in the University of Geneva. Our material, which was acquired between 1925 and the end of 1969, consists of 2700 brains of patients who died in the clinic and on whom autopsies were carried out. We have studied standard samples taken from the hippocampus, and from the temporal, frontal, and occipital cortex of these brains, using silver-staining (a modified Globus technique). In this way we have been able to collect a group of cases with SP and NFC. We eliminated from the series all those cases which showed additional macroscopic or microscopic vascular foci, traumatic lesions, tumours, or toxic or infectious lesions, as well as some other cases of rare disorders. We were left with 576 brains in which the only lesions consisted of SP and NFC. Continuing the same process, we picked out the brains of patients who had died after the age of 65 without showing any vascular lesions, whether degenerative or not. In this group we found a certain number of cases showing very marked ventricular dilation, probably corresponding to the disease entity described by Adams *et al.* (1965) as normotensive senile hydrocephalus. We eliminated these patients from our series and shall report on them elsewhere. We were thus left with a group of 72 ageing brains of psychiatric patients 'without lesions' which, added to the 526 cases with SP and NFC, gave us a total of 648 brains. In a high proportion of these cases we had determined the weight of the fresh brain as well as Reichardt's coefficient. We studied the clinical records of these patients and in accordance with the description given there and with our own criteria we evaluated the presence or absence of disorders of memory, and of so called instrumental disorders (aphasia–apraxia–agnosia). Wherever possible, we noted the age of onset of the dysmnesia and of the instrumental disorders. Where we knew the age of onset of the dysmnesia, we also knew the survival period. Where we knew the age of onset of the instrumental disorders, we also calculated the time that elapsed between onset of dysmnesia and the appearance of the instrumental disorders.

Histologically, the samples were all taken from the same cerebral areas, using the same technique. Some 2500 histological preparations were examined microscopically by the same worker. In view of the large number of preparations involved, we did not make a quantitative count. So far as SP were concerned, we noted only their presence or absence. For NFC we estimated their density (low density (+); average density + ; high density + +) in the hippocampal isocortex and neighbouring temporal neocortex as well as in the frontal and occipital neocortex. According to the topographic density of NFC and the presence of SP, we then established seven groups:

I. High density of neucortical NFC (frontal, occipital) with NFC present in the hippocampus and with SP.
II. Average density of NFC in the neocortex, with NFC also present in the hippocampus and with SP.
III. Low density of NFC in the neocortex, with NFC also present in the hippocampus and with SP.
IV. Average or high density of NFC in the hippocampal isocortex (and possibly also in the neighbouring temporal neocortex), with NFC also present in the allocortex, and with SP, but with no NFC in the frontal or occipital neocortex.
V. SP and NFC present in the allocortex, but few, if any, in the hippocampal isocortex.
VI. SP present but no NFC.
VII. Neither SP nor NFC.

Some anatomical and clinical data on these seven groups are given in Table 6.4, on which the following observations may be made:

(1) Brain weight shows a decrease and Reichardt's coefficient an increase which both run parallel to the density and diffusion of these lesions.
(2) When NFC are present in the frontal and occipital neocortex, all cases show disorders of memory. When the NFC are limited to the hippocampus, 87 per cent of cases show such disturbances. But if only SP are present, with no NFC, 72 per cent of patients show slight, discrete disturbances of memory, as do 30 per cent of the cases with neither SP nor NFC.
(3) The disorders which we call instrumental are present in 90 per cent of the cases which have a high neocortical density of NFC, in two-thirds of the cases which have an average density of NFC, and in half the cases in which neocortical density is low; when the NFC do not extend beyond the hippocampal isocortex and the

Table 6.4. Analysis of cases according to the degree of cortical degeneration

		Neurofibrillary lesions										
Group	SP	Allocortex hippocampal	Neocortex hippocampal	Neocortex frontal occipital	No. of cases	Average age at death (years)	Weight of brain (g)	Coefficient of Reichardt (%)	Incidence of dysmnesia (%)	Age of onset of dysmnesia (years)	Survival after onset of dysmnesia (years)	Incidence of instrumental disorders (%)
I	+	+	+,+ +	+ +	173	74.9	1102	16.15	100	67.57	6.8	91
II	+	+	+,+ +	+	77	80.7	1125	13.7	100	74.76	5.3	65
III	+	+	+,+ +	(+)	105	81.8	1142	14.6	100	76.16	5.1	51
IV	+	+	(+),−	−	58	83.0	1150	12.3	87.7	80.25	2.75	32
V	+	+	−	−	96	81.3	1168	11.4	84.0	79.60	1.7	16
VI	+	−	−	−	67	78.8	1175	11.3	72.5	78.1	0.7	12
VII	−	−	−	−	72	73.9	1248	8.8	30	73.3	0.6	3

Table 6.5. Analysis of cases according to intensity of neocortical Alzheimerization

	High (a) No. of cases	High (a) Values	Average (b) No. of cases	Average (b) Values	Low (c) No. of cases	Low (c) Values	Significance (a) vs (b) + (c)
Age of onset of dysmnesia (years)	147	67.57 ± 8.41	65	74.76 ± 7.77	73	76.16 ± 0.01	$p < 0.001$
Proportion of cases with instrumental disorders	158–173	0.91 ± 0.02	50–77	0.65 ± 0.05	50–105	0.51 ± 0.05	$p < 0.001$
Interval between onset of dysmnesia and appearance of instrumental disorders (years)	106	3.21 ± 2.68	31	3.88 ± 2.31	28	3.92 ± 3.15	NS

neighbouring temporal neocortex, and when their density there is average or high, a third of the cases show instrumental disorders, while only one-sixth are affected when the density of NFC in the hippocampal isocortex is low. Finally, when SP are present, but there are no NFC, twelve per cent of cases show instrumental disorders, as compared with only three per cent when neither of these lesions is observed. There is thus a correlation between the incidence of instrumental disorders and the density and diffusion of NFC, particularly in the neocortex.

(4) The average age of onset of dysmnesia is lower when there is a very high density of NFC. As we have already pointed out, it is in this group that most of the presenile cases are found (Constantinidis, 1968).

(5) When the onset of dementia is senile, there is a parallel between the survival period and the density and diffusion of the NFC. It seems that in the senile group, those who become 'Alzheimerized' live longer.

(6) There is a very clear correlation between histological 'Alzheimerization' (intensity and diffusion of NFC) and clinical 'Alzheimerization' (instrumental disorders). This correlation is not absolute, since nine per cent of the cases which showed strong histological 'Alzheimerization' showed no instrumental disorders, while twelve per cent of the cases which showed SP and no NFC did have such disorders.

These findings led us to make a more detailed statistical analysis of cases in the first three groups characterized by diffuse NFC in the frontal and occipital neocortex (Constantinidis, 1973). Table 6.5 shows that the onset of dysmnesia occurs at a significantly earlier age in the group with strong 'Alzheimerization' than in the rest. The proportion of cases with instrumental disturbances is also significantly higher. The time that elapses between the onset of dysmnesia and the appearance of instrumental disorders is shorter in the highly 'Alzheimerized' group, though the difference is not significant.

As soon as we realized that these histological groups varied according to the age of onset of the dysmnesia, we analysed our cases from this point of view. The bell-shaped curve of group I cases (highly 'Alzheimerized') when analysed according to age of onset of the dysmnesia, shows a peak between 60 and 74 years, that of groups II and III (average and slight 'Alzheimerization') occurring between 70 and 84 years. The two curves meet around 70 years. Having established this, we divided our cases into two groups: the first showing onset of dysmnesia at up to 69 years, (presenile cases), the second at 70 or over (senile cases). Table 6.6 shows that 80 per cent of presenile cases have strong neocortical 'Alzheimerization', while only one-third of the senile cases are highly 'Alzheimerized'. Instrumental disorders are present in 90 per cent of the presenile cases and two-thirds of the senile cases (a significant difference). In presenile cases the illness progresses more rapidly towards these symptoms than in senile cases, but the difference is not significant.

We may conclude that early onset of the disease is related to more intense neocortical 'Alzheimerization', and that there is an almost constant and relatively rapid progression towards the instrumental disorders. This last fact emerges very clearly from Table 6.7, in which our cases are analysed according to the presence or absence of these instrumental disorders. The average age of onset of

TABLE 6.6. Analysis of cases according to age of onset of dysmnesia

	up to 69 years (a)		70 years and over (b)		Significance (a) vs (b)
	No. of cases	Values	No. of cases	Values	
Proportion of cases with high neocortical Alzheimerization	88–108	0·81 ± 0·03	59–177	0·33 ± 0·03	p < 0·001
Proportion of cases with instrumental disorders	100–108	0·92 ± 0·02	116–177	0·65 ± 0·03	p < 0·001
Interval between onset of dysmnesia and appearance of instrumental disorders	78	3·12 ± 2·84	87	3·76 ± 2·56	NS

TABLE 6.7. Analysis of cases according to presence or absence of instrumental disorders

	Present (a)		Absent (b)		Significance (a) vs (b)
	No. of cases	Values	No. of cases	Values	
Proportion of cases with high neocortical Alzheimerization	158–269	0·60 ± 0·03	15–93	0·16 ± 0·03	p < 0·001
Age of onset of dysmnesia (years)	216	69·71 ± 8·61	69	76·75 ± 6·41	p < 0·001
Survival after onset of illness (years)					
Total	216	6·56 ± 3·80	69	4·42 ± 3·44	p < 0·001
Presenile	100	7·78 ± 4·30	8	4·75 ± 4·02	NS
Senile	116	5·51 ± 2·96	61	4·38 ± 3·40	p < 0·05
Group I	137	7·04 ± 3·96	10	4·30 ± 2·83	p < 0·05
Group II	41	5·92 ± 3·55	24	4·12 ± 2·92	p < 0·05
Group III	38	5·52 ± 3·22	35	4·67 ± 3·96	NS

dysmnesia is significantly lower in the group with instrumental disorders; similarly the proportion of cases with strong neocortical 'Alzheimerization' is higher in this group.

It is a curious fact that the cases with no instrumental disorders, and therefore less seriously affected clinically, show a shorter average survival period, and this applies both to the series as a whole and separately to the senile group and the groups with strong and average 'Alzheimerization'. It is possible that if these patients have not shown instrumental disturbances, in spite of the presence of diffuse NFC, this because they have not lived long enough to do so, and perhaps it is necessary for a certain period of time to elapse before a given density of NFC gives rise clinically to instrumental disturbances.

In conclusion, SP and NFC represent the morphological substratum of simple senile dementia, of 'Alzheimerized' senile dementia, and of Alzheimer's presenile dementia. These lesions may occur in small quantities in non-dementing elderly persons. It is their quantity and their localization that correlate with dementing disorders, and the closest anatomo-clinical correlation seems to us to be with NFC. Their presence at the level of the hippocampus is related to dysmnesia and their diffusion in the frontal and occipital neocortex is related to instrumental disturbances. These lesions have to reach a certain density and a certain period of time must elapse after their appearance, before clinical signs appear. The age of onset of the disturbances (presenile and senile) is related to the density of the lesions. Presenile cases show more severe degeneracy than senile. Presenile illnesses also progress more rapidly towards instrumental disorders. With these differences thus more sharply defined, we may, in agreement with Newton (1948), Arab (1960, Albert (1964) and Lauter and Meyer (1968) continue to accept the nosological and clinico-anatomical unity of these three forms of disorder.

Acknowledgement

This chapter was translated from the original French by Miss Helen Marshall.

References

Only references since 1960 have been given; for earlier references see C. Müller: *Alterspsychiatrie*, Georg Thieme, Stuttgart, 1967; *Manuel de gérontopsychiatrie*, Masson, Paris, 1969; *Bibliographia gerontopsychiatrica*, Huber, Bern, 1973.

Adams, R.D., Fisher, C.M., Hakim, S., Ojemann, R.G., and Sweet, W.H. (1965) 'Symptomatic occult hydrocephalus with abnormal cerebrospinal fluid pressure', *New Engl. J. Med.*, **273**, 117–126.

Ajuriaguerra, J. de, Boehme, M., Richard, J., Sinclair, H., and Tissot, R. (1967a) 'Désintégration des notions de temps dans les démences dégénératives du grand âge', *Encéphale*, **56**, 385–438.

Ajuriaguerra, J. de, Dias Cordeiro, J., Steeb, U., Fot, K., Tissot, R., and Richard, J. (1969) 'A propos de la désintégration des capacités d'anticipation des déments dégénératifs du grand âge', *Neuropsychologia*, **7**, 301–311.

Ajuriaguerra, J. de, and Gauthier, G. (1964) 'Etude de la désorganisation motrice dans un groupe de déments séniles "alzheimérisés" ', *Méd. Hyg. (Genève)*, **22**, 409–410.

Ajuriaguerra, J. de, and Kluser, J.P. (1965) 'Praxies idéatoires et permanence de l'objet.

Quelques aspects de leur désintégration conjointe dans les syndromes du grand âge', *Psychiat. Neurol. (Basel)*, **150**, 306–319.

Ajuriaguerra, J. de, Muller, M., and Tissot, R. (1960) 'A propos de quelques problèmes posés par l'apraxie dans la démence', *Rev. neurol.*, **102**, 640–642.

Ajuriaguerra, J. de, Rego, A., Richard, J., and Tissot, R. (1970a) 'Psychologie et psychométrie du vieillard', *Confront. psychiat. (Paris)*, **5**, 27–37.

Ajuriaguerra, J. de, Rego, A., Richard, J., and Tissot, R. (1967b) 'De quelques aspects des troubles de l'habillage dans des démences tardives dégénératives ou à lésions vasculaires diffuses', *Ann. méd. psychol.*, **125**, 189–218.

Ajuriaguerra, J. de, Rego, A., and Tissot, R. (1963a) 'Activités motrices stéréotypées dans les démences du grand âge', *Ann. méd. psychol.*, **121**, 641–664.

Ajuriaguerra, J. de, Rego, A., and Tissot, R. (1963b) 'Le réflexe oral et quelques activités orales dans les syndromes démentiels du grand âge. Leur signification dans la désintégration psycho-motrice', *Encéphale*, **52**, 189–219.

Ajuriaguerra, J. de, Rey-Bellet-Muller, M., and Tissot, R. (1964) 'A propos de quelques problèmes posés par le déficit opératoire de vieillards atteints de démence dégénérative en début d'évolution', *Cortex*, **1**, 232–256.

Ajuriaguerra, J. de, Steeb, U., Richard, J., and Tissot, R. (1970b) 'Processus d'induction dans les démences dégénératives du grand âge', *Encéphale*, **59**, 239–268.

Ajuriaguerra, J. de, and Tissot, R. (1966) 'Application clinique de la psychologie génétique', in *Psychologie et épistémologie génétique, thèmes Piagétiens*, Dunod, ed., Paris, pp. 333–338.

Ajuriaguerra, J. de, and Tissot, R. (1968) 'Some aspects of psycho-neurologic disintegration in senile dementia', in *Senile dementia*, (Ed. C. Muller and L. Ciompi), Berne, Huber, pp. 69–79.

Albert, E. (1964) 'Senile Demenz und Alzheimerache Krankheit als Ausdruck des gleichen Krankheitsgeschehens', *Fortschr. Neurol. Psychiat.*, **32**, 625–673.

Arab, A. (1960) 'Unité nosologique entre démence sénile et maladie d'Alzheimer d'après une étude statistique et anatomo-clinique', *Sist. nerv.*, **12**, 189–201.

Arie, T. (1973) 'Dementia in the elderly: management', *Br. Med. J.*, **4**, 602–604.

Bhasker, P.A. (1974) 'Medical management of dementia', *Antiseptic*, **71**, 45–47.

Blessed, G., Tomlinson, B.E., and Roth, M. (1968) 'The association between quantitative measures of dementia and of senile change in the cerebral grey matter of elderly subjects', *Br. J. Psychiat.*, **114**, 797–811.

Brion, S. (1966) 'Atrophies et scléroses cérébrales tardives', in *Encyclop. Méd. chir. Syst. Nerveux*, 17.056, A10.

Burnand, Y., Richard, J., Tissot, R., and Ajuriaguerra, J. de (1972) 'Nature du déficit opératoire des vieillards atteints de démence dégénérative: conservation des quantités physiques, épreuves de causalité et de transitivité, *Encéphale*, **61**, 5–31.

Collard, M. (1972) 'Etude micro-angiographique du cortex cérébral dans le syndrome de la démence sénile', *Acta Radiol. Ser. Diagn.*, **13**, 66–73.

Constantinidis, J. (1960) 'Proteines sériques dans les différentes démences de l'âge avancé', *Ann. méd. psychol.*, **118**, 129–137.

Constantinidis, J. (1962a) 'Indications fournies par différents examens sériques dans l'étude des syndromes démentiels des vieillards', *Psychiat. Neurol. (Basel)*, **144**, 193–211.

Constantinidis, J. (1962b) 'Le fer sérique et les dépôts ferreux cérébraux chez les vieillards déments', *Rev. franç. Géront.*, **8**, 267–284.

Constantinidis, J. (1965) 'L'incidence familiale des lésions cérébrales vasculaires et dégénératives de l'âge avancé', *Encéphale*, **54**, 204–239.

Constantinidis, J. (1968) 'Correlations between the age of onset of dysmnesia and the degree of cerebral degeneration', in *Senile dementia*, (Ed. C. Muller, and L. Ciompi) Bern, H. Huber, pp. 29–33.

Constantinidis, J. (1973) 'Démence présénile d'Alzheimer et démence sénile "alzheimérisée" (étude statistique des corrélations anatomo-cliniques)', *Proc. Vth World Congress Psychiatry*, Mexico 1971, Excerpta Med. (Amsterdam), *Intern. Congr. Series*, **274**, pp. 831–838.

Constantinidis, J. and Ajuriaguerra, J. de (1965) 'L'incidence familiale des plaques séniles', *Confin. psychiat. (Basel)*, **8**, 130–137.

Constantinidis, J. and Ajuriaguerra, J. de (1968) 'Les altérations cérébrales au cours du vieillissement', *Acta neurol. psychiat. hellen.*, **7**, 79–115.

Constantinidis, J., Garrone, G., Tissot, R., and Ajuriaguerra, J. de (1965a) 'L'incidence familiale des altérations neurofibrillaires corticales d'Alzheimer', *Psychiat. Neurol. (Basel)*, **150**, 235–247.

Constantinidis, J., Garrone, G., and Wildi, E. (1962) 'Relations entre les lésions cérébrales dégénératives séniles et l'élimination urinaire des hormones stéroïdes', *Schweiz. Arch. Neurol. Psychiat.*, **89**, 384–413.

Constantinidis, J., Krassoievitch, M., and Tissot, R. (1969) 'Corrélations entre les perturbations électro-encéphalographiques et les lésions anatomo-histologiques dans les démences', *Encéphale*, **58**, 19–52.

Constantinidis, J., Richard, J., and Ajuriaguerra, J. de (1965b) 'L'incidence familiale de l'angiopathie dyshorique du cortex cérébral', *Internat. J. Neuropsychiat. (Chic.)*, **1**, 118–124.

Constantinidis, J., Richard, J., and Tissot, R. (1974) 'Pick's disease. Histological and clinical correlations', *Europ. Neurol.*, **11**, 208–217.

Constantinidis, J., Tissot, R., Richard, J., and Ajuriaguerra, J. de (1972) 'Le rôle de l'hérédité dans le développement de la démence présénile d'Alzheimer et de la démence sénile "alzheimérisée"', in *Dimensiones de la paiquiatria contemporanea*, (Ed. C. P. de Francesco), Pren. méd. mex. (Mexico), p. 328–339.

Cornu, F. (1974) *Comportements des déments dégénératifs vis-à-vis de la douleur et asymbolie à la douleur*, Thesis (Med.), Geneva, No. 3391.

Crapper, D.R. (1973) 'Experimental neurofibrillary degeneration and altered electrical activity', *Electroenceph. clin. Neurophysiol.*, **35**, 575–588.

Crapper, D.R., Krishnan, S.S., and Dalton, A.J. (1973) 'Brain aluminium distribution in Alzheimer's disease and experimental neurofibrillary degeneration', *Science*, **180**, 511–513.

Dago-Akribi, A. (1969) 'Etude anatomo-pathologique et statistique des altérations cérébrales de la sénescence physiologique', *Encéphale*, **6**, 539–577.

Dayan, A.D. (1970a) 'Quantitative histological studies on the aged human brain. I. Senile plaques and neurofibrillary tangles in "normal" patients', *Acta neuropath. (Berl.)*, **16**, 85–94.

Dayan, A.D. (1970b) 'Quantitative histological studies on the aged human brain. II. Senile plaques and neurofibrillary tangles in senile dementia', *Acta neuropath. (Berl.)*, **16**, 95–102.

Dejaiffe, G., Constantinidis, J., Rey-Bellet, J., and Tissot, R. (1964) 'Corrélations électro-cliniques dans les démences de l'âge avancé', *Acta neurol. belg.*, **64**, 677–707.

Delay, J., and Brion, S. (1962) *Les démences tardives*, Masson, Paris.

Duheille, J., Cuny, G., Penin, F., and Peroz, F. (1973) 'Anticorps antitissu nerveux dans les démences séniles', *Ann. Med. Nancy*, **12**, 441–442.

Dusheiko, S.D. (1972) 'Senile plaques and Alzheimer changes in the neurofibrillae in mental patients dying at an advanced age', *Zh. Nevropat. Psikhiat.*, **72**, 1029–1033.

Duval, F. (1966) *Désintégration du langage au cours des démences séniles dégénératives. Ses rapports avec les données de l'acquisition chez l'enfant*, Thesis (Med), Paris.

Ferm, L. (1974) 'Behavioural activities in demented geriatric patients', *Geront. clin.* (Basel), **16**, 185–194.

Fot, K. Richard, J., Tissot, R., and Ajuriaguerra, J. de (1970) 'Le phénomène de l'extinction dans la double stimulation tactile de la face et de la main chez les déments dégénératifs du grand âge', *Neuropsychologia*, **8**, 493–500.

Gaillard, J.-M. (1970) 'Désintégration du schéma corporel dans les états démentiels du grand âge', *J. Psychol. norm. path.*, **67**, 443–472.

Gainotti, G. (1970) 'Deterioramento intellettivo e desintegraziōne psico-motrice nelle demenze', *Acta neurol., Napoli*, **25**, 607–627.

Gontas, N.K., Gambetti, P. (1970) 'The pathology of the synapse in Alzheimer's disease', in *Alzheimer's disease*, London, Churchill, p. 169.

Guilleminault, C. (1968) *Désintégration de la perception stéréognosique dans les démences dégénératives du grand âge*, Thesis, Paris.

Gustafson, L., and Risberg, J. (1974) 'Regional cerebral blood flow related to psychiatric symptoms in dementia with onset in the presenile period', *Acta psychiat. scand.*, **50**, 516–538.

Hirano, A. (1970) 'Neurofibrillary changes in conditions related to Alzheimer's disease', in *Alzheimer's disease*, London, Churchill, pp. 185–207.

Hirano, A., Dembitzer, H.M., Kurland, L.T., and Zimmerman, H.M. (1968) *The fine structure of some intraganglionic alterations'*, *J. Neuropath. exp. Neurol.*, **27**, 167–182.

Irving, G., Robinson, R.A., McAdam, W. (1970) 'The validity of some cognitive tests in the diagnosis of dementia', *Br. J. Psychiat.*, **117**, 149–156.

Jonsson, C.O., Waldton, S., and Malhammar, G. (1972) 'The psychiatric symptomatology in senile dementia assessed by means of an interview', *Acta psychiat. scand.*, **48**, 103–121.

Kidd, M. (1963) 'Paired helical filaments in electron microscopy of Alzheimer's disease', *Nature*, **197**, 192–193.

Kidd, M. (1964) 'Alzheimer's disease. An electron microscopic study', *Brain*, **87**, 307–320.

Lampert, P. (1971) 'Fine structural changes of neurites in Alzheimer's disease', *Acta neuropath. (Berl.)*, suppl. 5, 49–53.

Lauter, H., and Meyer, J.E. (1968) 'Clinical and nosological concepts of senile dementia', in *Senile dementia*, (Ed. C. Müller and L. Ciompi.) Berne, H. Huber, pp. 13–27.

Levy, R., Isaacs, A., and Behrman, J. (1971) 'Neurophysiological correlates of senile dementia. II. The somatosensory evoked response', *Psychol. Med.*, **1**, 159–165.

Levy, R., Isaacs, A., and Hawks, G. (1970) 'Neurophysiological correlates of senile dementia. I. Motor and sensory nerve conduction velocity', *Psychol. Med.*, **1**, 40–47.

Luke, A.S. (1973) 'L'étude des interactions sociales chez les déments du grand âge', *Ann. méd. psychol.*, **131**, 349–385.

Malamud, N. (1965) 'A comparative study of the neuropathologic findings in senile psychoses and in "normal" senility', *J. Am. Geriat. Soc.*, **13**, 113–117.

Mark, J., and Brun, A. (1973) 'Chromosomal deviations in Alzheimer's disease compared to those in senescence and senile dementia', *Geront. Clin. (Basel)*, **15**, 253–258.

Matsuyama, H., Namiki, H., and Watanabe, S. (1965) 'Senile changes in the brain in the Japanese' in *Proc. Vth Internat. Congr. Neuropath.*, Amsterdam, Excerpta Med. Found., pp. 979–980.

Miller, E. (1971) 'On the nature of the memory disorder in presenile dementia', *Neuropsychologia*, **9**, 75–81.

Miyakawa, T., Sumiyoshi, S., Murayama, E., and Deshimaru, M. (1974) 'Ultrastructure of capillary plaque-like degeneration in senile dementia. Mechanism of amyloid production', *Acta neuropath. (Berl.)*, **29**, 229–236.

Müller, M. (1961) 'Apport de certaines épreuves psychologiques à l'étude de la désintégration sénile', *Méd. Hyg.*, **19**, 502.

Nielson, J. (1968) 'Chromosomes in senile dementia', *Br. J. Psychiat.*, **114**, 303–309.

Nikaido, T., Austin, J., Rinehart, T., Trueb, L., Hutchinson, J., Stukenbrok, H., and Miles, B. (1971) 'Studies in ageing of the brain. I. Isolation and preliminary characterization of Alzheimer plaques and cores', *Arch. Neurol (Chic.)*, **25**, 198–211.

Nikaido, T., Austin, J., Trueb, L., and Rinehart, R. (1972) 'Studies in ageing of the brain. II. Microchemical analyses of the nervous system in Alzheimer patients', *Arch. Neurol. (Chic.)*, **27**, 549–554.

Obrist, W.D., Chivan, E., Cronqvist, S., and Ingvar, D.N. (1970) 'Regional cerebral blood flow in senile and presenile dementia', *Neurology (Minneap.)*, **20**, 315–322.

Paulson, G., and Gottlieb, G. (1968) 'Development reflexes: the reappearance of foetal and neo-natal reflexes in aged patients', *Brain*, **91**, 37–52.

Pratt, R.T.C. (1970) 'The genetics of Alzheimer's disease', in *Alzheimer's disease*, London, Churchill, pp. 137–143.

Richard, J. (1964) 'De quelques aspects de la désintégration des fonctions supérieures du système nerveux central dans les démences tardives', *Med. Hyg. (Genève)*, **22**, 411–412.

Richard, J. (1968) 'On institutional therapy and the integration of intra and extra-hospital rehabilitation', in *Senile dementia*, Ed. C. Muller, and L. Ciompi, Berne, H Huber, pp. 145–149.

Richard, J. (1970) 'A propos de problèmes institutionnels hospitaliers en gériatrie', *Fortbildungskurse schweiz. Ges. Psych.*, **3**, 76–88.

Richard, J. (1971) 'Démences séniles et comportements', *Fortbildungskurse schweiz, Ges. Psych.*, **4**, 85–100.

Richard, J. (1974) 'Neuro-psychologie et gériatrie', *Med. Hyg. (Genève)*, **32**, 1189–1193.

Richard, J. (1975) 'De l'application et de l'intérêt des méthodes de la psychologie génétique en gériatrie avec un exemple sur la désintégration de la stéréognosie dans les démences dégénératives du grand âge', *Psychol. Med.*, **7**, 9.

Richard, J., and Constantinidis, J. (1970) 'Les démences de la vieillesse', *Confront. psychiat.*, **5**, 39–61.

Richard, J., and Constantinidis, J. (1975) 'Les démences organiques de l'adulte', in *Pathologie médicale*, (Ed. H. Pequignot,) Paris, Masson, pp. 1354–1369.

Richard, J., and De Bus, P. (1973) 'Principi generali d'organizzazione dell'assistenza psichiatrica in geriatria', in *Gerontologia e Geriatria* Vol 1, (Ed. F.M. Antonini, and C. Funagalli, Milan, Wassermann, pp. 437–455.

Richard, J., Eisenring, J.-J., and Feder, M. (1970) 'L'application des techniques de mobilisation en gériatrie intra-hospitalière', *Méd. Hyg. (Genève)*, **28**, 1719–1723.

Richard, J., and Tissot, R. (1974) 'Mémoire et intelligence dans les syndromes démentials dégénératifs de l'âge avancé', *Rev. Méd. Dijon*, **9**, 475–479.

Roth, M., Tomlinson, B.E., and Blessed, G. (1966) 'Correlation between scores for dementia and counts of "senile plaques" in cerebral grey matter of elderly subjects', *Nature* **209**, 109–110.

Rotin, L.Y. (1972) 'Examination of the activity of certain hydrolytic enzymes in the so-called Alzheimer's change of neurofibrillae', *Byull. éksp. Biol. Med.*, **74**, 110–113.

Savage, R.D. and Bolton, M. (1968) 'A factor analysis of learning impairment and intellectual deterioration in the elderly', *J. genet. Psychol.*, **113**, 177–182.

Schlote, W. (1965) 'Die Amyloidnatur der kongophilen, drüsigen Entartung der Hirnarterien (Scholz) im Senium', *Acta neuropath. (Berl.)*, **4**, 449–468.

Seitelberger, F. (1969) 'Neurology and pathology of non vascular cerebral processes of ageing', *Wien. Klin. Wachr.*, **81**, 509–516.

Shelanski, M.L., and Taylor, E.W. (1970) 'Biochemistry of neurofilaments and neuro-tubules', in *Alzheimer's disease*, London, Churchill. pp. 249–266.

Sim, M. Turner, E., and Smith, W.T. (1966) 'Cerebral biopsy in the investigation of presenile dementia', *Br. J. Psychiat.*, **112**, 119–125.

Suzuki, K., and Terry, R.D. (1967) 'Fine structural localization of acid phosphatase in senile plaques in Alzheimer's presenile dementia. *Acta neuropath. (Berl.)*, **8**, 276–284.

Terry, R.D. (1963) 'The fine structure of neurofibrillary tangles in Alzheimer's disease', *J. Neuropat. exp. Neurol.*, **22**, 629–642.

Tissot, R. (1973) 'Démences et mémoire', *Encéphale*, **62**, 491–505.

Tissot, R., Constantinidis, J., and Richard, J. (1975) *La maladie de Pick*, Vol.1, Paris, Masson, pp. 1–122.

Tissot, R., Joannides, A., Richard, J., and Ajuriaguerra, J. de (1972) 'Activités perceptives visuelles dans les démences dégénératives du grand âge', *Rev. oto-neuro-ophtal.*, **44**, 205–212.

Tissot, R., Richard, J., Duval, F., and Ajuriaguerra, J. de (1967) 'Quelques aspects du langage des démences dégénératives du grand âge', *Acta neurol. belg.*, **67**, 911–923.

Todorov, A.B., GO, R.C.P., Constantinidis, J., and Elston, R.C. (1975) 'Specificity of the clinical diagnosis of dementia', *J. Neurol. Sci.*, **26**, 81–98.

Tomlinson, B.E., Blessed, G., and Roth, M. (1968) 'Observations on the brains of non-demented old people', *J. Neurol. Sci.*, **7**, 331–356.

Tomlinson, B.E., Blessed, G., and Roth, M. (1970) 'Observations on the brains of demented old people', *J. Neurol. Sci.*, **11**, 205–242.

Tomlinson, B.E., and Kitchener, D. (1972) 'Granulovacuolar degeneration of hippocampal pyramidal cells', *J. Path. Bact.*, **106**, 165–185.

Vernea, J. (1973) 'Pathological reflexes in presenile dementia', *Proc. Austr. Ass. Neurol.*, **9**, 105–109.

Wang, H.S. (1975) 'Somato-psycho-social view of senile dementia—a positive approach', *Proc. 10th Internat. Congress of Gerontology*, Jerusalem, Israel.

Wildi, E., and Dago-Akribi, A. (1968) 'Altérations cérébrales chez l'homme âgé', *Bull. schweiz. Akad. med. Wiss.*, **24**, 107–132.

Wildi, E., Linder, A., and Costoulas, G. (1964) 'Etude statistique des altérations dégénératives cérébrales apparaissant au cours de vieillissement', *Psychiat. Neurol. (Basel)*, **148**, 41–68.

Wildi, E., Linder, A., and Costoulas, G. (1967) 'Schizophrénie et involution cérébrale sénile', *Psychiat, Neurol, (Basel)*, **154**, 1–26.

Wisniewski, H.M., and Terry, R.D. (1973) 'Re-examination of the pathogenesis of the senile plaque', in *Progress in neuropathology* Vol.2 (Ed. H.M. Zimmerman) New York, Grune and Stratton, 1–26.

7

THE CLINICAL PSYCHOLOGIST'S ROLE IN ASSESSMENT AND MANAGEMENT

A. Whitehead

Introduction

The practice of clinical psychology with the elderly is considered something of a speciality. In part this is related to the elderly manifesting pathological processes that are somewhat different from those seen in earlier life; but probably of greater importance is the development that occurs with normal ageing. The older individual differs in terms of level of functioning, attitudes, and lifestyle from the younger; and in the assessment, treatment, and rehabilitation of elderly patient, it is necessary to take this into account. These changes do, of course, develop throughout life; with the possible exception of retirement, there is no one stepwise change that occurs at the start of, or during, the senium. However, it is during old age that these changes become sufficiently notable and widespread, that account must be taken of them and a person considered by comparison with the normal functioning and expectancies of his age peers. Some individuals, at their best, may be barely coping with the complexities of living and any process that diminishes functional capacity, by however little, may be sufficient to produce a gross collapse, a much less likely occurrence in a younger person with more in reserve.

This chapter is concerned with both assessment and management but it is on the former that the majority of the interest and research has been focused, as will be witnessed by the proportion of the chapter devoted to it. It will be clear also that the emphasis has been on the consideration of the deficits and disabilities of these patients; little attention has been paid to the possibilities of assessing a patient's strengths and relating these to the success of a positive programme of rehabilitation. It seems that clinical psychologists have tended to share a general pessimism that if disorders of the elderly failed to respond to physical treatments, there was nothing to be done—a counsel of despair that has tended to dissipate with increased involvement and the movement way from solely hospital-based services.

A final point that should be made is that this chapter will concentrate on those aspects of clinical practice with the elderly that are specific to that age group. In the practical situation, problems and techniques will frequently be the same as those encountered with younger adults and within the constraints of allowing for the different functional level of the older patient, they will be dealt with in the same way. It is intended here, however, to consider only areas specific to psychogeriatrics.

Psychometric evaluation

It has long been considered that psychometrics have an essential role to play in the assessment of the elderly psychiatric patient. Some of the reasons for this are easily apparent; such individuals frequently demonstrate measurable impairments and some of the disorders of the senium are actually characterized by diminished levels of functioning. Not surprisingly the focus of interest in both research and clinical practice has been on cognitive functioning, especially general intellectual ability, learning, and memory function—and in view of this it is intended to concentrate the present consideration to these areas.

Three research strategies have been adopted. These attempt to relate level of functioning to:

(a) Membership of some group, defined clinically, usually by diagnosis;
(b) Outcome;
(c) Changes over time.

Each of these research areas will be considered, together with their practical applications to differential diagnosis, prognosis, and the assessment of treatment effects. Unless stated otherwise, in all the reported work the subjects will have been elderly, normally over the age of 60 or 65.

Studies of clinically defined groups

Four questions can be considered:

(a) To what extent do members of specific clinical groups give evidence of impairment?
(b) Are the impairments general or are they specific to certain types of task?
(c) Do similar impairments exist in all members of the clinical group?
(d) What differences occur between different clinical groups?

In a series of studies, Savage and his colleagues (summarized by Savage *et al.*, 1973) have looked at the structure of cognitive functioning in elderly people and attempted to assess the effects of ageing and pathology. Their sample has consisted of both normal community residents and hospitalized psychotics carrying diagnoses of schizophrenia, affective psychosis, or organic psychosis. Savage and Bolton (1968) subjected scores from the Wechsler adult intelligence scale (WAIS) and two verbal learning tests, the Modified new word learning test (MWLT) and the Inglis paired associates learning test (PALT) to principal components analysis. They found four independent factors and came to the conclusion that age and diagnosis were affecting different areas of functioning. Changes in general intellectual level and in verbal performance discrepancy appeared to be related more notably to ageing than to diagnosis while the reverse was true for intellectual deterioration and verbal learning impairment.

Intellectual deterioration implies more than just differences between individuals in general level of functioning. There is evidence that, where there has been a decline from a previously higher level of function, some types of task will show a greater performance decrement than others; in particular, tasks involving much old 'crystallized' ability, such as vocabulary knowledge, will be little affected while those needing a new problem-solving approach, 'fluid' ability, will show more effect. Deterioration is thus measurable by indices taking into account differential level of performance on various types of task and several such measures have been developed that may be derived from the WAIS. Bolton *et al.* (1966) extracted some of these indices for the sample already mentioned and found some differences between subgroups but there was a great deal of overlap. For example, for the WAIS deterioration quotient, scores in the 'organic' range were obtained by seven per cent of normals, 23 per cent of functional psychotics and 52 per cent of organics.

These results suggest that there are similarities in the impairments shown on the WAIS by various types of patient. Whitehead (1973a) looked at whether this was explicable in terms of total subtest pattern. She tested depressives and dements on the WAIS and found that, although the dementing patients scored at a lower level over all, there was no difference in the pattern of subtest scores; both groups tended to have better or worse scores on the same subtests. Although age-corrected subtest scores were used in the analysis and so ageing decline was not of itself responsible for the similarities in the pattern of impairment, nevertheless it was on those subtests known to be most affected by ageing that the two groups of subjects performed least well.

Both these studies are consistent with a rather general tendency towards intellectual deterioration; similar tasks show impairments whatever the process involved in causing the decline. Material mainly involving the use of 'crystallized' ability is little affected by ageing or by pathological processes but where 'fluid' ability is required, impairments will be noted.

In the study of Savage and Bolton (1968), the other component of diagnostic importance was that relating to verbal learning. This is hardly surprising since memory difficulties are so notable an accompaniment of the dementing processes. There is no dearth of experimental investigation of the nature of the impairment involved, in both ageing and dementia.

In the Savage and Bolton study, although verbal learning could be established as an independent factor, scores on the learning tasks also loaded on the general intelligence factor; and this relationship between learning scores and intelligence has been generally found. Thus in making comparisons between groups, it is normally thought worthwhile to ensure that differences in performance are specific to the learning or memory task and not merely a function of differences in general intellectual level, and this is best done by equating groups. This does, however, raise problems with dementing subjects for whom some lowering of intellectual level is likely to have occurred. The solution normally adopted is to use measures that will be relatively unaffected by deterioration, such as verbal IQ or an estimate of vocabulary knowledge and all comparative studies to be reported here will have some such control. This does have the effect that these investigations deal mainly with individuals in an early stage of dementia, which may not give an adequate picture of what happens later in the process. However, in the early stages, differences in specific functions may well be more easily demonstrable.

Ageing does of itself produce substantial changes in the acquisition and retention of complex material. A full consideration is not possible here (for a review, see Botwinick, 1970). In brief, the evidence suggests that there is little decline in the span of immediate recall, usually estimated by the digit span, nor for the long term retention of fully acquired material. On most other tasks, such as the familiar rote learning tests, ageing deficits are demonstrable; but it has been shown that the type of material involved in the task determines the extent of the ageing deficit. Older subjects are comparatively less impaired with familiar, meaningful, high association material and with self paced learning.

In clinical practice, the focus of interest has been on dementia or clinical memory disorder, a term suggested by Inglis (1957) to avoid problems associated with the use of the diagnostic term (a fuller consideration of this difficulty will be made in a later section). There is ample evidence that such patients show considerable deficits on rote learning tasks by comparison with functional patients or normal controls (e.g. Kendrick and Post, 1967). Studies designed to elucidate the nature of the difficulty have found that, on most testable aspects, deficits may be seen, a notable exception being that, as with normal ageing, deficits are not found in the span of immediate recall (e.g. Whitehead, 1973b).

The dichotic digits technique is a way of comparing the accuracy of immediate and slightly delayed recall of digits; different series of digits are played simultaneously through earphones to the two ears (e.g. 5,7,1 to the right and 4,3,6 to the left). Typically a subject reports the whole of one message before starting the other, which is thus delayed slightly. With this method, Inglis (1960) found that only for the delayed message were memory disordered patients worse than controls. Long term retention has been studied by Newcombe and Steinberg (1964) who showed greater forgetting of narrative texts over periods of up to 28 days by dementing than by functional patients. Unfortunately, the dements performed at a lower level even on immediate testing and this may have affected the long term retention, since it has been shown that with normal ageing, long term retention is impaired for partially but not for fully acquired material (Hulicka and Weiss, 1965).

Retrieval processes have been studied and the results suggest that faulty retrieval could not be a sufficient explanation for the deficits found, since the use of a recognition format does not eliminate the defects of dementing or memory disordered subjects (Inglis, 1957; Whitehead, 1973b).

Ease of association has been found to be an important variable in determining the extent of the deficit of ageing individuals. For memory disordered subjects, Inglis (1959a) found no impairment on a task involving high association material; but this result may have been an artefact of the material being too easy since performance of both groups was near perfect. There have been a few studies involving non-verbal material. Whitehead (1975) demonstrated that dements showed similar deficits for recognition memory of complex pictorial material as for familiar words. Perceptuomotor learning has been shown to be impaired in dements compared with depressives (Crookes and McDonald, 1972) and in organics compared with functional psychotics (Savage *et al.*, 1973). Neither of these two last studies is fully comparable with those considered earlier since in the first only a proportion of the subjects were elderly and in the second the groups were not matched for verbal intelligence, but the experimenters were able to demonstrate that no correlation existed between performance and intellectual level.

Thus, for patients with early dementia, the picture is one of fairly general impairment on tasks involving learning or memory ability, with only the span of immediate recall remaining intact. Differences between individuals have not been widely studied, but it will be seen in a later section, that as dementia progresses levels of performance will tend to decline; but nothing is known about changing patterns of deficit.

For depressives, the picture is more complex. Deficits are demonstrable on some rote learning tasks; for the Synonym learning test (SLT), 16 per cent of a sample of depressed patients gained scores in the same range as dementing subjects (Kendrick *et al.*, 1965); yet no normal elderly subject performed at such a low level (Kendrick and Post, 1967).

As with dementia, attempts have been made to specify the deficits of the depressive subjects. Comparing ill and recovered patients, Whitehead (1973b) could find no deficits for digit span; recognition of verbal material; or immediate or delayed (half-hour) recall of a narrative text. For rote learning tasks, impairments were demonstrable for the SLT and on a serial learning task involving familiar words; on the other hand, there was no evidence of deficit on two tasks based on the Inglis PALT, using either the standard 'hard' low association pairs or on the 'mediate' pairs (Inglis, 1959a). Similar results had been found for rote learning tasks by Irving *et al.* (1970); their functional sample, most of whom were depressives, scored at a similar level to normals on the PALT and on a high association 'name learning test'; on the SLT, although no direct comparison was made with the normal sample, there was evidence of impairment in the functional patients. The defective performance of the ill depressives on the SLT was not merely a result of refusal to complete the test, since it was demonstrable over fewer trials or where scores from those who refused to complete were excluded.

In view of the lesser deficit found in normal ageing subjects when material is familar and unpaced, Whitehead (1974) looked at the effects of altering these two variables. Only familiarity was successfully manipulated using the criterion of over-all changes in level of performance but no differential effects was found; the depressive deficit was no less with familiar than with unfamiliar material.

Thus, the evidence to date suggests that the deficit of elderly depressives is confined to certain types of rote learning task. The exact parameters of material on which defective performance will be demonstrable have not been determined but it has been suggested that it may be where large quantities of low association material are involved (Whitehead, 1974).

Given that deficits are demonstrable for groups of depressives, are all such patients similarly impaired? Post (1966) reviewed some of the clinical features of those depressives who gained scores on the SLT in the 'organic' range and showed that such patients tended to be female, to have low verbal intelligence, to suffer from severe especially delusional depression and to have a poor knowledge of general events. With serial learning tasks, Whitehead (1974) found that patients with low vocabulary scores gained lower learning scores but this was true for both ill and for recovered depressives; the less intelligent subjects showed no increased tendency to impaired learning function while ill. This result is not discrepant with that of Post, since he was looking at those scoring below a cut-off point; less intelligent subjects would be closer to that level and would therefore be more likely to descend below it while ill. Whitehead found supportive evidence that degree of deficit was related to the severity of depressed mood.

These results are, then, consistent with a position that all elderly depressives are prone to exhibit impairments in their performance on certain rote learning tasks, the degree of decline being related to the severity of the depressive disorder. Those of lower intelligence, starting from a lower level, are more likely to function psychometrically and possibly also clinically in a way similar to dements.

Over all, it appears that the deficit shown in depression is both less severe and more circumscribed than that shown in dementia. There has been some interest in the pattern of impairment of the two groups. Whitehead (1973b) failed to demonstrate differential deficits in rote learning tasks but found that there were notable differences between the two groups in the type of error made. On the serial

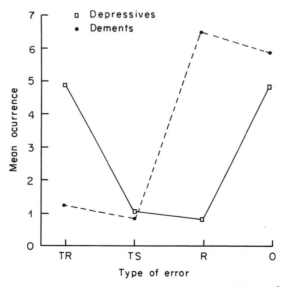

FIGURE 7.1. Comparison of errors made by depressives on Inglis hard and dements on Inglis mediate (TR and TS are transposition errors of response and stimulus words respectively; R are random errors; and O are omission errors). Reproduced by permission of the editor, *British Journal of Psychiatry*, from *idem*, **123,** 207

learning task, it was noted that, compared with depressives, dementing patients made a larger number of both omission and random errors (words irrelevant to the task) but a smaller number of transposition errors (words relevant to the task but misplaced within it). Similarly, on a recognition task, no difference occured for the number of false negative responses (failing to respons to a word previously seen) but the dements made substantially more false positive responses (responding affirmatively to a word not previously seen).

There was a possibility that these differences were not indicative of different types of learning disorder but merely reflected the greater difficulty experienced by the dements with the material to be learned. This could be tested by holding difficulty ✻ level constant—comparing the performance of depressive patients on the Inglis hard pairs with that of the dements on the Inglis mediate pairs, a tactic which approximately equalized the total number of errors made. The pattern of errors may be seen in Figure 7.1 There is a significant tendency for the dementing subjects to make an excessive number of random errors and for the depressives to make more transposition errors.

In summary, the results do not paint an entirely consistent picture, but for both general intellectual performance and for learning and memory ability, the deficits of dementing subjects seem to be both more severe and more diffuse than for functional patients. Depressives also show impairments that, although less marked and possibly less widespread than those found in dements, nevertheless have much in common in terms of performance on standard tests. More research is obviously required to determine the extent to which the two groups differ in their pattern of impairment but the types of error made is suggestive of some differences in the processes responsible for the deficits.

Differential diagnosis

Since the most frequently required discrimination in clinical practice is that between dementia and functional conditions, any of the tasks upon which differences in performance have been found would be of potential value in the assessment of the individual patient. However, it is necessary first to establish that the level of discrimination is at a sufficiently high level to justify its use. Ideally such validation would be against a definitive biological demonstration of diffuse brain changes but, since this is not practical, the normal method involves the extent of agreement with psychiatric diagnosis which itself is made to a large extent on the basis of observed intellectual and behavioural deficits. As clinician and psychometrician are using similar criteria to establish diagnosis, there is the danger of apparent close agreement depending not so much on each attaining accurate diagnosis but rather agreeing on the extent of the cognitive disorder. This problem has been called 'criterion contamination' by Shapiro *et al.* (1956) who demonstrated that several tasks involving learning and memory function were good diagnostic discriminators, provided that the clincian made his diagnosis in the normal fashion. If instead, he had to diagnose using only information not pertaining to cognitive function, then these tasks no longer discriminated between the groups.

To insist that the clinician make an essentially inefficient diagnosis has its obvious disadvantages and Inglis (1957) has suggested that, instead of using the diagnosis of dementia, the operational description of memory disorder is of heuristic value. Yet this approach offers no solution to the differentiation of the mild impairments which, if occurring in early dementia must be supposed irreversible and progressive but if in depression to carry a more hopeful prognosis. The stability of diagnosis over time is itself a way of reducing 'criterion contamination' classification of such patients.

The diffuse nature of deterioration in intellectual performance has ensured that this type of function has been of little practical use in the development of diagnostic tools. Most of those of demonstrated validity have been based on verbal learning tests; and the MWLT, SLT, and Inglis PALT have all been shown to discriminate at a high level between dementing and functional patients.

Kendrick and his colleagues (Kendrick, 1965) have developed a battery designed to discriminate between elderly depressives and dements of similar vocabulary level. It contains tasks assessing not only verbal learning ability (the SLT and PALT) but also psychomotor speed (Digit copying test (DCT) and the WAIS Digit symbol subtest). On all these tasks, dementing subjects perform at a lower mean level than depressives; but the battery is designed also to take into account the pattern of performance. A further feature is the validation of a six weeks test–retest sequence based on the SLT and DCT.

The original standardization yielded very high levels of discrimination—94 per cent correct at initial testing which increased to 97 per cent on retest.

In a later study (Kendrick, 1967), a more realistic and difficult discrimination was attempted. A sample of depressives was chosen that contained a high proportion of individuals characterized by 'pseudodementia' and an attempt made to differentiate these from dementing patients. Slight alternations had to be made to the earlier cut-off points; but the results were promising in that for this very difficult discrimination, 93 per cent could be correctly identified.

Kendrick adds the rider that the battery is not suitable for those of low vocabulary level. This was confirmed by Whitehead (1971) who showed that of those with IQ equivalent over 95, two-thirds of depressives were correctly assigned but of those below this level, only one-third were. Following a reanalysis of part of his data, Kendrick (1972) has suggested that the battery might be modified to improve discrimination for those of lower ability; but it is likely that different and simpler tasks, such as the Inglis mediate pairs would be more appropriate for use with duller subjects for whom the SLT in particular tends to be extremely difficult.

No study has yet attempted to look systematically at the relative efficiency of diagnostic tools. There would be especial interest in comparing the relative effectiveness of the clinical psychologists' tests and psychiatrists' objective but less formal screening tasks, such as the clinical sensorium of Post (1965). It is clear that as the assessment made by the psychiatrist increases in sophistication, in order to provide useful additional information, that of the clinical psychologist might also have to change.

In summary, there is evidence that psychometric evaluation can aid differential diagnosis, even in the realistically difficult discrimination between early dementia and depressive 'pseudodementia'. As yet, though, these methods appear less adequate for patients of lower verbal intelligence.

Prediction of outcome

Much of the interest in psychometric evaluation has been directed towards the recognition of dementing processes; and one of the major reasons for requiring the differential diagnosis is its implications for prognosis. Yet Payne (1958) has pointed out that a test can be a very efficient diagnostic tool; and a diagnosis can be highly correlated with outcome without test performance necessarily being of prognostic significance. A practical demonstration of this was provided by results of Inglis *et al.* (1960) who found that scores on a simple perceptual task, although giving very good diagnostic discrimination between functional and organic diagnoses, failed to adequately predict two year outcome in terms of death of degree of invalidism; although clinical diagnosis was related to outcome.

Rather more successful levels of prediction have been found with verbal learning tasks. Walton (1958) showed that MWLT scores were predictive of changes in diagnosis despite the clinician having no access to the results; Inglis (1959b) suggested that these changes of diagnosis were indicative of outcome not fulfilling earlier expectancy. Sanderson and Inglis (1961) showed that poor performance on the MWLT and Inglis PALT could significantly predict dying within 16 months; diagnosis was marginally less efficient.

Whitehead (1976) has attempted to predict the one year outcome of a series of consecutive admissions to psychiatric beds and has found that unfavourable outcome (i.e. dying or a heavy reliance on the hospital based services) was capable of significant prediction by clinical and psychometric measures. Some of the relevant psychological tasks were those measuring learning and memory function, but others were estimates of intellectual level. Principal component analysis of the data showed that almost all the successful predictor variables loaded on one general factor, a result which suggests that outcome may be related to rather generalized and non-specific decline of level of functioning.

The findings of Savage *et al.* (1973) are also consistent with this. They showed that, of their total sample, subjects who failed to survive for six and a half years functioned at a generally lower level on initial testing, even when age differences had been taken into account. This was not merely a result of the impaired organic patients showing poor survival since it was demonstrable even for the normal subjects taken on their own, but not at a significant level for the functional psychotics.

Relatively little has been done in assessing the practical value of assessment in prediction of outcome but some results of Whitehead (1976) are suggestive that unfavourable outcome at one year can be predicted with an accuracy higher than base rates. This raises the possibility that accuracy of prognosis may, like diagnosis, be increased by the use of psychometric tools.

Changes over time

In order to assess the effects of increasing age and of psychoses on the intellectual functioning of the elderly, Savage *et al.* (1973) have followed their sample for six and a half years during which time they have been tested on four occasions. To prevent distortion of the data by selective attrition of subjects, they considered only the results from those subjects who survived the full period. As only one dementing subject was alive even at the second testing (i.e., after three years), developmental data were not obtained for that clinical subsample. The other results are, however, of some interest. For the normal community residents, there was a significant tendency for decreased scores on the verbal subtests of the WAIS and for increased scores on the performance subtests. The changes in the psychotic subjects were less marked, but increases in performance scores were demonstrable in the affective group while decreases in the verbal scores could be shown for the schizophrenics. The reasons for the pattern of change are undoubtedly complex and apart from differential practice effects, Savage *et al.* suggest that their results might be related to the highly selected nature of a group of very elderly subjects who survive for six and a half years. A full discussion may be found in their book.

These workers looked also at performance on the MWLT and a perceptuomotor learning test on two occasions with an interval of 18 months and found little evidence of change for normals or for psychotics.

The present author has, as yet, unpublished data from patients who had been tested soon after admission and were re-tested after one year. In order to be available for re-test, the patient had to be attending hospital as an in- or a day-patient and so the group contained a high proportion of patients with longer term difficulties; about one-third were considered to be suffering from chronic brain syndrome. Scores were obtained on a variety of tasks including WAIS vocabulary, digits forwards, and verbal learning tests. The most notable result was of the stability of scores over time. For none of the measures was there evidence of shift in the mean score and the correlations of scores across the two occasions of testing were high, ranging from 0·54 to 0·84.

For this mixed clinical group, there was thus stability of scores over time. However, a small group of patients could be selected to give information about changes occurring in dementing processes. These patients were of unequivocal diagnosis of chronic brain syndrome at the end of one year and on neither occasion of testing had any other disorder, such as acute brain syndrome, likely to affect their scores. For these patients, there was a significant decline in mean scores on each of the tasks considered. Thus, for this carefully selected clinical group, there was evidence of progressive decline in tasks relying on intellectual ability or learning and memory function.

The most probable practical application of results such as these is in the assessment of the individual patient, examining the differences between his expected and attained level of functioning and relating this to changes in his clinical condition.

For general evaluation of the effects of specific treatments on cognitive functioning, it would of course, be necessary to employ a control group. The problem is then one of adequate measurement—choosing tasks on which relevant deficits should be apparent; of an appropriate difficulty level that scores will be free to move in either direction; and of sufficient reliability that changes will be demonstrable. Especially for treatments purporting to improve the functioning of dementing subjects, a psychometric evaluation is likely to add considerably to the assessment of the patients.

General overview

This review has covered material related to diagnosis, prognosis and changes over time; and not all the findings appear consistent. In particular, there is evidence that general intellectual impairment might be as adequate a prognostic indicator as learning impairment, a result difficult to reconcile with the latter being more efficient in the diagnosis of dementia. It renders untenable a simple model that the major cause of differences in prognosis between elderly subjects is related to dementia. Yet the results are explicable in terms of development over time. Impairments in learning and memory are measurable at a much earlier stage of a dementing process than intellectual decline, and such sensitivity is essential for efficient diagnosis. Yet it may be that at this stage, the prognosis of the dement is not substantially worse than that of the functional patient, anyway in the short term. It is only when dementia has progressed to a level where intellectual impairments are also apparent, that prognosis becomes notably worse.

Some support for this model can be mentioned. McDonald (1969) found differences in short term mortality in patients with senile dementia, with those scoring poorly on tasks involving simple perceptuomotor function tending to die. The present author has data indicating that patients with mixed or equivocal diagnosis of chronic brain syndrome (a group assumed to contain a large proportion of early dements) were distinguishable from functional patients on verbal learning tasks but not on the WAIS vocabulary; whereas those with unequivocal and unmixed diagnoses (presumed to be later dements) performed at a lower level on both types of task. Developmental evidence has already been mentioned; those with definite chronic brain syndrome showed evidence of decline over a year for both intellectual ability and learning.

However, it should be said that these results could be artefactual. Criterion difficulties are maximized in the diagnosis of early dementia; verbal learning tasks might appear optimal only because clinicians are also putting prime emphasis on learning and memory function. Ageing is a further complicating factor since it both produces declining levels of function and increases the likelihood of dying.

In the practical field, the useful application of psychometric tasks has been demonstrated. Currently, the major problem to which they are applied is in differential diagnosis but there is evidence that a wider range of problems could be usefully probed with standardized psychological tests.

Management

In general clinical practice, the psychologist's role in management is most often concerned with behavioural approaches to assessment and treatment. Many of the difficulties of the elderly are similar to those found also in the mentally handicapped and chronic psychotics and this has led to the publication of several theoretical papers concerning the feasibility of applying some of the same methods of treatment (e.g. Lindsley, 1964). On the other hand, there have been surprisingly few accounts of practical applications and of those, the majority give insufficient detail of the general functional level of the patients (sometimes even whether they are clinically demented, aged chronic schizophrenics, or merely very old). The treatment methods employed are also not always adequately described.

Many of the behavioural deficits found in the elderly involve not so much a loss of ability but merely a failure to emit adequately preserved behaviour—that patients are capable of the required activites, such as physical or social recreation, but rarely or never perform them spontaneously. With this kind of problem an operant treatment paradigm would appear ideal, since it involves increasing the frequency of emission of responses by the use of contingent positive reinforcement. Loosely, this means rewarding the occurrence of a response or some approximation to it, but it should be stressed that this is a loose interpretation. Positive reinforcement is actually defined in terms of its tendency to increase the probability of occurrence of the preceding response and contingency implies that the reinforcer will normally only occur following that response; not all the empirical findings are consistent with merely regarding positive reinforcement as equivalent to reward, although it will serve for the present purposes.

Even for the severely memory disordered, there is evidence that simple responses can be increased in frequency provided a suitable positive reinforcement is found (Ankus and Quarrington, 1972). There are several studies looking at the effects of such treatment on increasing social interaction and walking activity (e.g. Sachs, 1975; Mueller and Atlas, 1972); but, although these studies do provide evidence of beneficial changes in the patients' behaviour, there is no convincing demonstration that it is the deliberately controlled positive reinforcement of the desired behaviour that is primarily responsible. Social reinforcement in the form of interest and attention, together with the cueing of behaviour, might be sufficient. MacDonald and Butler (1974) intended to use verbal reinforcement to increase walking behaviour in normally wheelchair-bound patients; but found that just suggesting that the person walk and offering a hand up from the chair were sufficient. This indicates that improved results might be found only by comparison with inadequate non-specific care; with good nursing, such patients would have already been encouraged to walk, and the effectiveness of normally available facilities has already been demonstrated. Cosin et al. (1958) showed beneficial, if transient, effects with occupational therapy in confused patients; and Sommer and Ross (1958) demonstrated that suitable grouping of chairs substantially increased the amount of social interaction among patients. Thus, it would be necessary to demonstrate that operant techniques are of value not in vacuo but rather as a useful addition to the existing facilities.

There is one report of a study comparing an operant approach with another form of treatment (Winkler, W. H., personal communication). The behaviours to be increased were activity and social interaction and the comparison treatments were positive reinforcement, reality orientation and a 'present treatment' control. Reality orientation has been gaining in popularity in the United States although no demonstration has been made of its specific effectiveness. The premise is that the confused patient suffers unfavourable non-specific effects, such as low morale and lack of ability to communicate, through his poor orientation in time and place. Thus reality orientation seeks to correct his orientation and this is done in small groups in a classroom type of situation with back-up displays provided on the ward. Information that the patients are required to 'learn' includes the day of the week, time of the next meal, the weather and so forth.

Most of the patients in Winkler's study were ageing long stay psychotics. During the eight week treatment period, the reinforcement group showed substantial increases in general activity and social interaction while the reality orientation patients were no better than the controls. After the end of treatment, most of the gains disappeared but the reinforcement group were still slightly better than the rest. Unfortunately, the experimental design was such that the reinforcement therapy had staff involvement for 63 hours per week, compared with only three hours for reality orientation, a possibly crucial difference since recent work by Brook *et al.* (1975) with dements suggests that the beneficial effects of reality orientation might be related in large part to the active encouragement of staff.

Thus it is possible that, in Winkler's study, the extra effectiveness of the reinforcement treatment was an artefact of greater staff involvement. It will also be noted that the main gains were only apparent during the active treatment phase. This is a property of operant treatments—that unless changes occur so that the activity becomes rewarding in itself or is maintained by the normal environment, then the operant programme will have to continue indefinitely. For those in long stay institutions, a feasible solution is the use of a token economy. This has not been investigated for elderly patients specificially, although it may be noted that in the early reported token system of Atthowe and Krasner (1968), a substantial proportion of the patients were elderly and although many were chronic schizophrenics, the remainder were suffering from organic processes and there is no suggestion of the latter responding less well. In a similar programme, Macpherson (Macpherson, E.L.R., personal communication) noted that elderly dements seemed to respond better than chronic schizophrenics. Clearly this is an area worthy of further study.

So far, the consideration has been of increasing the frequency of occurrence of intact behaviours. Operant techniques have also been tried to reinstate lost behaviours, in particular for the treatment of incontinence. Pollock and Liberman (1974) attempted to treat daytime incontinence in six men with chronic brain syndrome. The main feature of the treatment was the positive reinforcement of dryness. The programme was largely unsuccessful and this they ascribe to their over simple analysis of the problem. After their study they found that one subject benefited by a line drawn for him to follow to the lavatory; and they suggest that a process of shaping towards approaching and using the toilet would be more appropriate. This is supported by others (Woods, R., and Britton, P.G., personal communication) who found that of eight incontinent women, only two had difficulty in micturating appropriately in the toilet; it was the approach response that was lacking. These workers also report two men, one a severe dement, successfully treated for nocturnal enuresis using the 'dry bed' technique developed by Azrin *et al.* (1973) for subnormals; this is a more complex treatment package but is also based on operant principles.

This short review suggests that there has finally been a stirring of interest in the behavioural management of elderly patients; the results so far are patchy and inconclusive but it is likely that there will be more substantial contributions in the near future.

Prospects for future development

It is clear that the clinical psychologist has a major part to play in the care of the elderly patient. Assessment techniques are available that can add useful information concerning diagnosis, prognosis and the measurement of treatment effects. Operant treatment approaches appear sufficiently in promising to justify their experimental use for the individual case.

Some of the likely immediate developments have already been mentioned; there will be continuing improvements in the efficacy of the psychometric methods. More systematic research into the application of behaviour modification techniques would be justified and in particular the possibilities of applying token economy systems with those in institutions of various kinds. In the longer term, the general shift of emphasis away from the hospital will increase the range of problems that confront the psychologist. Like his colleagues, he will be less concerned with 'medical' problems such as diagnosis and more involved with the problems in living encountered by old people in various types of residential facility. In particular, both assessment and treatment are likely to be increasingly concerned with maximizing old people's capacity to cope with and enjoy living in optimal circumstances.

References

Ankus, M., and Quarrington, B. (1972) 'Operant behaviour in the memory disordered', *J. Gerontology*, **27**, 500–510.

Atthowe, J.M., and Krasner, L. (1968) 'Preliminary report on the application of contingent reinforcement procedures (token economy) on a "chronic" psychiatric ward', *J. Abnorm. Psychol.*, **73**, 37–43.

Azrin, N.H., Sneed, T.J., and Foxx, R.M. (1973) 'Dry bed: a rapid method of eliminating bedwetting (enuresis) of the retarded', *Behav. Res. Ther.* **2**, 427–434.

Bolton, N., Britton, P.G., and Savage, R.D. (1966) 'Some normative data on the WAIS and its indices in an aged population', *J. Clin. Psychol.*, **22**, 184–188.

Botwinick, J. (1970) 'Geropsychology', *Ann. Rev. Psychol.*, **21**, 239–272.

Brook, P., Degun, G., and Mather, M. (1975) 'Reality orientation, a therapy for psychogeriatric patients: a controlled study', *Br. J. Psychiat.*, **127**, 42–45.

Cosin, L.Z., Mort, M., Post, F., Westropp, C., and Williams, M. (1958) 'Experimental treatment of persistent senile confusion', *Internat. J. Soc. Psychiat.*, **4**, 24–42.

Crookes, T.G., and McDonald, K.G. (1972) 'Benton's Visual Retention Test in the differentiation of depression and early dementia', *Br. J. Soc. Clin. Psychol.*, **11**, 66–69.

Hulicka, I.M., and Weiss, R.L. (1965) 'Age differences in retention as a function of learning', *J. Consult. Psychol.*, **29**, 125–129.

Inglis, J. (1957) 'An experimental study of learning and memory function in elderly psychiatric patients', *J. Ment. Sci.*, **103**, 796–803.

Inglis, J. (1959a) 'Learning, retention, and conceptual usage in elderly patients with memory disorders', *J. Abnorm. Psychol.*, **59**, 210–215.

Inglis, J. (1959b) 'On the prognostic value of the modified word learning test in psychiatric patients over 65', *J. Ment. Sci.*, 1100–1101.

Inglis, J. (1960) 'Dichotic stimulation and memory disorder, *Nature*, **186**, 181.

Inglis, J., Colwell, C., and Post, F. (1960) 'An evaluation of the predictive power of a test known to differentiate between elderly "functional" and "organic" psychiatric patients', *J. Ment. Sci.*, **106**, 1486–1492.

Irving, G., Robinson, R.A., and McAdam, W. (1970) 'The validity of some cognitive tests in the diagnosis of dementia', *Br. J. Psychiat.*, **117**, 149–156.

Kendrick, D.C. (1965) 'Speed and learning in the diagnosis of diffuse brain damage in elderly subjects: a Bayesian statistical approach', *Br. J. Soc. Clin. Psychol.*, **4**, 141–148.

Kendrick, D.C. (1967) 'A cross-validation of the use of the SLT and DCT in screening for diffuse brain pathology in elderly subjects', *Br. J. Med. Psychol.*, **40**, 173–178.

Kendrick, D.C. (1972) 'The Kendrick battery of tests: theoretical assumptions and clinical uses', *Br. J. Soc. Clin. Psychol.*, **11**, 373–386.

Kendrick, D.C., Parboosingh, R.C., and Post, F. (1965) 'A synonym learning test for use with elderly psychiatric subjects: a validation study', *Br. J. Soc. Clin. Psychol*, **4**, 63–71.

Kendrick, D.C. and Post, F. (1967) 'Differences in cognitive status between healthy, psychiatrically ill and diffusely brain-damaged elderly subjects', *Br. J. Psychiat.*, **113**, 75–81.

Lindsley, O.R. (1964) 'Geriatric behavioural prosthetics', in *New thoughts on old age* (Ed. R. Kastenbaum) New York, Springer, 41–60.

Macdonald, M.L., and Butler, A.K. (1974) 'Reversal of helplessness: producing walking behaviour in nursing home wheelchair residents using behaviour modification procedures', *J. Gerontology*, **29**, 97–101.

McDonald, C. (1969) 'Clinical heterogeneity in senile dementia', *Br. J. Psychiat.*, **115**, 267–271.

Mueller, D.J., and Atlas, L. (1972) 'Resocialization of regressed elderly residents: a behavioural management approach', *J. Gerontology*, **27**, 390–392.

Newcombe, F., and Steinberg, B. (1964) 'Some aspects of learning and memory functions in older psychiatric patients', *J. Gerontology*, **19**, 490–493.

Payne, R.W. (1958) 'Diagnostic and personality testing in clinical psychology', *Am. J. Psychiat.*, **115**, 25–29.

Pollock, D.D., and Liberman, R.P. (1974) 'Behaviour therapy of incontinence in demented inpatients', *Gerontologist*, **14**, 488–491.

Post, F. (1965) *The clinical psychiatry of late life*, Oxford, Pergamon.

Post, F. (1966) 'Somatic and psychic factors in the treatment of elderly psychiatric patients', *J. Psychosom. Res.*, **10**, 13–18.

Sachs, D.A. (1975) 'Behavioural techniques in a residential nursing home facility', *J. Behav. Ther. Exp. Psychiat.*, **6**, 123–127.

Sanderson, R.E., and Inglis, J. (1961) 'Learning and mortality in elderly psychiatric patients', *J. Gerontology*, **16**, 375–376.

Savage, R.D., and Bolton, N. (1968) 'A factor analysis of learning impairment and intellectual deterioration in the elderly', *J. Gen. Psychol.*, **113**, 177–182.

Savage, R.D., Britton, P.G., Bolton, N., and Hall, E.H. (1973) *Intellectual functioning in the aged*, London, Methuen.

Shapiro, M.B., Post, F., Lofving, B. and Inglis, J. (1956) ' "Memory function" in psychiatric patients over 60: some methodological and diagnostic implications', *J. Ment. Sci.*, **102**, 233–246.

Sommer, R., and Ross, H. (1958) 'Social interaction on a geriatric ward', *Internat. J. Soc. Psychiat.*, **4**, 128–133.

Walton, D. (1958) 'The diagnostic and predictive accuracy of the MWLT in psychiatric patients over 65', *J. Ment. Sci.*, **104**, 1119–1122.

Whitehead, A. (1971) *An investigation of learning in elderly psychiatric patients*, Unpublished Ph.D. thesis, University of London.

Whitehead, A. (1973a) 'The pattern of WAIS performance in elderly psychiatric patients', *Br. J. Soc. Clin. Psychol.*, **12**, 435–436.

Whitehead, A. (1973b) 'Verbal learning and memory in elderly depressives', *Br. J. Psychiat.*, **123**, 203–208.

Whitehead, A (1974) 'Factors in the learning deficit of elderly depressives', *Br. J. Soc. Clin. Psychol.*, **13**, 201–208.

Whitehead, A. (1975) 'Recognition memory in dementia', *Br. J. Soc. Clin. Psychol.*, **14**, 191–194.

Whitehead, A. (1976) 'Prediction of outcome in elderly psychiatric patients', *Psychol. Med.*, **6**, 469–479.

8

NEUROPHYSIOLOGICAL DISTURBANCES ASSOCIATED WITH PSYCHIATRIC DISORDERS IN OLD AGE

R. Levy

Although the changes in the nervous system associated with ageing and their relationship to mental illness have attracted a good deal of attention over the years and have been studied by a variety of techniques there is comparatively little neurophysiological data pertaining to this subject.

While it is true that the fifties and early sixties saw the appearance of a spate of papers on the EEG in dementia (reviewed by Levy, 1969) and more recently the group at Duke University (Wang *et al.*, 1970) have carried out more sophisticated correlations between EEG, cerebral blood flow, and intellectual performance in groups of healthy elderly volunteers, traditional techniques have yielded disappointing results. Few would disagree that some patients with grossly disturbed mental states may have normal EEGs and that apparently normal subjects may have very abnormal recordings.

It is also striking that such studies as have been carried out have focused particularly on organic mental deterioration in the form of dementia and have generally ignored affective disorders and schizophrenia. Although the title of this paper suggests that this deficiency might be remedied, this is not the case. The studies to be described have been limited to patients with dementia and have only used depressives and schizophrenics as controls.

My interest in this field started with the realization that although considerable attention had been paid to the state of the central nervous system of demented patients, I was unable to discover any investigations whether clinical, pathological, or physiological on the peripheral nervous system. It seemed to me that in the study of ageing processes and associated clinical disorders it is worth considering whether abnormalities in one part of a body system occur in relative isolation or are associated with multiple defects elsewhere in the same or in other systems. In this way it may be possible to define the contribution of both general and specific disturbing factors to the various clinical syndromes associated with ageing. It is important to consider whether the dementia of elderly patients results from some special selective disturbance in an otherwise intact and well preserved nervous system, or whether alternatively, it might merely represent one prominent facet of disturbance in a nervous system with multiple widespread defects arising from a generalized degenerative process.

In the first study (Levy and Poole, 1966) an attempt was made to determine whether patients with central nervous abnormalities presenting as senile or arteriosclerotic dementia showed evidence also of peripheral nerve dysfunction and differed from non-demented aged patients in this respect.

The measurement of peripheral nerve conduction velocity was selected as a method of studying the peripheral nerves which would overcome the disadvantages of clinical examination and avoid the difficulties of a histopathological study by providing reliable and reasonably reproduceable results.

The method used was a modification of that described by Simpson (1956). The median nerve was stimulated by means of square pulses of 1 ms duration produced by a 'Medelec' EMG-stimulator unit. The stimulation sites were (a) at the elbow, (b) at the wrist. Recording electrodes were applied to the abductor pollicis brevis. The traces were displayed on a twin-beam oscilloscope, one beam providing a ms time marker. These traces were photographed, ten traces being superimposed.

The conduction velocity between the two points of stimulation was calculated in the usual way. The subjects were obtained from two hospitals.

(1) The 'B' series from a small psychogeriatric investigation unit at the Bethlem Royal Hospital.

Eight dements and eight depressed patients were seen and tested. The mean ages were 71·0 (SD 9·0) and 71·2 (SD 7·6) respectively and there were three men and five women in each group.

(2) The 'T' series from the wards of a large mental hospital with a special interest in geriatric patients (Tooting Bec Hospital). It consisted of 21 dements and 21 'controls' (depressives and schizophrenics) all of whom were males. The mean ages were 73·4 (SD 6·8) for the dements and 73·1 (SD 6·7) for the 'controls'.

The demented patients in both series had unequivocal evidence of dementia based on a detailed clinical appraisal with supporting evidence from psychological tests in the 'B' series. They were considered to be suffering from senile or arteriosclerotic dementia, and no attempt was made in this study to distinguish between these two diagnoses. The 'T' series were less fully documented but the dementia was always well established indeed, the dementia in the 'T' series was generally more longstanding and more advanced than in the 'B' series and the patients had been hospitalized longer. Because of such differences, the results from each series were evaluated separately.

Both non-demented 'control' groups consisted of patients diagnosed as having functional psychoses considered after detailed clinical appraisal to have no evidence of organic disorder. In each series they were matched in age and sex with the demented patients.

At the outset it was decided to exclude patients on the following grounds:

(1) Those with a history or signs of overt peripheral neuropathy
(2) Those who were bedridden or ill in other respects
(3) Those suffering from metabolic or toxic disorders likely to affect peripheral nerve function or those known to have had a grossly inadequate diet.

One patient was rejected from the 'B' series. She was a woman who had been living on her own for a long time and had evidence of multiple vitamin deficiencies. In the 'T' series three dements were rejected. Two were bedridden and grossly incapacitated and the third had a history of heavy drinking. Drug administration presented a problem since it was considered unjustifiable to disturb drug regimes for this study. However, in the 'B' series all patients were tested before having drug therapy and the drugs employed (phenothiazines or antidepressants) are not known to depress peripheral nerve function.

The patients selected were examined clinically from both physical and psychiatric viewpoints and then tested as described.

The essential findings of this study are shown in Figure 8.1 and Table 8.1. In Figure 8.1a forearm conduction velocities have been plotted against the age of the patients in each of the two dement and control groups. In both series the majority of the demented patients have slower forearm conduction velocities and fall to the left of the 'control' patients. However, this is not the case with the latencies of muscle response following wrist stimulation which appear plotted in the same way against age in Figure 8.1b.

MOTOR CONDUCTION IN MEDIAN NERVE

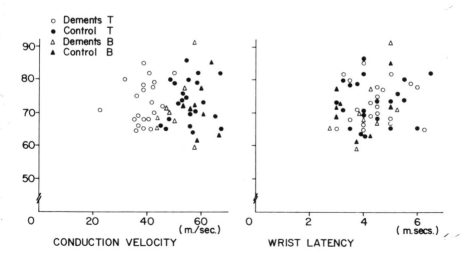

FIGURE 8.1. (a) Conduction velocity in m s^{-1} plotted against age of patient for each series; (b) latency in ms of muscle response following stimulation at wrist plotted against age of patient for each series as in (a)

TABLE 8.1. Age and conduction velocity data in demented and non-demented control subjects

Series	No.	Age (y)		Forearm conduction velocity (ms⁻¹)		Wrist latency (ms)		Correlation coefficients (r)		
		Mean	SD	Mean	SD	Mean	SD	Age/ conduction velocity	Age/ latency	Conduction velocity/ latency
B controls	8	71·2	7·6	59·4	4·7	3·8	0·8			+ 0·16
B dements	8	71·0	9·0	50·1	5·2	4·2	0·7			+ 0·32
T controls	21	73·4	6·8	55·4	6·1	4·4	0·9			− 0·09
T dements	21	73·1	6·7	38·4	5·4	4·4	0·8			+ 0·45
Total controls	29	72·8	7·0	56·5	6·1	4·2	0·9	+ 0·07	+ 0·14	− 0·12
Total dements	29	72·6	6·6	41·6	7·5	4·4	0·8	+ 0·20	+ 0·21	+ 0·19
Grand total	58	72·7	6·8	49·1	10·1	4·3	0·9	+ 0·10	+ 0·18	− 0·04

The actual mean values and standard deviations for each group are shown in Table 8.1. These results were compared statistically using analysis of variance, and correlation coefficients were calculated for both conduction velocity and wrist latency with respect to age.

The statistical analysis confirms that:

(1) Mean conduction velocities in both dementia groups were lower than in both control groups. ($p < 0.01$ for 'B' series; $p < 0.001$ for 'T' series.)
(2) The demented patients in the 'T' group had a substantially lower mean conduction velocity than those in the 'B' groups ($p < 0.001$). The 'T' control groups had a slightly lower mean conduction velocity than the 'B' control group but this difference was not statistically significant ($p < 0.1$).

Considering wrist latencies, there were, in contrast, only slight differences between each of the groups (p values < 0.1). The wrist latency results were, however, consistent with the conduction velocity results to the extent that the latencies were shortest in the 'B' controls who had the fastest conduction velocities and were slightly longer in the dementia series than in the control series. In both series it is also noteworthy that there was no suggestion of a much wider scatter of values in any one group such as might occur if the differences were dependent on gross lesions in a few patients.

In view of the reported correlation between age and motor nerve conduction (Wagman and Lesse, 1952; Norris et al., 1953) correlation coefficients were calculated for age in relation to forearm conduction and wrist latency. These all gave small positive values (shown in Table 8.1), none being statistically significant.

This first experiment then suggested that there was a definite decrease in motor nerve conduction velocity in the median nerve of patients with dementia as compared with patients of similar age who were not demented and although no attempt was made to rate the severity of the dementia there appeared to be a possible correlation between this and the degree of slowing of nerve conduction.

The next investigation (Levy et al., 1970) was designed with the following aims in view:

(1) To focus more specifically on the possible relationship between the severity of mental impairment and the slowing of peripheral motor nerve conduction.
(2) To follow the changes that might occur in this relationship after a period of one year.
(3) To investigate *sensory* nerve function which had been omitted from previous study owing to lack of adequate instrumentation.
(4) To examine the possibility that differences in peripheral temperature might act as contributory factors.
(5) To look into the possible role of deficiencies of vitamin B_{12}, folic acid and other vitamins of the B group in view of suggestions that psychogeriatric patients often show abnormal serum levels of these vitamins.

The subjects tested consisted of a group diagnosed as suffering from senile dementia. They were obtained from a large psychiatric hospital (Cane Hill) and from a day centre for elderly demented patients (Page's Walk Centre). The latter were included in order to obtain a wider range of severity of dementia than would be expected from an investigation of inpatients only. There were 28 patients (18 females and ten males). The control group consisted of 19 patients (eleven females and eight males) suffering from functional psychoses without organic impairment who had been admitted to a small psychogeriatric unit (Bethlem Royal Hospital).

The demented and control groups were matched for age, the mean ages being 77·1 and 75·3 respectively. An attempt was also made to match for sex but it will be noticed that there was a higher proportion of females in the demented group. This was not thought to be important as it should, if anything, militate against finding any significant differences between the groups since conduction velocity in women is reported to be higher than in men (Wagman and Lesse, 1952; Norris et al., 1953).

Certain patients were excluded on the same grounds as those given above.

Psychiatric evaluation was carried out by an independent psychiatrist (A.D.I.) who rated patients using a dementia rating scale (Blessed et al., 1968) which was slightly modified.

In addition, a series of rough psychological tests were administered. This proved difficult as demented patients tended to score zero on standard tests. Since we wished to obtain a suitable spread of scores a set of simple but relatively unstandardized tests was adapted. These were:

(1) The memory and concentration questionnaire (Blessed et al., 1968).
(2) Immediate recall of sentences (IRS). Two sentences each containing seven scorable items were composed taking as a basis the paragraphs of immediate recall subtest of the Wechsler memory scale form 1, procedure was as for the original. The sentences were administered on two separate occasions about a week apart since it was thought that the performance of the demented subjects might be very variable as was their general state of health. The product–moment correlation obtained was high ($r = 0.01$, $n = 34$) indicating that there was in fact little variability and also providing evidence for the test–retest reliability of the procedure.
(3) Design copying (DC). Two designs for copying were taken from Benton's visual retention test using administration 'C'. A further two were selected from the Bender gestalt test as being those shown to provide the most effective discrimination between samples of patients diagnosed as 'organic', 'functional', and 'doubtful' in one series of studies (Shapiro et al., 1956, 1957). Standard scoring procedures had to be abandoned and a point was given if the copy was a recognizable version of most of the original. No retesting was attempted for this task.
(4) Immediate recall—designs (IRD). Designs used in the widely used standard tests of visual retention (e.g. Benton, 1955) were too complicated or too small for our demented subjects. Six extremely simple shapes were chosen which were drawn on cards and shown to the subject for ten seconds, after which he was asked to

draw them from memory. A simple scoring system was devised. The six designs were usually administered in two groups of three to allow for variability as with IRS. The correlation between occasions was 0·85 (n = 35) which is high considering that different, not necessarily equivalent, forms were used. Again this indicates that variability in performance was not marked and suggests that the task is fairly reliable.

Measures of nerve conduction

At the beginning of the recording session the patient's peripheral temperature was measured over the ulnar nerve at the wrist and elbow using an electrical skin thermometer (Light Laboratories Ltd.). Conduction velocity measurements were then made on the left ulnar nerve.

(1) Motor nerve conduction: the technique used was a modification of that described by Simpson (1956). It is fully described elsewhere (Levy et al., 1970).
(2) Sensory nerve conduction: this was determined by recording nerve action potentials over the ulnar nerve at the elbow following peripheral stimulation of the digital branches of the ulnar nerve by means of ring electrodes placed round the little finger. The recording was done by means of saddle-shaped electrodes mounted on a Perspex plate. The method was that described by Gilliatt et al. (1965) modified in so far as the averaging was performed by a digital averaging computer rather than by a barrier-grid storage tube. An average of 64 responses was recorded and this was, in turn, written out by an X–Y plotter.

All tests were carried out in a warm room after the patients had had time to get accustomed to the conditions of the experiment.

Approximately a year after these tests had been carried out the motor nerve measurements were repeated on those of the Cane Hill patients who were still available. Unfortunately because of the high mortality and general morbidity rate in these patients, this only proved possible in nine of the 21 original cases.

Vitamin levels

Serum B_{12} and folate levels, and red cell folate content were also estimated in these patients. They were also given three tablets a day of thiamine compound, strong BPC (each containing thiamine hydrochloride 5 mg, riboflavine 2 mg, nicotinamide 20 mg, and pyridoxine hydrochloride 2 mg) for three months after which the motor nerve conduction tests were repeated. These investigations were only introduced late in the study and only nine of the demented patients and none of the controls were tested.

Motor nerve conduction velocity

The findings are expressed in Table 8.2 which shows that motor nerve conduction velocity was lower in demented patients (46·6 ms^{-1}) than in controls (57·2 ms^{-1}) and that inpatient dements had slower motor nerve conduction (44·5) than outpatient dements (53 ms^{-1}). However, although the trend was in the expected direction none of these differences were statistically significant.

TABLE 8.2. Motor nerve conduction velocity in three groups of patients

Series	No.	Mean age	Conduction velocity (motor)	
			Mean	SD
Inpatient dements	21	78·0	44·5	12·4
Outpatient dements	7	76·7	53·0	4·9
Total dements	28	77·1	44·4	9·89
Controls	19	75·3	57·2	10·3

Closer examination of the dementia ratings revealed the fact that some of the patients originally classified as 'controls' had symptoms of dementia and some of the outpatient dements who were assumed to have only mild symptoms had in fact rather high dementia scores but were able to live out of hospital because of good family support. In view of this, it was thought reasonable to reclassify all the subjects into two groups, those with low dementia scores (below seven) and those with high dementia scores (seven or above). Table 8.3 shows the results of the reclassified patients. Motor nerve conduction velocity was significantly lower in those with higher dementia scores than in those with low dementia scores (p = 0·01).

TABLE 8.3. Motor nerve conduction velocity in relation to dementia score

Series	No.	Mean age	Conduction velocity (motor)	
			Mean	SD
Dementia score < 7	15	79·6 ± 5·5	41·7	9·9
Dementia score > 7	32	75·0 ± 2·9	55·2	9·5

These results are expressed in Figure 8.2 which shows clearly that although there was a good deal of overlap, all subjects with conduction velocities of less than 44 m s^{-1} were demented, the majority of them seriously so.

Table 8.4 shows the results of intercorrelation between motor nerve conduction, dementia scores, psychological tests, and age for 27 demented patients (one patient with a dementia score of zero was omitted). It will be seen that conduction velocity was significantly correlated with dementia scores (p < 0·02), immediate recall of sentences (p < 0·05), design copying (p < 0·02) and immediate recall of designs (p

< 0·05). The psychological tests and dementia score were all significantly intercorrelated but there were no significant age correlations.

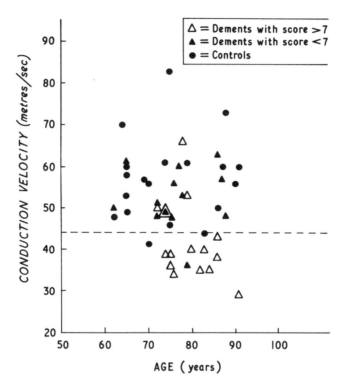

FIGURE 8.2. Distribution of motor nerve conduction velocity in demented subjects and controls

TABLE 8.4. Intercorrelation matrix (Pearson's product—Moment correlation coefficient)

	Conduction velocity	Dementia score	Memory and concentration	IRS	DC	IRD	Age
Conduction velocity							
dementia score	−0·51[2]						
Memory and concentration	0·29	−0·68[3]					
IRS	0·39[1]	−0·59[2]	0·81[3]				
DC	0·57[2]	−0·69[3]	0·67[3]	−0·52[2]			
IRD	0·40[1]	−0·75[3]	0·80[3]	−0·71[3]	0·83[3]		
Age	−0·30	0·22	−0·05	−0·21	−0·02	0·01	

[1] < 0·05 (1-tail); [2] < 0·02 (1-tail); [3] < 0·01 (1-tail).

Sensory nerve conduction

There were no appreciable differences between the groups on this measure. The mean velocity was 46·8 ms⁻¹ for dements and 48·1 ms⁻¹ for controls. In the reclassified subjects it was 47·5 (SD 11) for those with low dementia scores and 51·1 (SD 15·6) for those with high scores. This measure did not correlate significantly with any of the psychological measures.

Retests at follow-up (one year)

It only proved possible to retest nine of the Cane Hill patients a year after the original tests. Three had had an increase in dementia score and this was in every case associated with a fall in conduction velocity. The changes in motor nerve conduction and dementia scores were significantly correlated ($r = 0·73$) at the two per cent level. However, although the changes in the psychological scores were in the expected direction the figures were too small to yield significant correlations.

Changes after three months of vitamin B therapy

In most patients there was no change in conduction velocity after administration of vitamin B complex. The mean value for the group remained unchanged. One patient however did show a marked increase in velocity (from 49 ms⁻¹ to 71 ms⁻¹). This change was also accompanied by an improvement in mental state. However, as patients were not rated again at this stage no systematic comparison of this can be made.

Vitamin B_{12} and folate levels

None of the patients had serum vitamin B_{12} levels below the lower limit of normal for the laboratory (150 pg ml⁻¹). One patient had an abnormally low serum folate of 4·5 pg ml⁻¹ (normal range 5–20) and a red cell folate of 143 ng ml⁻¹ (normal range 160–640 ng ml⁻¹). There were in addition three patients with abnormally low red cell folates but normal serum folates.

Peripheral skin temperature

There were no significant differences in skin temperature at the wrist or elbow between the various groups of subjects. The results of this second study therefore seemed to confirm those of the first in regard to the motor nerve conduction velocity in patients suffering from senile dementia.

The slowing of conduction was of a degree usually associated with primary neuronal or axonal degeneration rather than with segmental demyelienation (Gilliatt, 1966). The fact that the slowing was restricted to motor nerve conduction is of some interest as it suggests that the process may affect only the larger fibres. Sensory nerve conduction being dependent on smaller fibres did not seem to be affected. This lack of interference with sensory conduction also happened to be convenient in view of the later studies on the somatosensory evoked response with are discussed later.

The postulated large fibre degeneration may run parallel with large cell degeneration in the cerebral cortex and in this context the significant correlation between the degree of dementia and the degree of slowing is noteworthy. There also appeared to be some correspondence between the rapidity of progression of the mental impairment and the changes in conduction velocity.

The changes can clearly not be attributed to alterations in peripheral temperature but the possible effect of diet and vitamin deficiency is more difficult to resolve. Although obvious dietary deficiency was excluded and low B_{12} levels were not found, there remains a possibility that low folate levels may have been at least partly responsible for either the dementia or the peripheral nerve slowing or both. This is clearly a point worth investigating more systematically.

Having demonstrated a slowing of conduction in peripheral nerve fibres we then set about determining whether there might also be evidence of slowing of conduction in the central nervous system of patients suffering from senile dementia. Straumanis *et al.* (1965) had already reported delay in the later components of the visual evoked response in patients with 'chronic brain syndromes' and Shagass and Schwartz (1965) had described age-related changes in the somatosensory response. It was therefore of some interest to compare specific somatosensory cortical evoked response in our senile dements to that of a non-demented control group.

We were interested not only in the question of conduction rates in the nervous system but in trying to develop a technique which might help to discriminate between senile dementia and functional psychoses in old age.

By the time this investigation started only nine (six females and three males) of the original demented subjects were available for testing. These were not receiving any medication other than night sedation which had been given about 16 h before the test was carried out.

The control group consisted of eight elderly depressives (six females and two males), the majority of whom were receiving tricyclic antidepressants.

TABLE 8.5. Results for demented group

Patient	Age	Latency of evoked response					Amplitude of 5 Amplitude of 1
		1	2	3	4	5	
1	84	29	35	55	85	116	0·55
2	67	27	37	69	85	—	0
3	82	16	22	58	63	107	1·0
4	83	25	30	45	57	—	0
5	73	17	23	27	37	61	0·72
6	85	37	43	53	63	—	0
7	83	34	44	58	86	—	0
8	69	23	32	36	42	77	3·25
9	75	23	28	48	55	85	1·14
Mean	77·9	24·6	32·7	49·9	63·6	89·0	0·74
SD	6·9	9·1	8·0	12·6	18·6	—	1·0

They were evaluated clinically and by means of the psychological tests previously mentioned.

Cortical somatosensory responses evoked by ulnar nerve stimulation were recorded over the contralateral receiving area for the hand. The averaging of 64 sweeps was carried out by computer and the trace written out by our X–Y plotter. Latencies of the successive peaks were recorded. These have been numbered 1 to 5. This numbering corresponds to N_1, P_1, N_2, P_2, N_3 used by other authors.

The latencies of each component of the responses is given in Tables 8.5 and 8.6 and shown in the histograms in Figure 8.3. The latency of each peak was greater in the demented patients but the difference only reached an acceptable level of significance for peak 3 (p = 0·05).

TABLE 8.6. Results for control group

Patient	Age	\multicolumn{5}{c}{Latency of evoked response}	Amplitude of 5 Amplitude of 1
		1	2	3	4	5	
1	80	23	29	43	67	85	1·67
2	86	25	37	43	85	98	3·0
3	72	18	25	38	55	82	1·2
4	79	23	31	42	74	93	2·67
5	74	22	30	34	49	73	1·1
6	73	25	35	53	77	106	5·5
7	71	15	20	30	40	65	3·4
8	85	20	24	32	50	75	2·33
Mean	77·5	21·4	28·9	39·4	62·1	84·6	2·61
SD	5·9	3·5	5·7	7·5	15·9	13·8	1·43

Inspection of the records also showed that wave 5 was either very flat or absent altogether in the demented patients. Since measures of absolute amplitude are difficult to interpret in attempting to quantify this variable we chose to express it as a ratio of wave 5 to that of wave 1. In controls the ratio was always greater than one whereas this was only true of two of the demented subjects. Although the mean ratios were not significantly different when the T-test was applied to this small group, this test was not thought to be appropriate since the distribution was skewed by the high proportion of zero values. All ratios of greater than unity were therefore designated as 'normal' and the others as 'abnormal' and the results expressed in a two by two contingency table. The significance was tested by Fisher's test of exact probabilty and the differences were then found to be significant at the 0·005 level.

When an attempt was made to use the results to allocate patients to the correct group using a cut-off point of 44 ms for the latency of wave 3, one control and two dements were misclassified (Figure 8.4). If the amplitude ratio was used two dements and no controls were misclassified (Figure 8.5) combining the two measures resulted in the misclassification of one demented subject.

The results tend to support the prediction that senile dements would show a

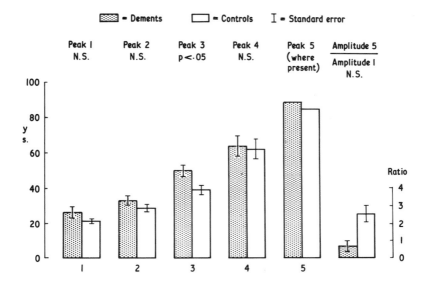

FIGURE 8.3. Histograms indicating mean latencies of respective peaks of the somatosensory evoked response and the ratio of peak 5 to that of peak 1 in nine demented patients and eight controls

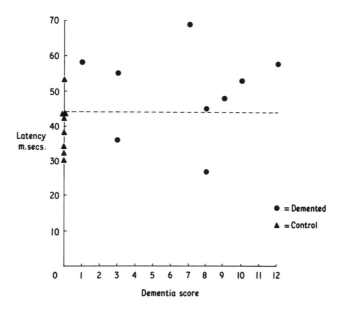

FIGURE 8.4. Scattergram of latency of peak 3 of the evoked response plotted against demention score in demented and control subjects. Dotted line indicates a cut-off point at 44 ms

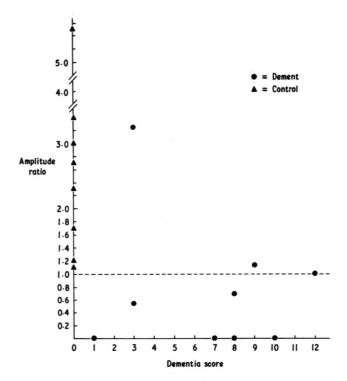

FIGURE 8.5. Scattergram of ratio of amplitude of peak 5 to that of peak 1 plotted against dementia score in demented and control subjects. Dotted line indicates a cut-off point at a ratio of 1

prolongation of the latency of the evoked response. The slowing may, of course, have occurred anywhere along the pathway from the ulnar nerve to the cerebral cortex but since the earlier study (Levy *et al.*, 1970) revealed no impairment of sensory as opposed to motor nerve conduction in demented subjects and since Straumanis *et al.* (1965) found similar delays in the visual evoked response it seems reasonable to suppose that the site of the slowing is likely to have been in the central nervous system and more probably in the brain.

The fact that the most significant changes were found in the later components of the response is of interest although it should be pointed out that what is referred to as 'late' in this chapter does not quite correspond to what other writers call 'late', since most of the responses which are described occurred in the first 100 ms. This is in keeping with the shorter latencies which are obtained for the somatosensory response as compared with the visual and auditory responses. However, with this proviso, the findings reported here are along the same lines as those of Straumanis *et al.* (1965) for the visual response. These workers found that the patients' responses differed from those of the controls mainly in the latencies of the later components. It is generally assumed that the somatosensory evoked responses represent cortical activity triggered by afferent input from two parallel projection systems: a specific lemniscal system mediating early components and a non-specific extralemniscal system mediating the later components. However, Williamson *et al.* (1958) studying groups of patients with unilateral cerebral lesions sited at different points from the thalamus and internal capsule to the cerebral cortex have questioned this view. They have shown that the integrity of the specific projection system is critical for the occurrence of the late components as well as the early components. Sutton *et al.* (1965) have suggested that the early components may be related to the arrival of the signal at the cerebral cortex and that the late components represent events associated with the processing of the information received. It would be tempting to suggest that the charges in the later components in demented patients represent a disorder of central processing rather than in conduction of the signal. However, in the present state of knowledge such a suggestion would be premature.

Also of relevance are the findings of Ertl and Schafer (1969) who have reported significant inverse correlations between latencies of the visual evoked response and the WISC and other psychological tests and those of Rhodes *et al.* (1969) who found differences between bright and dull children. Similar delays have been reported in cretinized rats (Bradley *et al.*, 1964) and hypothyroid patients (Nishitani and Kooi, 1968). Slowing of conduction may indeed be a very basic function which may underlie such well documented features as the slowing of the α-rhythm in ageing and dementia.

The somatosensory evoked response may in time become a helpful diagnostic aid in the differentiation of organic from functioning psychoses in old age. As compared with the more widely used visual and auditory responses it has the advantage of requiring less co-operation on the part of the patient, allowing a better differentiation between specific and non-specific responses and providing a method of testing the integrity of the peripheral pathway by monitoring the response higher up along the nerve. This latter point is of particular importance in elderly patients who suffer from impairment of vision and hearing which may be potent non-cerebral causes of alterations in the evoked response.

It is clear that the method is relatively effective in correctly categorizing already diagnosed patients, whether it can do so in patients in whom the diagnosis is in doubt will emerge from further studies.

In the chapter I have tried to show some of the ways in which neurophysiological techniques can be applied to the study of psychiatric disorders in old age. I have steered clear of the traditional EEG approach which has not been very useful or interesting and discussed methods which are still in their infancy. It remains to be seen whether they will survive into productive maturity and live to a ripe old age or whether it is their fate to end on the scrap heap of interesting but useless technological developments.

Summary

The contribution reports on three main studies which attempted to measure various neurophysiological variables in groups of patients suffering from dementia in old age and in non-demented control group.

The first study revealed a slowing in motor nerve conduction in peripheral nerves of demented patients and suggested the possibility that there might be a relationship between the severity of the dementia and the degree of slowing.

The second study confirmed the presence of impairment in motor nerve conduction but failed to show any slowing in sensory nerve conduction. It showed a significant negative correlation between cognitive impairment and motor nerve conduction velocity and traced the pattern of this correlation in a subgroup of patients followed up a year after the first testing. It appeared that increase in dementia went hand in hand with a further fall in conduction velocity.

The possibility that the changes might have been due to vitamin deficiency was also looked into. Loading doses of vitamin B complex only improved nerve conduction in one patient. No abnormalities in serum B_{12} were found but four out of nine patients had an abnormal red cell folate content and one of these also had a low serum folate.

The third study recorded the cortical somatosensory evoked response in demented and control subjects. This preliminary inquiry revealed that the latency of each component of the response was greater in the demented group but the difference only reached an acceptable level of significance for the second negative peak. There was in addition a tendency towards flattening of total absence of the later components of the response. An attempt was made to use these characteristics of the evoked response to categorize patients into either the demented or the control group. A measure of success was achieved but it is suggested that these indices will have to be studied in a larger group of borderline cases before their usefulness is established.

The significance of these results is discussed and it is suggested that slowing of conduction may be a very basic function in ageing and its related psychiatric disorders.

Postcript

A later study was conducted in order to obtain more information about the apparent delay in the cortical evoked response in a larger group of subjects which included a group of normal old people, a group of depressives, a group of senile dements and a smaller group consisting of patients with a combination of depression and dementia (referred to as 'mixed' cases). Since the somatosensory evoked response had not proved to be as sensitive an indicator as we would have wished, the further study included in the auditory response as well. Other aspects which were judged to be of interest were the relationship between the evoked potential variables and clinical variables such as cognitive function and effective state. The plan also included an examination of depressive patients after recovery. The results have not yet been published but they may be summarized as follows:

All components of the auditory response except the first differentiated significantly (at least at the one per cent level between controls, depressives and dements. The latencies for the depressives were intermediate between those of the controls and those of the dements and although the number of mixed cases was small the latencies of this group fell between those of the depressives and dements.

There were similar trends for the somatosensory response but these did not reach an acceptable level of significance. In other words, elderly depressives showed changes that were similar to but milder than those found in dements. Furthermore, and rather surprisingly, the scores for the depressives did not return to normal after clinical recovery, suggesting that the delayed responses might be related to suceptibility to depression rather than to the depression *per se* and re-opening the question of whether late onset depression may be facilitated by organic cerebral changes related to ageing. When the relationship between symptom scores and cognitive tests on the one hand and evoked potential latencies on the other were examined, it was found that in the subject population as a whole there were consistent negative correlations between scores on all cognitive tests and the latency of the auditory response. This was particularly strong in the case of the Gresham Ward questionnaire and the digit symbol substitution sub test of the WAIS. However, when the group of dements was examined separately a significant correlation was only found in the case of the digit symbol substitution Test i.e. although the evoked potential latency seemed to be a sensitive indicator of dementia, it did not seem to be a particularly good measure of the severity of the dementing process.

Within the group of depressives, there was no statistically significant relationship between symptom scores and evoked potential variables, although there was a tendency for those with high scores for depressive retardation to have longer evoked potential latencies.

The inter-relationships between clinical measures and physiological ones are being subjected to further analysis.

The neurophysiological measures described have therefore proved to be effective in distinguishing between normals, depressives, and dements, but preliminary analysis does not suggest that any very clear correlations emerge between the severity of the depression or dementia and the degree of slowing of the evoked responses. This is probably not surprising in view of the heterogeneity of the conditions studied and the relative crudeness of the available clinical measures of severity. The fact that in depression there appears to be no change with recovery means that the measures will not be of value in monitoring treatment of this condition although they have already helped to answer certain basic theoretical questions. As regard dementia it will be interesting to examine to what extent evoked potential latency changes with the progress of the disease, and whether it can be used as a method of assessing the effect of drugs which are claimed to affect this condition.

References

Bender, L. (1946) *Instructions for the use of the visual-motor gestalt test.* New York. American Orthopsychiatric Associations.

Benton, A.L. (1955) *The revised visual retention test. Clinical and experimental applications.* Iowa, Iowa State University.

Blessed, G., Tomlinson, B.E., and Roth, M. (1968). 'The association between quantitive measures of dementia and senile changes in the cerebral matter of elderly subjects', *Br. J. Psychiat.*, **114**, 797–812.

186

Bradley, P.B., Eayrs, J.T., and Richards, N.M. (1964) 'Factors influencing potentials in normal and cretinous rats', *Electroenceph. Clin. Neurophysiol.*, **17**, 308–313.

Ertl, J.P., and Schafer, E.W.P. (1969) 'Brain response correlates of psychometric intelligence', *Nature*, **223**, 421–422.

Gilliat, R.W., Melville, I.D., Velate, A.S., and Willison, R.G. (1965) 'A study of normal nerve action potentials using an average technique', *J. Neurol. Neurosurg. Psychiat.*, **28**, 191–200.

Gilliat, R.W. (1966) 'Applied electrophysiology in nerve and muscle disease' *Pro. Royal Soc. Med.*, **59**, 989–993.

Levy, R., and Poole, E. W. (1966), 'Peripheral motor nerve conduction in elderly demented and non-demented psychiatric patients', *J. Neurol. Neurosurg. Psychiat.*, **29**, 362–366.

Levy, R. (1969) 'The neurophysiology of dementia', *Br. J. Hos. Med.*, **2**, 688–690.

Levy, R. Isaacs, A.D., and Hawks, G. (1970) 'Neurophysiological correlates of senile dementia 1. Motor and sensory nerve conduction velocity', *Psychol. Med.*, **1**, 40–47.

Levy, R. Isaacs, A.D. and Behrman, J. (1971) 'Neurophysiological correlates of senile dementia II. The somatosensory evoked response'. *Psychol. Med*, **1**, 159–165.

Nishitani, H., and Kooi, K.A. (1968) 'Cerebral evoked responses in hypothyroidism', *Electroenceph. Clin. Neurophysiol.*, **27**, 554–560.

Norris, A.H., Shock, N.W., and Wagman, I.H. (1953) 'Age changes in the maximum conduction velocity of motor fibres of human ulnar nerves', *J. App. Physiol.*, **5**, 589–593.

Rhodes, L.E., Dustman, R.E., and Beck, E.C. (1969) 'The visual evoked response: a comparison of bright and dull children', *Electroenceph. Clin. Neurophysiol.*, **27**, 364–372.

Shagass, C., and Schwartz, M. (1965) 'Age, personality and somatosensory cerebral evoked responses', *Science*, **148**, 1359–1361.

Shapiro, M.B., Post, F., Loefving, B., and Inglis, J. (1956). 'Memory fuction in psychiatric patients over 60. Some methodological and diagnostic implications', *J. Ment. Sci.*, **102**, 233–246.

Shapiro, M.B., Field, J., and Post, F. (1957) 'An enquiry into the determinants of differentiation between elderly organic and non-organic patients on the Bender Gestalt Test', *J. Ment. Sci*, **103**, 364–374.

Simpson, J.A. (1956) 'Electrical signs in the diagnosis of carnal tunnel and related syndromes', *J. Neurol. Neurosurg. Psychiat.*, **19**, 275–280.

Straumanis, J.J., Shagass, C., and Schwartz, M. (1965) 'Visually evoked response changes associated with chronic brain syndromes and aging', *J. Gerontology*, **20**, 498–506.

Sutton, S., Braren, M. Zubin, J., and John, E.R. (1965) 'Evoked–potential correlates of stimulus uncertainty', *Science*, **150**, 1187–1188.

Wagman, I.H., and Lesse, H. (1952) 'Maximum conduction velocities of motor fibres of ulnar nerve in human subjects of various ages and sizes', *J. Neurophysiol.*, **15**, 235–244.

Wang, H.S., Obrist, W.D., and Busse, E.W. (1970) 'Neurophysiological correlates of the intellectual function of elderly persons living in the community', *Am. J. Psychiat.*, **126**, 1205–1212.

Williamson, P.D. Goff, W.H., Matsumiya, Y., and Allison, T. (1970) 'Somatosensory evoked potentials in patients with unilateral cerebral Lesions'. *Electroencephalography and Clinical Neurophysiology*, **28**, 91.

Acknowledgements

We wish to thank the editors of *Journal of Neurology, Neurosurgery and Psychiatry* and *Psychological Medicine* for their kind permission to use some figures and tables.

Journal of Neurology, Neurosurgery and Psychiatry: Figure 8.1 and Table 8.1.

Psychological Medicine: Figures 8.2, 8.3, 8.4 and 8.5, and Tables 8.2, 8.3, 8.4, 8.5 and 8.6.

This chapter is reproduced by permission of De Erven F. Bohn from *Ageing of the central nervous system* edited by van Praag and Kalverboer, Utrecht, Bohn, Scheltema and Holkema.

9

EVALUATION OF DIAGNOSTIC METHODS: AN INTERNATIONAL COMPARISON

J.R.M. Copeland

Introduction

It is incontrovertible that for the elderly accurate diagnosis can be life saving. The distinction between depressive illness and senile dementia may govern the decision between curative and palliative treatment. Even the more difficult distinction between senile and arteriosclerotic dementia may have prognostic implications. (Post, 1951; Roth and Morrisey, 1952). A number of questions can, therefore, be posed. Is it possible to improve diagnostic reliability and test its validity? To what extent do psychiatrists in different countries use the same diagnostic terms according to the same criteria? What is the prevalence in hospital and community practice of diagnoses made according to the terms of the International Classification of Disease and the World Health Organization Glossary of Mental Disorders? Are patients bearing these diagnoses recognized by doctors and treated? Finally, would a new diagnostic system serve us better?

The attempt to answer some of these questions has occupied the US–UK Project since 1970.

Standardization and reliability of psychiatric diagnoses and symptom recognition

Before psychiatric diagnosis can be made reliable the clinical interview itself must be standardized. This helps to ensure that key symptoms are not forgotten by the interviewer, and that style of interview and persistence do not result in either qualitative or quantitative differences in the symptoms recorded. Semi-structured interviews aiming at standardization, while retaining as far as possible the flexibility and judgement of a clinical interview, have been used for some years on younger age groups (Spitzer *et al.*, 1964; Wing *et al.*, 1967). A combined form of both the Wing and Spitzer interviews was used by the US–UK Project in its earlier studies of patients in the age group 19–59 years. To provide a similar interview for patients aged over 60 presented some difficulties. The nature of normal ageing was one. In previous studies the interviewer, a psychiatrist, had been required to rate the pathology of a piece of behaviour against his own experiential standard of normality. However, for the elderly it was not clear which of the patients' symptoms, if any, could be attributed to ageing alone and which to illness, while the nature of the relationship between previous cognitive level, present mental state and symptom variability between patients of the same age, added further uncertainty. The least unsatisfactory solution seemed to be to rate all behaviour variations irrespective of the patient's age.

The high level of physical disability in the elderly tended to confuse such ratings as, lack of energy, slowness, loss of appetite, sleep disturbance etc. In the younger age groups these symptoms were not rated if they had a clear physical cause. For the elderly such distinctions are less clear and the judgements required more numerous, suggesting that when present they should be rated positively and assessed later against a physical examination. Even if the latter is not feasible as in most community studies, they should probably still be rated; subjects' feeling of slowness, for example, has been shown to be correlated more highly with depression than with physical illness. (Gurland *et al.*, 1976).

Certain questions seem inappropriate for the elderly, but this assumption should not be made without testing. For example, 'How do you see your future?' was not necessarily answered pessimistically, even by patients of advanced age, unless they were also depressed.

The elderly appeared able to understand and respond appropriately to complex questions, provided these questions were broken up into short sentences and presented slowly. Neither lack of concentration nor tiredness was a problem. A patient capable of concentrating for 30 min could do so for three times that period. For the community elderly, interviews of two hours duration are well tolerated, fatigue affecting the interviewer rather than the patient who generally claims to enjoy the experience 'Thank you for taking so much trouble with me' or 'It's so nice to talk to somebody who listens'. Occasionally physical illness or cognitive impairment necessitate a short interview. In order to accommodate this possibility 36 key questions, important for diagnosis, the 'initial items', were selected to be rated early in the interviews. If diurnal fluctuation in the mental state of the aged occurs, as some suggest, it did not appear to interfere with the patient's ability to respond to the questions. Because old people were said to experience a period of disorientation shortly after a change of surroundings, those patients who showed cognitive impairment on the first interview after hospital admission were reinterviewed one week later.

The combined mental state (CMS) used for the 19–59 year olds had consisted of a mixture of most of the items of the present state examination (eighth edition) (Wing *et al.*, 1967), and nearly 200 items from the present status schedule (Spitzer *et al.*, 1964). In addition to the considerations already mentioned, items for the geriatric mental state (GMS) were selected according to the results of a factor analysis of data derived from the CMS used with 500 younger patients which provided 25 factors shown to be valid discriminators for the project diagnoses (Fleiss *et al.*, 1971). These factors had formed the basis of a classification scheme by which patients had been grouped into symptom profiles correlating with both project and hospital diagnoses, type of treatment received and duration of hospital stay. Thus the GMS retained the advantage of having been developed from both British and American sources.

Additional items thought to be of importance for the elderly were added, including more extensive cognitive sections dispersed between less stressful questions. Provision was made for examining and rating comatose and stuperose patients, and finally at the end of the interview for recording types of communication difficulty due to sensory and physical defects. In general, the interview aimed to follow a technique acceptable to a good clinician while minimizing the examiner variability existing between even the best clinicians.

It was necessary to show, to what proportion of unselected elderly admissions to a mental hospital, an interview of this kind could be given. A study of 100 consecutive admissions aged over 60 showed that 77 per cent completed the full interview and a further 13 per cent completed 'initial items', so that in only ten per cent did the structured interview have to be abandoned altogether. In 70 per cent, the interviewer was sufficiently content with his diagnosis to append no alternative possibility. When the difficult alternative diagnoses of senile and arteriosclerotic dementia were excluded by labelling them both 'dementia', the proportion without an alternative diagnosis rose to 86 per cent. There were no cases in this particular series where the main diagnosis was organic and the alternative functional or vice versa.

Having constructed the interview schedule, tried it out on a series of patients in both London and New York and made such modifications as were required, the next stage was to discover the reliability of the diagnoses made and the symptoms recorded by trained psychiatric interviewers. In other words, how reliable can psychiatric diagnosis be for elderly patients compared with a younger age group?

The two studies undertaken are summarized here. Study one used an earlier version of the interview which subsequently underwent minor modifications to become the definitive GMS. This study was performed by three project psychiatrists trained to use the schedule who interviewed a consecutive series of 18 mental hospital admissions in London. The three raters using the schedule, rated all the patients, each rater either interviewing a given patient, observing another rater interviewing or reinterviewing the next day. Using a balanced design 54 sets of ratings resulted from this method (Copeland et al., 1976), an independent provisional diagnosis based on the International Classification of Diseases (eighth edition) and using the descriptions of the WHO proposed Glossary of Mental Disorders was made by each rater at the end of the interview. It was not possible to complete the interviews for two patients, who were nevertheless given provisional diagnoses. For the item analysis they were replaced by two further patients. The second study (Study 2) which was done at the end of the main study, one year later, used the final version of the GMS and all five project psychiatrists from both the UK and US teams participated. One rater interviewed the patient while all the other psychiatrists observed. In this manner ten American and twelve British patients were interviewed.

Diagnostic agreement was studied first. As only the mental state of each patient was examined and no information made available on history, social situation, or physical state, the raters had only limited information with which to make a diagnosis. If anything, this ought to have restricted their agreement if it can be assumed that further information would have clarified rather than confused their task. The most stringent, but in the present state of knowledge, the most unrealistic agreement is that using the four digit code of the ICD. In Study one there was interviewer and observer agreement at this level on twelve of the 20 cases, but in Study 2 in only 38 per cent of diagnostic pairs (the interviewers diagnosis compared with that of each of his observing colleagues). The patients in Study 2, by common consent, posed exceptionally difficult diagnostic problems and tended to attract alternative diagnoses reflecting the rater's uncertainty. The diagnostic composition of the patients in these studies is reported elsewhere (Copeland *et al.*, 1976). Using six principal categories (affective disorder, schizophrenia and paranoid states, organic psychoses, alcoholism, neuroses and personality disorder, and 'other diagnoses'), agreement occurred in Study 1 for 17 out of the 20 patients and 69 per cent of pairs in Study 2. The participants were allowed to append an alternative diagnosis if they felt uncertain about the main diagnosis they had made. In the absence of additional data, especially history, distinctions between main and alternative diagnoses may be difficult. 'Partial' agreement was examined where one rater's main diagnosis was another's alternative diagnosis. For Study 1, at least partial agreement occurred for 19 of the 20 cases, and in Study 2 for 85 per cent of US pairs and 80 per cent of UK pairs. The equivalent figures for complete and partial agreements in the interview–reinterview comparison of Study 1 were eleven and 17 of the 20 cases respectively. On the whole diagnostic agreement was better for elderly patients than had been anticipated and was considered good in comparison with other studies of diagnostic reliability.

Next, the agreement on individual items or symptoms was examined. Using the total number of questions rated positively by each psychiatrist for each patient, the role taken by the psychiatrist, interviewer–observer or follow-up interviewer was shown to have little effect on the number of ratings made. The product–moment correlation coefficient between interviewer and observer for the total number of positive ratings was 0.87 and for the reinterview comparison 0.78. A multivariate analysis of variance carried out using the number of positive ratings made by each rater for each patient in the second study, showed no significant differences between American and British patients, between individual raters, nor between the US raters *versus* the UK raters in this respect, whereas a separate one way analysis treating the four sets of ratings for each patient as replicates, showed a highly significant difference between patients ($p < 0.001$).

In order to discover whether or not patient variables gave rise to a systematic lack of agreement between the raters, agreement indices, K, were calculated for each patient. K (Cohen, 1960) is defined as $K = (p_o - p_c)/(1 - p_c)p_o$ is the proportion of observed agreements between two raters, and pc the proportion of chance (expected) agreements; $+1$ represents perfect agreement between two raters; 0, chance agreement, and -1 complete disagreement, while a low K indicates a difficult case producing little inter-rater agreement.

For all items the mean value of K was 0.73, for the interviewer–observer comparison and 0.48 for interviewers *versus* reinterviewers, with ranges of

0·50–0·89 and 0·11–0·66 respectively. For elderly patients, whose mental state may fluctuate during the period immediately following admission to hospital, the initial *versus* the reinterview comparison was expected to produce less agreement. Behavioural and speech items produced less agreement than direct questions (the mean κ for the former were 0·56 and for the latter 0·80). There was a slight tendency for patients diagnosed as organic to produce more disagreements between raters than others.

No rater showed a consistent tendency to rate very high or very low on the number of positive ratings he made. But could the raters agree on which positive ratings to make? A calculation of the mean κ for all items within and between the teams, showed that agreement between teams was no worse than within teams and all κ were reasonably high. None of the differences between the mean figures for positive ratings was significant, so the five psychiatrists seemed to agree reasonably well between themselves.

It was likely that certain items in the schedule would consistently produce less agreement than others, to examine this weighted κ (Cohen, 1968) was used. This modification of κ takes into account the relative seriousness of particular disagreements, for example, if one rater had rated an item 'absent' and another 'present' in some degree, this would receive a higher disagreement weighting than if their ratings had agreed the item 'present', but they had rated different points on a quantitative scale. Similarly, differences involving adjacent points on a scale received a lower weighting than those involving non-adjacent points. Weighted κ were computed for each item, taken over the set of 18 patients. The mean values of weighted κ for the commonly used items with sufficient positive ratings were somewhat better for items in the main part of the schedule than those for the seventh edition of the present state examination used on patients aged 19–59 (Kendell *et al.*, 1968). As, in Kendell's study, reinterview κ were lower than those for the observer comparison and behavioural items lower than those in the main part of the schedule where only two questions had weighted κ of less than 0·50. Altogether the reliability of the individual items was considered satisfactory.

After the interview had been constructed and its reliability tested, it was used for a comparison of US and UK hospital admissions (to be described briefly below). A factor scoring procedure was developed using data from this study which enabled each patient's mental state to be described by determining his scores on 21 factors, approximating to the most important clinical symptoms. These factors provide an economical method, not only for examining the differences in symptoms between groups of patients and for their graphical display as symptom profiles but also for testing the clinical expectations regarding the clustering of symptoms against the more empirical findings of the factor analysis.

Because the sample of patients was comparatively small (100) a correlation procedure was used as well as a conventional factor analysis. Items in the GMS which had appeared in the factors in the original analysis of the combined mental state (younger age groups) were chosen as tentative factors. To these were added three more considered to be important for the elderly, and conveniently named, impaired memory, cortical dysfunction, and disorientation which were composed of

GMS items chosen by psychiatric judgement. Each patient received a score of the number of positive items for each tentative factor, and each item itself was correlated with each factor. The factor items were those which had the highest correlation with a given factor, provided that correlation reached at least 0·35, and its square was at least 50 per cent higher than the square of its correlation with any other factor. These new factors then replaced the tentative ones and the procedure was repeated. After five repetitions the change in factor items became small enough for the analysis to be stopped. The results were reviewed and any items completely at odds with clinical experience were eliminated, so that the remaining 21 factors represented clusters of items acceptable on both clinical and empirical grounds.

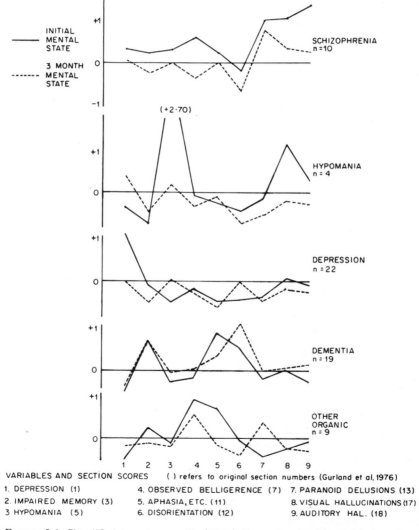

VARIABLES AND SECTION SCORES   ( ) refers to original section numbers (Gurland et al. 1976)

1. DEPRESSION (1)   4. OBSERVED BELLIGERENCE (7)   7. PARANOID DELUSIONS (13)
2. IMPAIRED MEMORY (3)   5. APHASIA, ETC. (11)   8. VISUAL HALLUCINATIONS (17)
3 HYPOMANIA (5)   6. DISORIENTATION (12)   9. AUDITORY HAL. (18)

FIGURE 9.1. Simplified symptom profile (GMS). Reproduced, with permission, from Gurland *et al.* (1976)

One example of the use of these derived factors can be given here and others will be referred to below. Figure 9.1 is drawn from the data from the study of US–UK hospital admissions. It shows the symptom profiles (much simplified by eliminating symptoms not relevant to the comparison) of two groups of patients, one diagnosed by the project as suffering from 'depressive illness' and the other from 'organic disorder'. The scores on each dimension are standardized on the geriatric sample to a mean score of 50.

The depression group shows more depressive mood, anxiety, somatic concerns, depersonalization and insight, and less non-social speech and cognitive dysfunction than the organic group. The scores on retardation of speech are nearly the same for each group and could be more a function of ageing, of illness, or of drug effects than of either depression or organic illness. The cognitive symptom which best separates the organic group from the depressive, is disorientation. This has been a consistent finding of these studies (Copeland et al., 1975a; Gurland et al., 1976).

Certain items sometimes regarded as features of normal ageing, such as the patients' assessment of difficulty with memory, concentration and recent slowness in thinking and bodily movement, are associated in these studies more with the factor of depression, rather than appearing as organic features, as are also loss of interest in entertainment and recreation, energy, sleep, and appetite disturbance. Thus, it would seem unwise to dismiss an elderly subject's complaints as simply being 'normal' for his age.

International agreement on psychiatric diagnosis

Having standardized a method for examining mental state and for making a diagnosis with acceptable reliability, it was now possible to study the reasons why certain countries, such as the United States and United Kingdom, differed in their reported statistics for mental illness. Such differences in the statistics could simply reflect different diagnostic criteria used by the psychiatrists who generated them, rather than true community differences, or the results of selective admission policies. If these differences between two countries sharing a common language and with many cultural similarities could be shown to arise because of different diagnostic criteria even more serious differences might be expected between psychiatrists working in more disparate cultures.

Similar studies had been carried out by the cross-national project for patients in the younger age group (19–59), between London and New York (Cooper et al., 1972) and between London and the West of Ireland (Kelleher et al., 1974). The first study had confirmed that Anglo-American differences had arisen because of different diagnostic criteria especially for the term schizophrenia but the second study had shown that Anglo-Irish differences were due to actual differences in hospital populations, thus requiring community studies for their further elucidation.

Over a decade and a half ago, Kramer (1961) had reported the important differences between the diagnostic frequencies for first admissions of the elderly to US and UK mental hospitals. Organic disorders appeared almost twice as frequently among US admissions than UK admissions, while functional diagnoses were apparently only about one-sixth the proportion found entering the UK hospitals. The possibility existed that numbers of functional, particularly depressed patients, were being diagnosed as organic in American hospitals. If diagnosis was used to indicate a regime of treatment, would the diagnosis of an organic condition in a patient suffering from depression tend to rule out antidepressant therapy or ECT and, therefore, lead to early deterioration, even death? In fact, death and discharge percentages within one year of admission to hospital for patients over 65, obtained from New York State (1968) and for 13 US states taken from an earlier unpublished study from the Biometrics Department of the NIMH (1960) tended to support this possibility. It appeared that patients admitted to US hospitals were twice as likely to die in the hospital within one year of admission than those admitted to British hospitals, and British elderly patients appeared three times more likely to be discharged within one year than their US counterparts. These figures could arise, either because the majority of patients entering US hospitals had a poor prognosis due to their being truly organic, or because misdiagnosis with a consequent failure to prescribe appropriate treatment led to early death. While discrepancies in the diagnostic frequencies for schizophrenia may be ascribed, in our present limited understanding, to differences in psychiatric definition, differences between organic and functional illness must reflect structural pathological changes and can be more confidently ascribed to 'misdiagnosis'.

In order to explore these questions further and also to provide data which would permit some validation of psychiatric diagnosis in this age group, the cross-national project undertook a comparative study of mental hospital admissions in two cities, New York and London. It was known that in London many elderly patients, particularly those with organic disorders, were admitted to geriatric hospitals only and, therefore, it was decided to take an additional sample of admissions from such a London hospital serving the same metropolitan area as the psychiatric hospitals. In New York these hospitals were generally not available and such patients, although often admitted to nursing homes were usually transferred to the mental hospitals eventually.

The measures and procedures adopted for the study have been described elsewhere (Copeland et al., 1975b) and, therefore, will only be briefly summarized here. The two areas chosen, Queens County in New York and the former Borough of Camberwell in London, tended to reflect their respective cities for the main demographic variables. The patients formed a consecutive series of admissions, 50 from Queens, but, in order to allow a comparison to be made between them, 75 each from psychiatric and geriatric facilities serving Camberwell. Each patient was interviewed by a project psychiatrist using the GMS and a history schedule. A series of psychological tests was selected (listed below) and given as a battery by a project psychologist. They were intended to validate the psychiatric diagnosis and so the results were not communicated to the psychiatric interviewers. The project social scientists collected sociocultural data and data on referral to hospital in subsequent interviews with both the patient and an informant. An independent physical examination was obtained on all patients in New York but on only 21 of the Camberwell psychiatric patients and eleven of the geriatric patients, for the rest, the physical examination performed by the hospital doctor was used, obtained from the case notes by a research worker without the hospital diagnosis being revealed to the project psychiatrists. A comparison between the project and hospital physical examinations for those patients who had received both, revealed only minor discrepancies.

Each patient was examined psychiatrically within 72 hours of admission to hospital and psychological and social measures were completed within a further few days. All measures were repeated one month and three months later, in hospital or at home if the patients had been discharged. In addition, those who showed evidence of organic symptoms during the first interview were reinterviewed using the GMS one week later in an attempt to distinguish transient confusional states from more chronic forms of organic illness. At each stage of the study a diagnosis for each patient was made using the criteria of the provisional WHO Glossary of Mental Disorders. In all, about 600 sets of interviews were undertaken. Each patient was discussed at two consensus meetings of the team, one at one month and one at three months after admission and a 'consensus diagnosis' agreed. At the second and final meeting the psychologists presented their evidence after the others had already reached a three month tentative diagnosis. The project and hospital diagnoses were kept separate at all stages and at no time were any findings discussed between the hospital and the project staff, except for two patients with seriously abnormal biochemical tests.

The results showed that the Camberwell, like the Queens sample, consisted mainly of white persons, but on the whole, tended to be a little older, to contain more women and to be of a slightly lower social class than the Queens sample.

A comparison of mental state items recalled the findings for the younger age group. The New York patients tended to have less pathology, possibly they under-reported their symptoms because they were more severely ill, and some had difficulty speaking English. The London patients had more depressive symptoms generally.

The diagnostic frequencies recorded by the hospitals on the study patients were not as extreme as those reported in the national statistics for the United States and the United Kingdom, as a whole, but are still considerable and significant (Table 9.1). 'Other diagnoses' includes personality disorder, alcoholism, neurotic conditions, and

TABLE 9.1. Percentage table. Comparison of diagnostic frequencies for patients over the age of 65 admitted to psychiatric hospitals in Queens County (New York) and Camberwell (London) compared with US and England and Wales

	US 1969 All admissions (%)	Queens hospitals (New York) (%)	Camberwell hospitals (London) (%)	England and Wales 1966 All admissions (%)
Organic	51·0	66·0	38·6	35·0
Affective	26·0	20·0	37·0	34·0
Schizophrenic	5·0	10·0	13·0	8·0
Others	18·0	4·0	11·0	23·0
Total	100·0	100·0	100·0	100·0

Reproduced by permission of *The British Journal of Psychiatry*.

in the UK 'paranoid' disorders. Table 9.2 shows a comparison of the project diagnoses for the same patients alongside those made by the hospitals. Apart from a tendency for there to be more organic cases in the Queens' sample, the differences between the project diagnoses are not significant. Differences in the national statistics are, therefore, not due to the patients but due to discrepancies between the terms used by their psychiatrists.

TABLE 9.2. Comparison of one-month Project consensus and hospital diagnoses for patients over the age of 65 admitted to psychiatric hospitals serving Queens (New York) and Camberwell (London)

| | Queens hospitals patients | | | | Camberwell hospitals patients | | | |
| | Hospital diagnoses | | Project diagnoses | | Project diagnoses | | Hospital diagnoses | |
	no.	%	no.	%	no.	%	no.	%
Organic	33	66·0	23	46·0	29	38·7	29	38·7
Affective	10	20·0	16	32·0	29	38·7	28	37·3
Schizo-								
phrenic	5	10·0	7	14·0	14	18·6	10	13·3
Other	2	4·0	4	8·0	3	4·0	8	10·7
Total	50	100·0	50	100·0	75	100·0	75	100·0

Reproduced by permission of *The British Journal of Psychiatry.*

Table 9.3 shows what happens if the psychiatric patients found in the geriatric hospital are added to the Camberwell psychiatric hospital sample. This cannot produce a group of patients entirely comparable to the US sample but goes some way towards it. It is remarkable how much closer the diagnostic frequencies between the two areas now become and emphasizes the importance of studies in the community in order to obtain true prevalence rates.

TABLE 9.3. Percentage table. All Camberwell geriatric patients with psychiatric diagnoses (including those in the geriatric wards), compared with Queens psychiatric patients

| • | Queens hospitals project diagnoses (psychiatric hospitals) $n = 50$ | | Camberwell hospitals project diagnoses (psychiatric and geriatric hospitals) $n = 123$ | |
	no.	%	no.	%
Organics	23	46·0	65	52·8
Affective	16	32·0	40	32·5
Schizophrenics	7	14·0	14	11·4
Others	4	8·0	4	3·3

Reproduced by permission of *The British Journal of Psychiatry.*

Where the diagnostic disagreements occur between hospital and project can be seen from Tables 9.4 and 9.5 which compare the results for the first 50 patients for each area (Copeland *et al.*, 1974). Table 9.4 shows the agreement between hospital and project in Camberwell. Although the proportions of each diagnostic group are similar, agreement on actual patients reached only 54 per cent. A finding similar to that of the earlier studies but never satisfactorily explained. Table 9.5 shows similar figures for Queens. Here the over-all agreement is slightly higher, 64 per cent. When the project makes a diagnosis of organic disorder, the hospital nearly always agrees.

TABLE 9.4. Comparison between project and hospital diagnoses for Camberwell

Project diagnosis	Hospital diagnoses				
	Organic	Affective	Schizophrenic	Other	Total
Organic	10	1	2	3	16
Affective	3	13	1	3	20
Schizophrenic	1	4	4	2	11
Other	1	2	—	—	3
Total	15	20	7	8	50

Reproduced by permission of The Canadian Psychiatric Association.

If the patients are simply divided into organic and non-organic, there is agreement between project and hospital diagnoses on over 75 per cent in both areas. Nevertheless, about one-quarter of those patients diagnosed by the Queens hospitals as organic were diagnosed by the project as either affective disorder or schizophrenia.

TABLE 9.5. Comparison between project and hospital diagnoses for Queens

Project diagnoses	Hospital diagnoses				
	Organic	Affective	Schizophrenic	Other	Total
Organic	22	—	—	1	23
Affective	5	8	3	—	16
Schizophrenic	3	1	2	1	7
Other	3	1	—	—	4
Total	33	10	5	2	50

Reproduced by permission of The Canadian Psychiatric Association.

Thus, further evidence has been adduced that sharp differences exist between US and UK psychiatrists in the diagnostic criteria they hold. Clearly US psychiatrists have a wider concept of organic illness or simply do not examine their patients with sufficient care to distinguish organic and functional conditions i.e. they make a misdiagnosis. Such a situation used to be more widespread in Britain before Post (1951), Roth and Morrisey (1952), and others drew attention to the importance of the distinction for both treatment and outcome. It is, of course, possible that US psychiatrists are guided more by the presence of certain symptoms to suggest treatment than the over-all diagnosis. For example, a patient showing depression could still receive appropriate antidepressant treatment even if the basic condition is misinterpreted as organic.

On the whole, the results of the follow-up study were equivocal, but in general there was a marked difference between the outcome of patients diagnosed by the project as organic, comparatively few of whom were discharged on either side, and who tended to have a higher death rate in the US hospitals, and those diagnosed as functional, 50 per cent of whom were discharged at three months when both samples are combined. However, rather more patients with functional illness were discharged in New York within three months of admission, 71 per cent compared to 23 per cent, and on the whole the scores for depressive mood fell further in New

York than the scores for similar patients in London. This could not be ascribed to specific treatment as only four of the 16 New York patients with a diagnosis by the project of affective disorder received antidepressant treatment, (Gurland *et al.*, 1976). The New York hospitals were geared to earlier discharge, possibly because some ten days after admission a decision must be made whether to discharge the patient home or transfer him to the local mental hospital.

The eight New York patients for whom there was serious diagnostic disagreement between project and hospital, the former ascribing a functional diagnosis, the latter organic, tended at three months to have an outcome like the other functional patients, thus lending support to the project diagnosis and to the notion that they were misdiagnosed by the Queens psychiatrists. However, although few of them seem to have received antidepressant treatment, this did not seem to prejudice their outcome, at least, for discharge.

Prevalence of diagnostic categories in hospital and community

Although psychiatrists from closely related cultures tend to disagree on the diagnostic criteria they use, psychiatrists in one part of London at least, seem to agree reasonably well. Two questions were now asked. To what extent do doctors who are aware of the need to recognize a psychiatric illness in the elderly, but who are not themselves psychiatrically trained, miss the diagnosis, and what is the actual prevalence of psychiatric diagnostic groups among the elderly in various clinical settings?

The study in the geriatric hospital has already been mentioned. It was conducted like the cross-natior.al study, except that the brisk admission rate dictated a random allocation of patients rather than a consecutive series. In addition, a consecutive series of 50 admissions to a geriatric day hospital and 50 to the general medical wards of a teaching hospital serving the same area of London as the geriatric and psychiatric hospitals were undertaken, followed by a pilot community study.

A diagnostic comparison of the psychiatric and geriatric hospitals for the 75 admissions to each can be seen in Table 9.6. In addition to physical illness there is a large proportion of psychiatric illness entering the geriatric hospital (65·9 per cent of new patients). The patients with senile dementia admitted to the psychiatric hospital had no physical illness requiring treatment while all but one admitted to the geriatric hospital did. Two-thirds of the patients diagnosed as having affective disorders entering the geriatric hospital were labelled depressive neurosis, whereas all such patients, except two entering the psychiatric hospital, were labelled manic depressive depressed. The patients in the geriatric facility tended to be discharged from hospital earlier than the others, probably because the depressive neurosis was reactive to the physical illness and recovered with it. Only one of the four patients labelled by the project, manic depressive depressed, and two of the eleven labelled depressive neurosis were diagnosed by the doctors in the geriatric hospital as depressed, two were given antidepressants and one minor tranquillizers. They were, however, those with more severe psychiatric illness.

This study provided an opportunity to examine to what extent psychiatric illness

TABLE 9.6. Percentage table. Comparison of psychiatric diagnostic frequencies found among patients aged over 65 admitted to a geriatric hospital, a geriatric day hospital, and general medicine wards with those entering the psychiatric hospitals serving the same area of London (Camberwell)

	Psychiatric hospitals $n = 75$	Geriatric hospitals $n = 73 + (2)^*$	Geriatric day hospital $n = 50$	General medical wards $n = 39 + (11)^*$
Affective disorder	38·7	15·1	30·0	30·8
Schizophrenia and paranoid states	18·7	0	0	0
Other functional	4·0	1·4	0	2·5
All functional	61·4	16·5	30·0	33·3
Senile dementia	22·6	13·7	30·0	2·5
Arteriosclerotic dementia	4·0	15·1	10·0	5·0
Other organic	12·0	20·6	2·0	13·0
All organic	38·6	49·4	42·0	20·5
No psychiatric diagnosis	0	34·1	28·0	46·2
All psychiatric illness	100	65·9	72·0	53·8

( )* No diagnosis possible due to severity of illness etc.

arising in the community tends to be misdiagnosed and elderly patients sent to the wrong hospital, geriatric or psychiatric, and whether such 'misplacement' adversely affected recovery. Using the same method of classification as that used by Kidd (1962) for convenience of comparison, only twelve per cent of patients in the geriatric hospital were considered 'probably misplaced', none 'definitely misplaced'; corresponding figures for the psychiatric hospital were 5·3 per cent and none respectively. The results of the one year follow-up study, consistent with the results of other studies (Mezey et al., 1968; Langley and Simpson, 1970) were unable to confirm that 'misplacement' prejudiced outcome. In fact, a review of the literature including Kidd's study seemed to indicate that there had never been convincing evidence to this effect. Kidd's original 'misplaced' patients were clearly very ill on all his measures and older than the others (Kidd, 1961), providing ample reason for their poor outcome without impugning different types of hospital care (Copeland et al., 1975a). It seems that given adequate pre-admission assessment, if necessary by both the psychiatric and geriatric team, an accurate diagnosis can be made for most patients and they can be correctly allotted to the appropriate facility. However, the geriatric staff while fully aware of the need to recognize depression were not always able to do so by themselves and treatment opportunities were lost. Thus, in service areas where geriatric and psychiatric facilities are adequate there is probably little need for psychogeriatric assessment units as such, while a strong case remains for joint treatment units. On the whole, a higher prevalence of psychiatric illness (mostly accompanying physical illness) was discovered than was expected among the geriatric admissions.

Similar results were obtained in a day hospital study. Although an active psychiatric day hospital exists in this part of London at the Maudsley Hospital, enquiry revealed that its treatment programmes did not cater for the elderly specifically and only a very few such patients had been admitted there of recent years. It seemed likely, therefore, that the geriatric day hospital serving the same catchment area was coping with a high proportion of psychiatric illness. One of the project's psychiatrists attended St. Francis Hospital each morning and interviewed a patient making his first attendance, using the geriatric screening schedule prepared by the project from the GMS. At his second attendance the patient was reinterviewed by another project psychiatrist using the GMS itself. Part of this exercise was to test the efficiency of the screening interview. In all 50 consecutive admissions were examined each by two psychiatrists (Copeland et al., 1973, 1976).

Once again a psychiatric diagnosis was made only when the group of symptoms fitted one of the descriptions to be found in the WHO Glossary of Mental Disorders. Table 9.6 shows that the proportion of patients given a psychiatric as well as a physical diagnosis (there are few persons of this age group to whom a physical diagnosis of some kind cannot be attached) was 72 per cent, not dissimilar to that found among admissions to the geriatric hospital. Affective disorders were more common in females, mainly as depressive neurosis. Manic depressive depressed diagnoses were similar for both sexes. As the proportion of elderly persons admitted to psychiatric day hospitals throughout the country is small (Department of Health and Social Security, 1969) it is likely that geriatric day hospitals are coping with considerable burdens of psychiatric illness. A strong case can be made both for increasing the psychiatric expertise available to the latter facility and for widening the scope of the psychiatric day hospital itself.

Because a large proportion of elderly persons are admitted to the general wards of any hospital, it is important to know to what proportion of these admissions a psychiatric diagnosis can be attached and whether such illnesses are recognized and treated. A random sample of 50 patients over the age of 65 with residence in the Camberwell area was selected from a consecutive series of admissions to medical wards of the Kings College Hospital group (Kings College, St. Giles, and Dulwich Hospitals). The proportion of patients taken from each hospital reflected the proportion of all elderly admissions to that hospital over the preceding year. Patients were interviewed within 72 hours of admission by a project psychiatrist using the GMS and a history schedule. The physical diagnosis, the findings of the physical examination and the medication prescribed were copied from the hospital case notes and ratings made of the degree of the patient's incapacity and the severity of his illness. The patients responses to the GMS initial items determined whether the rest of the interview was given. In eleven cases (22 per cent) either the severity of the physical illness or the patient's early death precluded a psychiatric diagnosis, leaving 39 patients in the study. Table 9.6 shows the diagnostic distributions. The proportion with a psychiatric illness is still high, about half the patients. As found in the day hospital about one-third have functional illnesses. In only two of the 21 cases diagnosed as having a psychiatric disorder was a psychiatric diagnosis recorded by the hospital in the case notes, and one of these did not agree with the project diagnosis. Only seven of the 21 cases were being treated with a psychotropic drug (two on antidepressants and five on minor tranquillizers). Thus, the majority of psychiatric disorders were unrecognized by the general physicians and as a consequence were not treated, at least in the early stages. The non-organic functional group had the highest rating for chronic physical incapacity. It is possible that psychiatric illness accompanying physical conditions may not respond well to drug therapy, nevertheless, it ought to be tried (Copeland *et al.*, 1973). Almost identical findings for the broad categories of psychiatric diagnoses in an 'acute medical unit in a general hospital' were found by Bergmann and Eastham (1974), dementia seven per cent, acute delusional states 19 per cent, and other functional 29 per cent, making a total morbidity of 52 per cent, compared with that of 53·8 per cent in the studies reported here.

The project, using its diagnostic procedures, is at present undertaking a comparative study of psychiatric illness and its relationship to physical illness, social factors and handicap among the elderly living in two communities, New York and London. Results for this study are not yet available but a pilot study carried out in London on a random sample of subjects taken from a sampling frame of family practioner lists yielded a tentative prevalence rate of for all types of mental illness in the community. This figure is 26 per cent.

Evaluation and validation of diagnostic procedures

The project asked four questions:

(1) Do the diagnostic groups recognized by psychiatrists, differ substantially from one another in their symptom patterns?
(2) Can they be tested against other methods of classification?
(3) Can they be used to predict outcome?
(4) Are groups derived mathematically similar to those derived by the psychiatrist from the same data: how do they, in turn, predict outcome?

Some partial answers to these questions can now be summarized.

The simplified symptom profiles for patients with schizophrenia, hypomania, depression, dementia, and 'other organic' illness can be seen in Figure 9.1. Insofar as the diagnosis was made by the same psychiatrist who recorded the symptoms, the two are not independent of one another. However, as the various symptoms are distributed throughout the interview and the rater is trained to assess each one in a standard manner, it is likely that some independence can be claimed. Sharp differences can be seen between the patterns for the diagnostic groups. The significance of differences between section scores for these groups was examined by an analysis of variance and a schaffe test procedure. The section scores for depression, hypomania, aphasia etc., disorientation, and paranoid delusions all reached the level of $p < 0.001$, auditory hallucinations $p < 0.002$, and impaired memory $p < 0.025$. The section scores for depression and disorientation showed differences between the diagnostic groups of depression and dementia at the $p < 0.001$ level and paranoid delusions distinguished between schizophrenia, dementia, other organic, and depression at $p < 0.001$ and auditory hallucinations between schizophrenia, dementia, and depression at p <0·002. Although appearing different graphically the diagnostic group hypomania contained too few patients for any comparison with other groups to reach significance. Figure 9.2 shows symptom profiles for patients on whom there was diagnostic disagreement between the project psychiatrists and the psychiatrists in the New York hospitals (Gurland *et al.*, 1976).

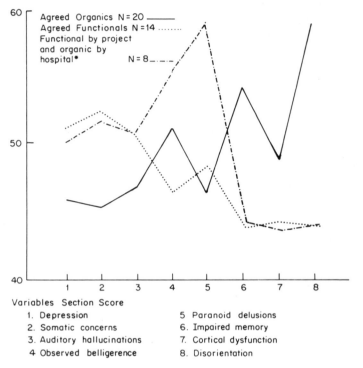

FIGURE 9.2. A comparison of patients agreed and disagreed to be either functional or organic by project and hospital psychiatrists in two New York hospitals. Reproduced, with permission, from Gurland *et al.* (1976)

On both the three cognitive components and the dimensions of depression, somatic concern, and auditory hallucinations, the disagreement group is seen to resemble the functional group, strongly suggesting that these cases are functional (as diagnosed by the project) and not organic (as diagnosed by the hospital). The disagreement group differs from the others by scoring highly on 'paranoid delusions' and 'observed belligerence'. The first may have been interpreted by the hospital psychiatrists as an organic symptom, for example, an elderly person who claims that others are stealing from him is judged to be actually losing his possessions as a result of his own forgetfulness, and the second, which generally indicates a hostile or unco-operative patient, may have made assessment difficult so that the hospital psychiatrists failed to elicit the functional symptoms. Thus, insofar as they can be regarded as independent, symptom profiles do show differences between the main diagnostic groups and can even help to indicate to the investigator why diagnostic disagreements arise.

The psychological tests used in the main study have already been mentioned. They were employed in order to test the validity of the psychiatric diagnoses in respect of organic and functional illness, firstly, by showing differences in test scores between the two groups and secondly, by revealing a differential improvement of those scores at follow-up. The study has been described in detail by Cowan and her colleagues (1975). Owing to the difficulty in testing the elderly and the need to have methods acceptable to both US and UK patients, only four psychological tests were used, the WAIS (vocabulary only, age-corrected subtest scores from this were transformed in order to give a rough index of pre-morbid intelligence level), Inglis paired associates learning test (PALT), the digit copying test (DCT) and the Bender gestalt test. Because many patients did not complete all the tests on all three assessments (refused, died etc.) the results were skewed and non-homogeneous in variance. For this reason non-parametric methods of analysis were used. The results showed that patients diagnosed by the psychiatrists as having dementia could be clearly distinguished from those diagnosed as suffering from affective disorders on both the PALT and DCT, while the Bender gestalt test discriminated both less consistently and less efficiently. An analysis of covariance, performed in order to take into account possible differences in score due to age and vocabulary, confirmed the original findings. A further analysis used the test scores themselves as independent criteria for allocating patients to diagnostic categories, subsequently comparing these allocations using M (Cohen, 1968), with those arrived at by the psychiatrists. A high rate of agreement was demonstrated. As expected, in the US disagreements were shown between psychological test results and hospital diagnosis for some of the dementing patients. The PALT classification disagreed with the hospital diagnosis on 32 per cent and 42 per cent of the patients called demented by the US hospital psychiatrists at initial and three month follow-up respectively. This, again, reflected the psychiatric results, in which the project psychiatrists disagreed with 48 per cent of the US hospital psychiatrists' diagnoses of dementia.

In all, the psychological test results successfully validate the psychiatric diagnosis by showing a highly significant difference between affective and demented patients as diagnosed by the project psychiatrists. There is also high agreement with their diagnoses when the patients were reallocated to diagnostic groups on the basis of their psychological test scores alone.

An attempt to validate the diagnosis of senile dementia by examining the hypo and hyper diploidy of genetic material in a joint study with the Genetics Unit at the Institute of Psychiatry, London, produced no confirmation of reports from smaller studies (Jarvik et al., 1962) that senile dementia in female patients could be distinguished by chromosomal fragmentation. The increasing prevalence of hyper diploidy with age was, however, confirmed and the chromosomes involved identified. This study will be reported in full elsewhere.

Can the outcome of the illness be predicted from its diagnosis? Post (1951), Roth and Morrisey (1952), showed in their studies that it could, that hospital death and discharge rates differentiate between effective and organic groups. It should be possible to demonstrate other changes over time. Quantifying symptoms at different time periods and displaying them in profile allows a graphic portrayal of their fluctuating intensities. For example, Figure 9.1 shows two profiles each for patients in five diagnostic groups, one for the initial interview and one for the three month follow-up. In general the fall in section scores after three months is in the direction expected. As anticipated the fall in the depression score over three months for the depression diagnostic group, and that for aphasia etc. for the 'other organic' group (mainly acute organic confusional states) were significant (both $p < 0.01$), whereas neither of these scores changed significantly for dementia.

Psychiatric diagnosis is, therefore, supported by changes in symptom profile over time. Although less dramatic, these changes received further support from the scores on the psychological tests recorded at follow-up. (Cowan et al., 1975). For the initial, nonparametric analysis, no greater improvement appeared in the change scores of patients with affective disorder than in those with organic disorder.

Some confirmation of psychiatric diagnosis was also obtained from a follow-up study using the Camberwell Register (Wing et al., 1968). During the first year 83 per cent of the patients admitted to the Camberwell psychiatric hospitals with affective disorders were discharged at least once during the year, compared with only 35 per cent of demented patients. In all, the mean number of days spent in hospital for the affective patients still alive at two years was 266, while that for the demented patients was 597 ($p < 0.002$). Death rates did not differentiate between the two groups at two years, probably because the demented patients tended to be only mildly ill on admission (Copeland et al., 1975).

The Wolfe formal mixture analysis procedure (NORMIX) was used to obtain preliminary clusters from the 75 patients admitted to the psychiatric hospital in London. After the elimination of nine patients with outlying scores (high on all forms of beligerence, alcohol abuse, and visual hallucinations), the remaining patients formed four clusters. This four group solution proved the best (the likelihood of there being more than these four groups was tested and found not to be significant, and discriminant function calculated between the groups revealed a remarkably high degree of separation). Of the 22 members of Group 1, 21 were organic (18 dementia and two confusional states), and of the five members of Group 3, four had a diagnosis of manic depressive depressed. Group 2 consisted mainly of mild depression but with some early dementia and schizophrenia. Group 4 was a mixture of patients, the members scoring highly on retarded speech or hypomania. Thus, most cases of dementia (90 per cent) and severe depression are clearly distinguished by the clustering procedure. A more complete analysis using a larger number of subjects and related outcome data will be reported.

Summary and conclusions

In common with other phenomena, mental illness must be identified before it can be classified and classified before it can be examined, or its aetiology and requirements determined. To achieve this, firstly, a hypothesis concerning the nature of the illness must be set up, which is open to empirical testing, and in turn to modification. The traditional model established by hospital based psychiatrists and formalized in the WHO International Classification of Disease and Glossary of Mental Disorders was chosen as the starting point. Evidence is available that this classification is clinically useful.

Secondly, reliable methods of qualitative and quantitative recording must be devised for illness behaviour. A structured interview following the pattern of those used by Wing, Spitzer, and their colleagues, for younger age groups, was drawn up and tested. Using this interview, further evidence was produced supporting the validity of these diagnostic groups by demonstrating distinctive and consistent symptom differences in their mean group profiles, differential outcome at follow-up and some correspondence between psychiatric and computer groupings. This interview is now used in other centres.

The success of psychiatrists and other doctors in identifying and classifying mental illness in the elderly using the model their forebears had developed was the subject of other studies described. The US–UK national statistics for the elderly showed a high proportion of organic cases among US first admissions to mental hospitals. The project working in one area of New York attributed this finding to the misdiagnosis of functional illness. Although this misdiagnosis probably results in a failure to treat many cases of depression in the New York hospitals it is not reflected in increased death rate within three months of admission or in delayed discharge. On the contrary, the New York hospitals discharged more patients within three months than their London counterparts, not that speed of discharge is necessarily evidence of therapeutic excellence. Further studies in London showed that a geriatric hospital, a geriatric day hospital and general medical wards handled many psychiatric conditions. Although the medical staff are aware of the problem, they fail both to recognize and to treat many of these conditions. Other studies made it clear that psychiatric illness can be recognized in the elderly and diagnosed accurately by both clinical psychiatrists and geriatric physicians, even on domiciliary visit, provided they make an adequate clinical assessment. A patient misdiagnosed and sent to the wrong type of hospital did not appear to suffer the catastrophic outcome reported by some earlier studies, based on what seems to have been a misinterpretation of data. It was concluded that for adequately staffed areas of the country, the evidence is against the usefulness of psychogeriatric assessment units of the kind suggested in Britain and in favour of treatment units administered jointly by geriatric and psychogeriatric staff.

To study mental illness in isolation from the many factors which influence it, is clearly unsatisfactory, and perpetuates the artifical divisions created for administrative convenience. A widower's painful knees which prevent him walking, restrict the people he sees and result in his feeling sad, failing to sleep at night, and requiring someone to do his shopping, represent a complex interaction of physical, psychological, and social factors, of cause and affect, which can only profitably be studied by the multidimensional attack. Outside hospital the need to intervene in order to prevent or treat an illness which has not yet emerged as a clear diagnosable syndrome may be judged by the social disability as well as the personal distress it causes and the success of its treatment by the degree of residual social handicap.

It follows that advances in psychiatric care and research into causality require reliable quantitative measures of social and physical disability, total handicap and degree of chronicity. With these measures it becomes possible to penetrate the other administrative divisions between institutional and community residence. In the community, untrammelled by extraneous selection procedures and by using repeatable methods, key questions can be asked about the meaning of illness. The cross-national project in its present studies is trying to tackle some of these. For example, to what extent can the concept of disease, useful in hospital practice, be applied outside? To what extent is both the cause and the form of a psychiatric illness determined by the social milieu of the patient and the life events which have occurred during the immediate or more distant periods of his lifespan. What are the criteria, social and otherwise, likely to play a part in deciding the level of disability necessitating care and what factors are associated with its becoming chronic? A study conducted as the cross-national project in two countries with basic cultural similarities but with striking differences in their social environment and health care facilities should help to elucidate those aspects of illness which are dependent and those which are independent of their respective cultures, suggest improvements to the services, and indicate areas for social change.

References

Bergmann, K., and Eastham, E.J. (1974) 'Psychogeriatric ascertainment and assessment for treatment in an acute medical ward setting', *Age and Ageing*, **3**, 174–188.

Cohen, J. (1960) 'A coefficient of agreement for nominal scales', *Educat. Psychol. Measur.*, **20**, 37–46.

Cohen J. (1968) 'Weighted kappa: nominal scale agreement with provision for scaled disagreement or partial credit', *Psychol. Bull.*, **70**, 213–220.

Cooper, J.E., Kendell, R.E., Gurland, B.J., Sharpe, L., Copeland, J.R.M., and Simon, R. (1972) *Psychiatric diagnosis in New York and London*, Maudsley Monograph No. 20, London, Oxford University Press.

Copeland, J.R.M., Kelleher, M.J., Kellett, J.M., Barron, G., Cowan, D.W., and Gourlay, A.J. (1975a) 'Evaluation of a psychogeriatric service: the distinction between psychogeriatric and geriatric patients', *Br. J. Psychiat.*, **126**, 21–29.

Copeland, J.R.M., Kelleher, M.J., Kellett, J.M., Gourlay, A.J., Cowan, D.W., Barron, G., and De Gruchy, J. (1973) 'Studies supported by the Department of Health and Social Security', US–UK Diagnostic Project 1971–1973, Submitted to the Department of Health, May 1973, pp.94 (not published).

Copeland, J.R.M., Kelleher, M.J., Kellett, J.M., Gourlay, A.J., Barron, G., Cowan, D.W., De Gruchy, J., Gurland, B.J., Sharpe, L., Simon, R., Kuriansky, J., and Stiller, P. (1974) 'Diagnostic differences in psychogeriatric patients in New York and London', *Canad. Psychiat. Assoc. J.*, **19**, 267–271.

Copeland, J.R.M., Kelleher, M.J., Kellett, J.M., Gourlay, A.J., Barron, G., Cowan, D.W., De Gruchy, J., Gurland, B.J., Sharpe, L., Simon, R., Kuriansky, J., and Stiller, P. (1975b) 'Cross-national study of diagnosis of the mental disorders: a comparison of the diagnosis of elderly psychiatric patients admitted to mental hospitals serving Queens County in New York and the old Borough of Camberwell, London', *Br. J. Psychiat.*, **126**, 11–20.

Copeland, J.R.M., Kelleher, M.J., Kellett, J.M., Gourlay, A.J., Gurland, B.J., Fleiss, J.L., and Sharpe, L. (1976) 'A semi-structured clinical interview for the assessment of diagnosis and mental state in the elderly. The geriatric mental state schedule. 1. Development and reliability', *Psychol. Med.*, **6**, 439–449.

Copeland, J.R.M., Kelleher, M.J., and Waring, E.H. (in press) 'Studies of elderly patients in hospital facilities in London, a general medical ward and a geriatric day hospital', *Internat. J. Ageing Hum. Develop.*, (in press).

Cowan, D.W., Copeland, J.R.M., Kelleher, M.J., Kellett, J.M., Gourlay, A.J., Smith, A., Barron, G., and De Gruchy, J., with Kuriansky, J., Gurland, B.J., Sharpe, L., Stiller, P., and Simon, R. (1975) 'Cross-national study of the diagnosis of the mental disorders: a comparative psychometric assessment of elderly patients admitted to mental hospitals serving Queens county New York, and the former Borough of Camberwell, London', *Br. J. Psychiat.*, **126**, 560–570.

Department of Health and Social Security (1969) Statistical Report series No. 7 *Pilot survey of patients attending day hospitals*, London, HMSO.

Fleiss, J.L., Gurland, B.J., and Cooper, J.E. (1971) 'Some contributions to the measurement of psychopathology', *Br. J. Psychiat.*, **119**, 647–656.

Gurland, B.J., Fleiss, J.L., Goldberg, K., Sharpe, L., Copeland, J.R.M., Kelleher, M.J., and Kellett, J.M. (1976) 'A semi-structured clinical interview for the assessment of diagnosis and mental state in the elderly. The geriatric mental state schedule. 2. A factor analysis', *Psychol. Med.*, **6**, 451–459.

Jarvik, L.F., Kallmann, F.J., and Falik, A. (1962) 'Psychiatric genetics and ageing', *The Gerontologist*, **2**, 164–166.

Kelleher, M.J., Copeland, J.R.M., and Smith, A.M.R. (1974) 'High first admission rates for schizophrenia in Ireland: their relationship to diagnosis', *Psychol. Med.*, **4**, 460–462.

Kendell, R.E., Everitt, B., Cooper, J.E., Sartorius, N., and David, M.E. (1968) 'The reliability of the present state examination', *Soc. Psychiat.*, **3**, 123–129.

Kidd, C.B. (1961) M.D. thesis, Queen's University, Belfast.

Kidd, C.B. (1962) 'Criteria for the admission of the elderly to geriatric and psychiatric units', *J. Ment. Sci.*, **108**, 68–74.

Kramer, M. (1961) 'Some problems for international research suggested by observations on difference in first admission rates to the mental hospitals of England, Wales and the United States', in *proceedings of the Third World Congress of Psychiatry*. Vol. 3, Montreal, pp.153–160.

Langley, G.E., and Simpson, J.H. (1970) 'Misplacement of the elderly in geriatric and psychiatric hospitals', *Geront. Clin. (Basel)*, **12**, 149–163.

Mezey, A.G., Hodkinson, H.M., and Evans, G.J., (1968) 'The elderly in the wrong unit', *Br. Med. J.*, **iii**, 16–18.

Post, F. (1951) 'The outcome of mental breakdown in old age', *Br. Med. J.*, **1**, 436–448.

Roth, M., and Morrisey, J.D. (1952) 'Problems in the diagnosis and classification of mental disorders in old age', *J. Ment. Sci.*, **98**, 66–80.

Spitzer, R.L., Fleiss, J.L., Burdock, E.J. and Hardesty, A.S. (1964) 'The mental status schedule: rationale, reliability and validity', *Comprehensive Psychiat.*, **5**, 384–395.

Wing, J.K., Birley, J.L.T., Cooper, J.E., Graham, P., and Isaacs, A.D. (1967) 'Reliability of a procedure for measuring and classifying "present psychiatric state" ', *Br. J. Psychiat.*, **113**, 499–515.

Wing, L., Bramley, C., Hayley, A., and Wing, J.K. (1968) 'Camberwell cumulative psychiatric case register. Part I, aims and methods', *Soc. Psychiat.*, **3**, 116–122.

Wolfe, J.H. (1970) 'Pattern clustering by multivarate mixture analysis', *Mult. Behav. Res.*, **5**, 329–350.

10

THE GERIATRIC PHYSICIAN'S ROLE IN ASSESSMENT AND MANAGEMENT

D.N. Prinsley

Geriatric medicine is all too often complicated by the presence in one patient of several disorders both of health and social surroundings. The geriatric physician recognizes that a multitude of factors are involved in the breakdown of health of old people. The failings of old age in the form of decreasing mobility and mental agility may be aggravated by new surroundings and lack of companions and the effects of isolation and loneliness may unmask mental deterioration to the extent that behaviour becomes abnormal. Old people living with relatives, when handled with lack of sympathy and understanding, may become unacceptable because of determined or defensive behaviour. Mental equilibrium is easily upset by a strange environment and admission to hospital for a valid physical disease may cause an intense behaviour disturbance. Brain failure due to neuronal degeneration or to arteriosclerotic disease is common; properly prescribed drugs may produce unexpected psychiatric responses, and failing faculties, especially hearing, may lead to aggression. The geriatrician becomes accustomed to patients who are disturbed or demented in addition to all their other problems.

The frequency of abnormal behaviour in old people is such that an organized service is necessary to enable accurate assessment to be made. Attempts to manage disturbed patients in ordinary acute wards or to manage physically ill patients in psychiatric units are not satisfactory. There is now a changing pattern in hospitals which indicates that geriatric units will play an increasing role in the care of cases of brain damage and psychiatric units will be involved mainly with functional disorders. In response to this development it is advantageous for a geriatric department to have an area allocated to the needs of psychogeriatric patients. Here it should be possible to carry out treatment of physical disease of all degrees of severity and, at the same time, manage any disturbance of behaviour. Patients suffering from brain failure can be admitted to such a unit in the first place and can, if necessary, be subsequently moved to other parts of the hospital when settled.

A geriatric patient may suffer from several diseases simultaneously, some of which are ignored or go unnoticed, but the presence of any organic disease must be taken into consideration when dealing with mental disturbance. Sudden onset of delirium should always prompt a search for a physical disorder. Correction, if possible, of physical disorders, in such circumstances will lead to rapid recovery from the delirium. Acute hospital wards can usually manage to cope successfully with short term disturbance associated with shock due to a coronary thrombosis or haemorrhage or acute retention of urine because these conditions respond readily to treatment with a rapid return of mental equilibrium. However, many diseases produce mental disturbance which is prolonged because the illness itself is likely to persist over many days. Congestive heart failure, pneumonia, severe anaemia, uraemia, and myxoedema come to mind as causes of mental disturbance which, although they may respond to treatment, will not recover rapidly. In such circumstances the general physician in a general medical ward may be faced with a difficult situation and, similarly, the geriatrician is equally embarrassed. Recognition of the physical disorder causing the disturbance is of prime importance but the management and treatment of such a patient may require specialized skills and equipment. Patients suffering severe illness may die before the disease comes under control but it is equally clear that many of these patients with mental disturbance, provided they can be nursed through their physical illness, will be restored to normal mental health. Mental disturbance in ill old people and the problems thus created in a general ward requires facilities which allow nursing care to continue without disturbing others.

The geriatrician must also treat a varying pattern of mental deterioration accompanying degenerative disorders. The effects of cerebral arteriosclerosis may be either dramatic and sudden or quite gradual in effect. The onset of a stroke occasionally causes a long continued psychiatric disturbance. There may be great intellectual loss but, apart from early restlessness and noisiness, the behaviour pattern does not often require special management. Many patients who have suffered a stroke become depressed and need suitable reassurance and the use of mood elevating drugs. Some stroke patients become over confident and unable to recognize their disability. Frustration due to aphasia may cause anger and resentment but, with intelligent recognition of the problem, this state can usually be relieved. A small number of stroke victims, usually with extensive paralysis, seem to lose all inhibitions and, although not demented in the true sense of the word, may become very demanding and noisy, having outbursts of temper which make their management difficult. Such patients, if in need of extended care, can be disturbing to other long term nursing cases and may need some form of segregation.

Arteriosclerotic dementia may be recognized by the history and the pattern of development of the dementia. There is usually evidence of widespread arteriosclerosis with abnormalities in the central nervous system and a history of repeated episodes, with or without minor paralysis, which suggest cerebral infarctions. Each episode, if it can be identified, tends to lead to a step-like deterioration in mental capacity although the progression of the disease is not always so clear cut. Nevertheless, patients with cerebral arteriosclerosis may have good periods, especially early in the day when they are quite rational and not confused or disturbed. As the day goes on the behaviour pattern tends to deteriorate until by teatime patients become confused and disorientated and incapable of coherent conversation. Assessment of dementia using dementia scales is somewhat unreliable as the results will vary so much with the state of the patient at the time the test is carried out. Patients with arteriosclerotic dementia are particularly prone to become acutely disturbed with some intercurrent illness, often of a quite minor nature such as an attack of diarrhoea or a head cold and come to the attention of the doctor only when such an episode occurs, although relatives and often the patient, have been well aware of progressive mental deterioration.

In senile dementia there is a steady and unremitting deterioration of intellectual powers until the patient is unable to put a sentence together and unable to recognize close relatives. The physical state may remain relatively good and the patient ambulant and continent but attention to personal hygiene soon disappears and lack of cleanliness and incontinence develops at a later stage. The length of history is several years and symptoms may have been noticed some four or five years before major behaviour problems are presented. A good caring family can cope with a case of slowly progressive senile dementia for a long time until elements of risk or danger are introduced by the patient's irrational and unsafe behaviour with fire and cookers, and in traffic. Night wandering in the house and wandering during the day can be the final straw which breaks the back of a caring family until they can no longer tolerate what has been an almost unbearable situation.

The behaviour of a case of senile dementia is constant and unvarying during the day when compared with arteriosclerotic dementia patients who often have long periods of relative lucidity. It is also noteworthy that the state of the central nervous system of patients with senile dementia is usually normal. Because the age group of senile dementia is the same as arteriosclerotic disease, arteriosclerosis and senile dementia may coexist and a patient with senile dementia can equally be affected by a sudden stroke or evidence of cerebral arteriosclerosis. It is however, important to differentiate between cases of arteriosclerotic dementia and senile dementia because the behaviour pattern can be predicted, the prognosis can be given to the family and the pattern of future care arranged. Arteriosclerotic cases tend to deteriorate steadily in general health and can be expected to have further episodes of cerebral infarction. Senile dementia patients, however, although the long term prognosis does not seem to be very different, may remain active and a management problem almost until their time of death. Active wandering senile dementia patients may need some form of secure environment to protect them from hazard and are less likely to respond to tranquillization.

Elderly patients with a prolonged preceding history of psychiatric illness who are under reasonable control in a domestic environment may become acutely disturbed when physical illness intervenes. The problem of management of the physical illness may then cause considerable concern in units more accustomed to dealing with acute medical and surgical problems. Emergency surgical treatment of elderly psychotic patients can also present problems of post operative management which may need removal from a surgical ward to a psychogeriatric unit.

Recognition of depression in the elderly is of great importance because relief from one or more of the many adverse factors involved in the onset of depression may be more effective than the exhibition of psychotropic drugs. It should also be remembered that agitation is often a feature of depression in old people. Whilst it is clear that the majority of cases of affective disorder in old age will be in the care of psychiatric units, the geriatrician should be able to manage affectively ill patients suffering from systemic illnesses which require general hospital facilities for investigation and treatment.

Organic neurological disease in old age may be accompanied by psychiatric abnormality. Epileptic fits can be differentiated from other causes of loss of consciousness, but temporal lobe attacks may be classified as dementia or otherwise wrongly diagnosed because the true nature of the disorder has not been recognized. Survival into old age is now occurring in cases of spastic diplegia and also cases of Down's syndrome. Finding a suitable ward for treatment when physical illness overtakes these patients can be a problem. The manifestations of organic disease affecting the brain can be quite bizarre. Elderly patients with primary or secondary cerebral tumours, neurosyphilis, subarachnoid haemorrhage and multiple sclerosis may become very disturbed. Huntington's chorea, a disease of middle age, may come under the management of a geriatrician largely because of the chronicity of the disorder. The long term management of these patients as they become increasingly disabled and demented is always difficult.

Recognition of drug intoxication is of importance because so many elderly patients are supplied with a vast armamentarium of tablets and may be on two or three psychotropic drugs in addition to other powerful and possibly disturbing drugs. This is not always the fault of the medical attendant. Elderly patients tend to keep supplies of tablets and become confused in self medication and take tablets in a haphazard fashion. Stopping all medication may well have completely curative effects. Antiparkinsonian drugs, now powerful and effective in combating the effects of the disease, are liable to cause hallucinations and agitation. Intoxication with tranquillizers comes about all too readily when a small dose is prescribed which is insufficient to achieve the desired therapeutic response and results in further agitation and subsequent overdose. Regrettably, barbiturates are still prescribed for old people because there has been failure to realize that excretion of barbiturates in the elderly is unreliable. Bromides are still very occasionally prescribed with the almost forgotten intoxication of bromism. Alcoholic intoxication is common and the results of treatment are as disappointing in the older age group as in the younger, with the inevitable subsequent relapse. The geriatrician is always aware that drugs given for good reasons may cause unsuspected disturbance of behaviour in the elderly. It is of key importance that, when a patient is seen as an outpatient or admitted to hospital, the entire drug supply in use should be brought to the hospital for identification and consideration.

Consultations with the geriatrician or admission to hospital may be the result of quite genuine mistakes. Deafness can result in the patient's apparently irrational behaviour and, similarly, blindness can also suggest the presence of dementia. Failure to recognize cerebral thrombosis with minimal paralysis but major speech disturbance can lead to error. Wilful misbehaviour by an elderly patient as a protest to unkindness or neglect can similarly lead to mistakes. It is advisable to assess the motivation of relatives who recount a florid story of misbehaviour of an elderly patient which proves, after observation in suitable surroundings, to be exaggerated. Hysterical illness in the elderly is rare, but a form of invalidism is well recognized where there is not physical reason for disability. This condition depends on the presence of an ever loving and caring relative in the household. The alleged sufferer relapses into a state of invalidism and only comes to attention, possibly years later, when the caring relative is struck down by a sudden illness and the long term invalid then requires admission to hospital. Full examination and investigation fails to reveal any disease. Nevertheless, rehabilitation of such a patient is virtually impossible. The condition seems to be more prevalent in rural communities when caring relatives are more common. Many titles have been given to this disorder. In North Yorkshire everyone is aware of what is meant by 'the Cleveland syndrome', referring particularly to the more rural districts.

The part played by the geriatrician in the medical management of a disturbed or demented patient in the early stages is concerned with advice and support, mainly for the family. Frequent supervision in an outpatient clinic or by home visit will give the relatives a feeling of security and at the same time will enable observation of the disease pattern to be more accurate. When tranquillizing drugs are necessary the dosage level is probably best worked out by a sensible relative who is able to assess the desired effect and is able to adjust the dose to avoid too much sleepiness. Hypnotics to ensure a good night's sleep should be of the simplest type and the use of alcohol in the evening should not be forgotten. Attendance of a disturbed or demented patient at the day hospital may be helpful in giving relatives some relief and a feeling that the patient is under supervision. However, day hospital attendance is not often successful and the patient may return home in the evening rather more disturbed than he would have been without the outing. Where management in the community becomes too difficult because of disturbed behaviour, aggressiveness, noisiness and nocturnal restless, admission to hospital for assessment and treatment is required. The benefits of management in a specialized psychogeriatric unit are derived from the skills and experience of staff accustomed to dealing with disturbed patients, in addition to application of treatment for the wide variety of physical disease which may coexist. More accurate diagnosis can be reached and treatment carried out unflustered by the patient's behaviour. Confident nursing produces a calming effect of great value in management. Assistance and advice from a psychiatrist may be required and must be available, but the main workload is carried by the geriatrician, treating the effects of physical and degenerative diseases.

Equipment and facilities for a psychogeriatric ward are comprehensive and comfortable but not complex. Single rooms assist in the early management of the patients. A few hospital beds of variable height type are needed for those with physical illness requiring much nursing care. The majority of the patients in the psychogeriatric unit are better supplied with beds of the divan type from which there is little danger of accidental falls. Cot sides should never be used for agitated patients as a means of restraint but may be needed for a patient who is restless during sleep and who may fall out of bed. Waist band restrainers are rarely needed for restless and insecure patients who may fall out of chairs. Geriatric chairs which can be tilted backwards at any angle are effective and more acceptable than retaining trays clamped across the front of upright geriatric chairs. The Buxton pattern chair manufactured by G. McLoughlin and Co Ltd, Victoria Works, Oldham Road, Rochdale, Lancashire, England, is comfortable and safe for patients and favourably regarded by nurses who are satisfied that the patient is not physically restrained but cannot fall out of the chair. Simplified eating utensils and crockery used in geriatric units for disabled patients are often appropriate as demented patients revert to a very primitive form of feeding, or may need feeding by nursing staff. Melaware Manoy tableware consisting of shaped plates with high sides and specially adapted cutlery is suitable and is manufactured by Antiference Ltd, Bicester Road, Aylesbury, Buckinghamshire, England. Use of non-slip mats under the plates gives further improvement in feeding arrangements. Dycem non-slip pads are obtainable from Dycem Plastics Ltd, Chapter Street, Portland Square, Bristol, BS2 8SE, England. Lavatories should be large, allowing nursing staff to accompany the patient where necessary and assist with toileting. Adequate stocks of attractive clothing will be needed to deal with the many incontinent patients in such a unit as personal appearance and cleanliness are of great importance in restoring the patient's self respect. The simplest form of security for such a unit should be available but rarely used and only brought into action where ingenious and persistent wandering causes danger to patients. A garden which is accessible from the ward and yet is securely but unobtrusively fenced can be a useful addition allowing patients to wander at will and avoid the disturbing effect of restlessness within the ward.

Nursing management in the psychogeriatric unit requires continuous maintenance of a calm, relaxed atmosphere. This can only be achieved if the nurses are confident of their own ability and know the nature of the problem and the disease pattern. Maximum reassurance of the patient by the nurses is given at all stages. Collection of information about the background and history of the disease is achieved by the nurses' skill in dealing with relatives, social workers, and other community staff. Maintenance of ambulation and activity and establishment of a regular pattern of the patient's day must take place as soon as possible. Simple persuasion is needed to help the patient deal with his frustrations. Special problems arise in nursing procedures particularly with administration of drugs, which should be given in fluid form, if possible. Where there is refusal by the patient the nurse should never argue but re-present the medicine some short time later when there is usually acceptance. Fluid intake must be kept at a high level especially when tranquillizers are in use. Observation of the patients must be meticulous because of the indifference to pain so often found in demented patients who may develop an acute condition without voicing any complaint. A nurse should see the relatives at frequent intervals to maintain contact with the home and to educate the family for future care of the patient. Visiting should be unlimited, outings encouraged, and family involvement maintained. Relatives visiting a demented patient will accept the disability of their own parent but are distressed by the sight of other patients with dementia. Arrangements should be available for visiting to take place in a small day room or the patient's own bedroom in this situation. As far as possible, patients should have their own personal marked clothing and all loose pieces of equipment such as dentures or calipers must be marked with the owner's name. The ratio of nursing staff to patients in a psychogeriatric unit should be at a higher level than any other acute ward (Prinsley, 1974).

Occupational therapists are essential in the management of psychogeriatric patients, especially in the establishment of regular patterns of behaviour, individually or in groups. Demented patients will, after a time, co-operate in ward activities and recreation, if encouraged with skill and patience. The benefits of sustained activity are then seen. It is helpful to have easily separated areas in day rooms to permit a variety of activities. Participation and assistance in ward activities by the patients' relatives should be encouraged. Passive entertainment is rarely helpful but increasing interest and attention to the television set is a sign of improvement. Physiotherapy and speech therapy should be available when necessary.

The aim of treatment by the geriatrician is to relieve physical disease and control psychiatric disturbance to make the patient manageable either at home or, if hospital care is required, in an ordinary ward. The majority of psychogeriatric patients admitted to a specialized unit can be discharged or moved to an ordinary geriatric ward. In a study of 700 admissions to a psychogeriatric unit 196 deaths took place in the unit, 229 patients were discharged home or to convalescence awaiting admission to social services accommodation, 133 patients became fit for transfer to ordinary wards for continuing treatment and subsequent discharge, 126 patients required long term nursing care in geriatric long stay wards. Twenty-six patients had to be transferred to a psychiatric unit (Prinsley, 1973).

Many admissions to a psychogeriatric unit are suffering from such severe physical disease that they die within a short period of time. Patients who require continued nursing care after the initial period of treatment in the psychogeriatric unit do so for reasons of physical disability rather than psychiatric disturbance. If the psychogeriatric unit is used as an admission and initial treatment unit which had ready access to other acute wards then the turnover will be high because the response to treatment is usually quite rapid and patients can be moved to ordinary wards as soon as the psychiatric disturbance is over. Experience has shown that a 24 bed unit is able to deal with the psychogeriatric cases in the average district general hospital catchment area covering a population of 250 000 to 300 000 with approximately eleven per cent over the age of 65. Few elderly patients admitted to a psychogeriatric unit are so unmanageable that removal to a psychiatric hospital is necessary. The troublesome group which might require more secure surroundings consists of the persistent wanderers, the very aggressive, strong patients, and male strippers.

The points of improvement which have been noted in the psychogeriatric patients have been obvious diminution of noisiness, wandering tendency and aggressive behaviour with control of the presenting breakdown symptoms. Lessening incontinence and pride in cleanliness and personal appearance and clothing are signs of improvement as well as an increased interest in surroundings, conversation with neighbours and attention to diversional therapy and television programmes. After a period in the psychogeriatric unit where the psychiatric disturbance has been controlled the patient may require further prolonged treatment in a geriatric ward with subsequently follow up. Patients discharged from the psychogeriatric unit to their own home surroundings need follow-up management at frequent intervals. Some may need day hospital attendance. The family must be reassured that help will always be available. Repeated admissions and holiday admissions help to maintain the family unit. The drug regime may require modification. Rehousing or supervision in warden accommodation may have to be arranged. Discharge to institutional care under the social services may be appropriate where family support is lacking.

The wide variety of problems which are presented will clearly have a varying pattern of development. Patients who need admission because of an acute psychiatric disturbance brought on by physical illness have a poor prognosis mainly due to the severity of the physical illness. If they survive the physical illness the outlook for their mental health is usually reasonably good. Cases of arteriosclerotic dementia and senile dementia can often be returned to the community when the breakdown symptom has been controlled but survival for both groups of patients is only poor and there will be inevitable deterioration requiring readmission. The aim must always be to control symptoms to produce a worthwhile life, not just to achieve survival. Provided that a policy is maintained of using the psychogeriatric unit as an acute admission and assessment ward for initial treatment, constantly aiming for improvement and discharge of the patient either home or to an ordinary ward, then there will be continuous effectiveness.

A geriatrician has always under his care a large number of mentally frail patients, either in acute and rehabilitation wards, or in long stay extended care wards. Mental frailty by itself needs sympathetic and understanding care from nursing staff and presents few problems to competent geriatric nurses. Assessment of the extent of brain failure and the management of the patient while still in the community is part of the geriatrician's consultation activity. Assessment and management during a disturbed period or when the position is not clear, is also part of the geriatrician's work and it should not be necessary during this phase to pass the patient over to another department. A complete geriatric unit should include an area for assessment and treatment of psychogeriatric patients where all the necessary skills can be concentrated for the benefit of the patient. Where such facilities are available many of the apparent difficulties of assessment and management are vastly simplified.

References

Prinsley, D.M. (1973) 'Psychogeriatric ward for mentally disturbed elderly patients'; *British Medical Journal*, **iii**, 574–577.
Prinsley, D.M. (1974) 'Nursing in a psychogeriatric ward', *The Nursing Times*, June 27, **70**, 994–997.

11

THE ACADEMIC TASKS IN GERONTOPSYCHIATRY

S. Kanowski

In gerontopsychiatric literature there is much talk of the urgent need for improving the care and treatment of mentally ill elderly persons, but little or none of the academic tasks of this young discipline.

At first sight this situation actually seems to be justified, since in many countries the treatment and rehabilitation of mental disorders in old age is very poorly developed. Although, in an ever growing number of publications, accounts are given, partly in an enthusiastic manner, of successful treatment possibilities and treatment results, the situation in daily practice is still rather depressing in many respects. This is true at least for the Federal Republic of Germany. Primary and tertiary prevention in gerontopsychiatry is barely or not at all developed, and secondary prevention, particularly in the ambulant sector, is far from offering all patients an optimal therapy—even with the restriction of economics. This present situation is dependent on various factors, but one may be that gerontopsychiatry is not very well established within academic institutions. The role which it could have in this field will be discussed in this chapter. The discussion will be based on related literature, but without claiming to be complete, as well as on the personal experiences of the author made in the gerontopsychiatric department of the Freie Universität Berlin and on the conceptions developed for the establishment of this department.

In view of the three-fold responsibilities of medicoacademic institutions—research, teaching, and medical care (Gruenberg, 1972)—we must contemplate which tasks gerontopsychiatry is to accomplish. Finally, it might be useful to ask if gerontopsychiatry is actually justified in being a subspeciality. One might possibly think it would be better to ask this question at the beginning of the discussion; however, the answer might possibly be more concrete if the tasks of gerontopsychiatry are outlined more closely as seen from the academic horizon.

Gerontopsychiatric research

The primary motive of any research is the gain of knowledge. This, of course, also applies to gerontopsychiatric research. Besides that, however, successful research may also result in a strategic gain, particularly, where the discipline concerned is not yet firmly established. Relevant research results demonstrate the existence and justify the claim of recognizing its independence. Moreover, active research stimulates young trainees to devote themselves to working in a new field; it expands research capacity and intensifies the impact to the young discipline. Gerontopsychiatry still, to a considerable degree, needs to gain both understanding and prestige. True, one cannot overlook the fact that the number of relevant publications has increased considerably, however, the number of active gerontopsychiatric centres is still small in comparison to the practical significance of mental diseases in old age. On the whole this observation is valid, even though the conditions in each country vary greatly. In the German Federal Republic systematic gerontopsychiatric research is being practised, at most, at three of 25 universities with medical faculties; however, the extent of such research has had to remain very small so far due to limited personnel capacities.

Nonetheless, the internationally increasing research activity has resulted in the establishment, in 1966 of a gerontopsychiatry section within *Excerpta Medica*. In the first year there were only 41 references, but this rose to 112 in 1974. In the same years the *British Journal of Psychiatry* had published respectively six and nine articles and the *American Journal of Psychiatry* one and three articles devoted to questions concerning psychiatric problems in old age. Of course, quantity tells nothing about quality, and a complete survey of literature would be extremely difficult. This sample, however, might be accepted as a representative one. According to the author's own opinion the quality of the articles varies extraordinarily which is not very surprising with a new discipline, since on one hand researchers or research teams must first gain some experience, and on the other less qualified researchers occasionally switch over to less well filled fields in order to find a niche for themselves. Goldman (1970) came to similar conclusions and considerations regarding clinical gerontology at an International Colloquium in Austria.

If one refrains from merely counting the number of publications and directs one's attention to the white areas still existing on the 'gerontopsychiatric map', one will observe that more speculations than reliable knowledge still exist about the true incidence and prevalence, the nosological definition, aetiology and the development of the most frequent mental diseases in old age.

For the purposes of illustration the following questions are given as examples.

Do genuine psychosomatic diseases and first manifestations of neuroses in old age exist? What is the cause of presenile and senile dementia? Is there any warranted connection between organic psychoses and social factors, and if so, of which kind is it? The number of questions still open could be easily multiplied. Kraepelin's observation that old age psychiatry is the darkest field of psychiatry still seems to be justified.

In asking for reasons why uncertainties are still so great in the field of mental diseases in old age, a few may be supplied. First and foremost is the still unresolved fundamental question concerning the nature of the ageing process itself. However, it is not only that its nature is unknown to us, but also that a satisfactory description of its manifestations is possible at neither the somatic, the psychiatric nor the social level. Particularly in the psychosocial field many questions are still open to discussion. With regard to the intellectual performance, is the ageing process best described by a deficit model or not? Does ageing in sociological terms mean engagement or disengagement?

Another problem is that of 'accumulation'. The longer an individual lives, the more he may have experienced meaningful situations of social, psychological, and somatic stress. But which situations are related to the present state of disorder? This holds true especially for psychiatric disorders. How can one find the traces throughout decades?

Next is the problem of multiple interactions between social, somatic, and psychiatric influences. The pure influence of each can hardly be separated, as it would be desirable for scientific analyses as well as for planning good therapy.

The last problem to be mentioned arises from the fact that whenever we study old persons in any way, we find only the survivors and do not know very much about those who died or escaped our screening programmes. This fact is important, especially in studies of long term character and is difficult to overcome.

So, in gerontologic research we are confronted with a highly complex matter and complicated problems of research strategy. A barrier for clinically orientated gerontologic research is built up by the complex questions of multiple pathology and the fact that most of the geriatric diseases are chronic ones.

But all these problems and difficulties give us a good chance to learn a lot about research techniques, strategies, and persistence which are so often necessary for achieving very small results after prolonged efforts. The main benefits which clinical gerontology is likely to contribute to medical science are the following.

(1) Clinical, gerontologic research demands an holistic approach to human existence in a manifold sense. It should not stick to the last period of life because this period is only the sum of lifelong changes; therefore, the geriatrician, as well as the gerontologist, has to explore the total life of any aged person he is concerned with and try to find some integrating view. He not only has to consider the social, psychological, or somatic dimension of a given biography, but focus on them simultaneously and see all their inter-relations, including the economic aspects. Thus gerontology may be apt to reverse to some degree overskilled specialization and fragmentation as seen in medicine during the last decades. In this relation gerontopsychiatry may give an impulse to reintegrate medicine into an anthropological science.

The ageing process by itself presents a broad area for research where biochemists pharmacologists, geneticists, psychologists, sociologists, and medical scientists of different branches can meet each other very productively in common work of research. It is by no means clear how the complex problems of multidisciplinary research could be solved, nor that this could be done easily, but from this arises a very stimulating challenge. In gerontopsychiatry questions concerning neuropathology and neurochemistry come into direct contact with those having psychosocial dimensions, as for example in the case of dementing processes when one wonders how it happens that one and the same degree of cerebral atrophy in two patients produces an entirely different impairment of intellectual performance. Here, the borders disappear between experimental and clinical research on the one hand as well as between the two fields and primarily practice orientated research on the other.

(2) Clinical gerontologic research opens the view for the significance and necessity of primary prevention, since numerous diseases in old age are based on seemingly irreversible processes, which at this stage are not accessible to curative treatment. Thus clinical gerontology supports the presently indispensable tendency for medical research to devote itself more to the question of how to prevent chronic diseases rather than, as it has been done until now, concerning itself—admittedly very successfully—more with the prevention and treatment of acute diseases, thus improving the chances of survival. The medical education of students still reflects the fact that medical acting and thinking concentrates on acute diseases. Thus, at least unconsciously, resistance is being induced in young doctors to working with geriatric and chronic patients. Since mental diseases *per se* are labelled by laymen and professionals alike as being 'chronic' and 'incurable', gerontopsychiatric patients must bear the double burden produced by the prejudice. Here, only successful research can finally effect a change in attitudes.

(3) 'Geropathology' can be considered with good reason as 'adaptation pathology' (Busse and Pfeiffer, 1969; Groh, 1970). This again is true in a very particular way for gerontopsychiatry (Kanowski, 1974). The question of the basic processes of ageing can also be formulated as concerning the respective specific factors which increasingly restrict, with advancing age, the adaptation ability of the various organic systems, as for example vigilance regulation. In the field of gerontopsychiatry and gerontopsychology social influences are also involved. Adaptation presupposes the concept of the physiological equilibrium as the aim of the adapting process. Translating this definition into analogous terms in other disciplines relating the adaptation capacity to the ageing process is a problem still broadly unresolved.

Thus clinical gerontologic research is a science concentrating on dynamic concepts, being by no means merely statically descriptive. It is to be considered as that field of basic research concerned with the processes of ageing which deals with problems bordering between physiological and pathological ageing.

(4) This problem of differentiating physiological ageing from pathological forms opens up another perspective for clinically oriented gerontologic research. Here, the identification of the phenomena characteristic of each form has not been achieved. The question is open whether the transition follows a continuum model or whether a threshold–value–model is more in agreement with reality, as for instance the transition from physiological ageing to senile dementia.

These fascinating questions have been asked for a long time now in medical history. Is age *per se* a pathogenetic factor ('*senectus ipsa morbus*') or is the time of occurrence and the speed of development of individual ageing determined by the combination and accumulation of previous pathological processes? Although medicine is compelled to make an autochthonous contribution in order to solve the difficulties concerning the borderline definition of ageing under physiological and pathological conditions, it surely cannot cope with this question alone. Medicine takes its place here as a partner of the humanities *sensu strictu*, namely psychology and sociology. Together they form a 'triad' having equal rights, but are strongly secularized in accordance with our times. However, neither philosophy and religious sciences nor other humanities should be excluded from the scientific body 'gerontology'. On the contrary, precisely the transcendental references of 'getting old' and 'being old' deserve to be constantly considered. However, psychology and sociology as neighbouring sciences surely relate closest to gerontopsychiatric problems.

In this context clinical gerontologic research can be considered as a re-integration of medicine into the association of anthropologic science disciplines, after it had become an almost purely technologically orientated science towards the close of the nineteenth and the beginning of the twentieth century.

(5) Before bringing this section on research to an end, let me make another general remark. Current geriatric and gerontopsychiatric literature is confined mainly to a descriptive level. Now it is true that one cannot overlook the fact that not all observable phenomena of ageing have been recognized and described so far. And yet it seems feasible and desirable that clinical research should shift its emphasis increasingly towards the formation and testing of hypotheses about the development of specific age processes.

Education

The primary aim of academic education is the academic professions. Besides that, universities also participate nowadays in the vocational training of non-academic vocations, as for example, social workers, nurses, etc. Finally, in many places universities contribute considerably to adult education. All these fields are dealt with in Ross (1975).

Linked with this rather formal differentiation of gerontologic education are relevant substantial aspects. In the broadest sense gerontologic education means information of every member of a given society about the process of ageing, the obstacles of successful ageing and the means to overcome the problems (Bunzel, 1973). So far gerontologic education is directed mainly at primary prevention. Apparently this is best done on a community level. Preretirement courses are a well known example. Teaching of lay people and even some professional groups, for example clergy, district nurses, etc., should facilitate secondary prevention. Those people should be able to detect old adults in need of some help. They should be skilled in giving over-all help and instruction to the old on how to help and instruction to the old on how to help themselves and each other. The gerontopsychiatric education of highly trained occupational groups is aimed at extending and deepening knowledge and skills in care, therapy and rehabilitation techniques. From their level of experience and knowledge the professionals should be aware of their role as multiplicators of skills and information to the public as a whole. Thus they work directly in the field of secondary and tertiary prevention and, indirectly, as mentioned before, in primary prevention.

Gerontopsychiatric education in academic professions

Medical students. Almost worldwide, complaints are heard that the geriatric education of medical students is insufficient, and when offered, it meets with little enthusiasm from the students (Bayne, 1974; Dawson, 1965; Deutsches Zentrum für Altersfragen, 1975/76; Freeman, 1971; Kimsey and Roberts, 1969; Geriscope, 1967; Harris, 1975; Kaiser, 1973; Kanowski, 1973). This situation stands in strong contradiction to the well known increase of the proportion of the population over 65 years of age in the highly industrialized countries, the consequence of which is that doctors of all medical disciplines, particularly psychiatrists, see themselves confronted with steadily growing tasks in geriatric care in the office practice as well as in the clinics (Busse and Dovermuehle, 1960; Kay *et al.*, 1964; Lauter, 1972, 1974; Hippius and Kanowski, 1974). Taking all methodical uncertainties into consideration, one must proceed from the fact that the mental over-all morbidity (prevalence) amounts to at least 30 per cent in the population over 65 years of age. Extreme estimates go as far as 60 per cent (Busse and Dovenmuehle 1960). The percentage of severe disturbances lies at 10–15 per cent with a rather good agreement on this point of almost all authors. In contrast to this, it is a fact that mentally ill old people are comparatively under represented among the outpatients. In the state mental hospitals, however, their numbers have been rising disproportionately for years. Under the heading of education it is of particular consequence that mental geriatric patients are found only in a small number in the university clinics (see Table 11.1). This demonstrates, among other things, the small interest which university medicine has shown in studying chronic disease processes, in particular geriatric diseases. This certainly holds for the Federal Republic of Germany.

TABLE 11.1. Comparison between the percentage of over 50 year olds in the population of Berlin (West) and various patient populations

	50–65	> 65
Berlin population*	21·8 %	21·2 %
Psychiatric practice	24·3 %	11·1 %
University Clinic (1968)	outpatient 20·2 %	8·8 %
	inpatient 24·8 %	8·9 %

* Information according to the Statistical Landesamt Berlin for the year 1968.

It is not surprising then, to often hear about iatrogenic complications as a consequence of wrong treatment (Rudd, 1972) and that the negative attitudes of students towards ageing reflect those of society as a whole (Spence *et al*, 1968; Sharma and Bhandari, 1970). The therapeutic pessimism which is felt towards geriatric diseases is widespread among medical staffs (Bunzel, 1973; Udelman, 1973). Diagnostic labelling of mental geriatric diseases occurs much too often globally as 'senility', 'senile dementia' or 'arteriosclerotic insufficiency'. Such labelling often results in compulsory accommodation in a state mental hospital without a thorough clinical assessment having been previously carried out (Bergener *et al*, 1974). The dignity and integrity of gerontopsychiatric patients are much too often thoughtlessly neglected on account of negative attitudes.

Another consequence of insufficient gerontopsychiatric education of doctors is the frequent failure to recognize somatic and psychic diseases is geriatric patients (Lauter, 1974; Williamson *et al.*, 1964; Williamson, 1967). They may be passed off as inevitable signs of ageing and treatment is not attempted. The question then arises in which way gerontopsychiatry can be integrated into the curriculum of the medical students in order that practical knowledge may be conveyed.

Among didactic points of view one can differentiate between two information fields which are to be co-ordinated and integrated as well as possible with each other, namely, the conveyance of:

(1) Gerontologic basic knowledge.
(2) Specific knowledge about mental diseases in old age.

In the first category can be included the presentation of human development in the customary medical curriculum. So far this has been mostly restricted to childhood and adolescence, and it is in need of extension to include the time of ageing and dying. Only then does the gestalt of the human life curve become visible as a whole, and the fact becomes increasingly evident that dynamic changes take place well into advanced age. In the same way the biological perspective prevailing hitherto in the development theory must be broadened by the psychic and social horizon and the intertwining of the three-dimensions be made visible. Maturation and involution with its critical phases can illustrate this as in a concave mirror. When the concept of biomorphosis which Bürger has introduced into gerontology (1965), is supplemented by psychomorphosis and sociomorphosis, the gestaltwandel of the total lifespan becomes evident.

Gerontologic basic knowledge, embedded in such a context, can be conveyed in a reasonable time probably only by way of a theoretic lecture. The most recent German regulations on education provide for medical sociology and psychology to be taken as preclinical, separate compulsory courses. This will probably mean that social and psychological gerontology should be treated separately, provided that they are considered in the curriculum at all. More desirable, without doubt, is an integrated form of instruction. This problem, however, will be referred to again in a later section.

In the second category, specific knowledge of mental diseases in old age it is essential to discuss the aetiology and pathogenetics as well as the pathoplastic influence of age on disease processes not specifically related to age. The presentation of the peculiarities in the therapy of mental diseases in old age and of ways of dealing with older patients demands detailed consideration, however. That includes knowing about age-dependent changes in the pharmacokinetics and pharmacodynamics as well as the knowledge of mechanisms of transference and countertransference which experience their specific modifications when the patient is of considerably higher age than the doctor (Radebold, 1976). Furthermore, gerontopsychiatry is a very suitable field for learning about the aims and problems of family therapy, because the inter-relations between the patient and his relatives are very complex and of great importance for the therapeutic process as well as the therapeutic outcome. In a similarly intensive way the manner of dealing with community agents and agencies can be taught. Knowledge of the general and local facilities and their optimal utilization for therapy and rehabilitation is an indispensable prerequisite for their success. A practice related way of instruction is without doubt a prerequisite for transmitting this knowledge and these capabilities. It is preferable for instruction to take place with small groups of students, where they are given the opportunity to gain experience directly and face to face in exploration with patients and their relatives, as well as in discussion with members of the gerontopsychiatric team. In this context it would be of particular importance for gerontopsychiatry to offer the students a chance to become acquainted with one or more patients, not only that one time in the actual, given situation, but also to be able to observe the development of a diagnostic and therapeutic process over a longer period of time. Furthermore, it seems important that the students become familiar not only with the problems of gerontopsychiatric patients in clinical institutions, but also with the problems of outpatient care. Here, particularly those aspects so very important for geriatrics, regarding prevention—prophylaxis as well as intensive screening, after care and rehabilitation can be incorporated into the instruction plan. Gerontopsychiatric outpatient clinics and day clinics are suited for this purpose provided that they have enough personnel available who are trained in medical students' education.

Turning to the relationship between psychiatry and geriatrics some have argued that an integrated plan of instruction would be desirable in combining all significant facts pertaining to geriatric medicine to a homogenous subject 'geriatrics' (Isaacs, 1972; Pathy, 1974). This, however, presupposes a thorough knowledge in numerous branches of medicine and could thus almost be considered as running counter to previous medical developments which aimed at an ever increasing specialization (Gruenberg, 1972). In the opposite model a geriatric, interdisciplinary course of lectures with many disciplines participating is possible and realizable. This very model would take into consideration the perhaps unchecked tendency for a deepening knowledge in a branch getting narrower all the time; it would try, however, to achieve the integration of partial knowledge in programmes agreed among the teachers and the productive discussion of the participating specialized scientists.

With regard to the first model of uniform instruction in geriatrics, it must be doubtful whether a single person is still capable of possessing the required wealth of detailed knowledge in internal medicine, cardiology, psychology, urology, gynaecology, orthopaedics, to mention only the most important fields. Problems resulting from shortage of time, difficult co-ordination and the need for a never tiring organizer are inherent in the second model of multidisciplinary instruction. Moreover, there is the danger that the instruction will be too heterogenous for the students, forcing them to carry the main load in accomplishing an integration of the conveyed facts and of the wealth of information. As a compromise solution the possibility could be considered to transfer the emphasis of geriatric instruction to the two disciplines which are undeniably most important here; internal medicine and psychiatry.

These reflections made in connection with the education of medical students may strike as being a bit 'academic', that is, theoretical. However, it is unmistakable that they are highly relevant to the very practical question of how how the constantly increasing medical care of the ageing population can be optimally planned and mastered according to reality's demand.

Behind the discussion being carried on with factual arguments, are also concealed the fears of the concerned medical branches that they must turn over a large group of patients to a new specialized discipline and forfeit in the process part of their authority and reduce their own basis for existence. In the Federal Republic of Germany the willingness to allow such a development is apparently greater among psychiatrists than among internists (see, for instance, *Enquete*, 1975) which is perhaps connected not least with the fact that psychiatrists are still a 'scarce commodity in great demand'.

Which of the three different ways in geriatric and gerontopsychiatric education will be taken is probably very much dependent on national and local conditions. One could, however, propose generalizations with regard to two principles:

(1) The education must take into account the close, multiconditional network of somatic, psychic, and social factors of diseases of old age.
(2) Instruction should be realized as far as possible within the scope of obligatory teaching occasions (lectures, seminars, etc.)

The first principle is probably in no need of further explanation. With regard to the second, it is a fact that the majority of authors agree that the spontaneous interest the students have in geriatrics is too small to guarantee an adequate education when courses are made available. As a result facultative seminars and colloquia are attended only by a few specifically motivated students and do not constitute an efficient form of education in the sense of quantitative criteria.

Medical education in psychogeriatrics should not stop after graduation. Intensification of postgraduate training is urgently needed (Lawton, 1971). The author's impression is that geriatrics should be integrated into general medical congresses far more than it is done at present. Besides congresses and special symposia, university centres and psychogeriatric departments should develop short, perhaps weekend, courses of practical orientation using audiovisual methods of information. They should start with case presentation and discussion.

Other academic professional groups

Here there are two professional groups to differentiate between, namely those which stand in close relationship to gerontopsychiatry, since they come into contact in some way or other with the care of mentally ill old people and others who are in need of the gerontopsychiatric aspect only within the scope of a general gerontologic education.

The former include pharmacologists, psychologists, sociologists, ministers of religion, and architects, the latter, for example, political economists, managerial economists, pedagogues (adult education), jurists, political scientists. While gerontologic, and with that gerontopsychiatric, knowledge should be an obligatory part of the instruction for those two groups—though in greatly varying intensity—there is a third group for which perhaps the faculative information possibilities could be considered as adequate. These are the basic natural sciences, such as biology and biochemistry.

Common to all three groups, however, is the fact that gerontopsychiatric knowledge seems practical and can become effective for them only in the context of a general gerontologic education.

Out of such considerations, however, resulted the necessity for the universities to develop gerontologic study courses according to a unit construction principle. The realization of such a goal is dependent not least on the question of who feels responsible for it and who takes the initiative. The gerontopsychiatrist would seem to me a figure not unprepared for this kind of task. He belongs to a rare professional group that learns to combine the natural sciences and psychological education with socioscientific knowledge and experience. However, he would have to avoid to derive from this a claim to omnipotence.

In literature there is little to be obtained about the development or realization of such gerontologic educational models in the form of a unit construction system which is adjusted to numerous professional groups. The gerontopsychiatric educational programme at Duke Centre (Varner and Verwoerdt, 1975; Verwoerdt, 1969) could perhaps be considered as an attempt in this direction. Nevertheless an attempt fashioned in such a way would seem stimulating for numerous reasons.

Education of non-academic staff

The gerontopsychiatric education of non-academic staff is in terms of quantity a great problem. In the author's own experience the demand for education and advanced education reaches far beyond the actually existing offers and possibilities. The discrepancy becomes even larger when the need for additional nursing staff is taken into account. Real demand calculations have not yet been drawn up for the Federal Republic of Germany, however, it was estimated for the period up to 1971 that there was a shortage of in all 30–40 000 nursing staff personnel and that in addition to the existing number about 10 000 were needed for establishments of institutional aid to the aged (Hirsch, 1971; Informationsblätter, 1969; Müller, 1971; Adams, 1973). However, gerontopsychiatric educational offers in this field may not only confine themselves to the nursing staff, the assistant staff being included (Haag, 1967), but they must also incorporate social workers, occupational therapists and physiotherapists which means not only those who work in the limited sector of psychiatry, but who work in the field of medical care as a whole. This necessity results from the fact that the care of the chronic somatically ill also steadily demands the consideration of psychoreactive disturbances and organic psychoses which are very often encountered there. Otherwise, faulty approaches on the part of the nursing staff (Bergmann, 1974; Miller, 1975), based on ignorance and lacking experience, could result and because of this rehabilitative efforts be doomed to failure. As learned from experience, instruction must, therefore, not only convey knowledge about mental disorders, but must also include psychological basics about how to deal with the chronic ill.

Designing a programme of instruction depends on whether it concerns staff already engaged in practical work (advanced education) or 'students' (education), since in the first case it is certainly convenient for the course of instruction to take advantage as far as possible of the experiences made by those already working.

The development of the respective curricula must be effected with particular care and take into account the differing educational background of each person. As an example for this the respective programme of the Duke Centre can again be mentioned (Varner and Verwoerdt, 1975; Verwoerdt, 1969).

The education of nurses, social workers, etc. is certainly not the main task of gerontopsychiatry in the academic sector; however, the elaboration of curricula and instruction models as well as the education of educators is relevant to it.

Adult Education

On the background of the manifold obligations of gerontopsychiatry in education and advanced education, which have already become evident, adult education—measured in terms of the existing capacity—can at the present time scarcely have more than marginal significance. This may seem deplorable, particularly, since in this sector of activity a direct way to primary prevention can be opened; for primary prevention means information and advice about how to lead and organize one's life precisely with regard to mental health. The small number of gerontopsychiatrists existing everywhere in comparison to the population, however, allows direct communication at the most occasionally and to a practically insignificant degree, unless one makes use of the public information media.

However, tempting this might seem, one has to consider how difficult it is giving information about mental diseases by means which do not allow the addressee direct questioning. The question how transmitted 'messages' are assimilated by the 'recipient' has not yet been sufficiently investigated—at least not for this sector of health information. According to an investigation attempt in this direction, older test persons who had seen television broadcasts about problems of ageing, had afterwards a more negative picture of old age than a comparative group (Thomae, H, personal communication). Every doctor engaged in practice can report from his own experience about the negative effect of such medical informatory articles in magazines. The effect which information provokes depends on the knowledge and experience background of each person, and that cannot be assessed at all in 'information broadcasts' being of a purely passive character, without feedback; from there a false assimilation of information cannot be corrected.

Therefore, the more effective contribution of gerontopsychiatry in adult education consists with certainty in the information and education of multiplicators. Politicians, journalists, and teachers in particular come into consideration as such besides those already mentioned in the preceding sections. Conducting joint seminars and workshops proves to be a suitable form of communication. The co-operation of gerontopsychiatrists in local, national, and international committees is of a significance, not to be underestimated. Here everyone—politicians for example— learn from each other what should and could be done in order to improve the care mentally handicapped old people, the gerontopsychiatrist on the other hand learns about the limits imposed by budget and prejudice.

Institutional counselling

One task which the academically committed gerontopsychiatrist cannot and should not evade is the psychiatric counselling of institutions devoted to the care of the physically or mentally handicapped old people. Often the gerontopsychiatric consultant must begin with reducing negative stereotypes of directors and supporters of such institutions so much that they are actually willing to admit that mentally disturbed persons are living within their walls, or to accept such patients for the first time for admission. Only then can the consultant recommend special therapeutic techniques or be allowed to familiarize the staff of the institutions with the necessary techniques. Since according to the studies of Goldfarb and other authors as well (Bergener et al., 1974) even in general nursing homes as many as 90 per cent of the patients are found with mental disorders of various kinds and differing intensity, this cannot be seen as a task of slight importance.

The Department for Gerontopsychiatry at the Freie Universität Berlin

The author's local background, West Berlin, belongs to the cities accommodating the highest percentage of old people within its walls. At the present around 22·1 per cent are over 65 years of age. That is almost twice the average for the Federal Republic of Germany (about 14 per cent). The basic facts about their living situation can be drawn from a representative survey published in 1974 in which over 6000 of these older citizens participated (Blume and Kuhlmeyer, 1974). Only a few facts can be mentioned here.

Thirty-two per cent of the persons over 65 years of age are men, 68 per cent women. The marital status can be gathered from Table 11.2, the following three tables (Tables, 11.3, 11.4, and 11.5) give information about educational background, occupational groups, and standard of living. Since it was a sociological study, the judgment of the condition of health was very general using only the data given by the respondents themselves. Sixty-one per cent of the men questioned and 67 per

TABLE 11.2

Marital status	Men	Women
Married	76 %	25 %
Widowed	15 %	54 %
Divorced	5 %	7 %
Single	4 %	14 %

TABLE 11.3.

Education	Men	Women
Elementary school (8 years)	71 %	81 %
Secondary school (GCE O-level)	19 %	16 %
Secondary school (GCE A-level)	4 %	2 %
University	6 %	1 %

TABLE 11.4.

Present or previous occupation	
Freelance, self-employed professional	6 %
Self-employed in craftsmanship, commerce or trade	15 %
Farmer	1 %
Labourer	34 %
Salaried employees	28 %
Civil servant	16 %

TABLE 11.5.

Family income (monthly)	
Below 300 DM	5 %
Above 300 up to 400 DM	7 %
Above 400 up to 500 DM	8 %
Above 500 up to 600 DM	10 %
Above 600 up to 700 DM	10 %
Above 700 up to 800 DM	10 %
Above 800 up to 900 DM	8 %
Above 900 up to 1000 DM	9 %
Above 1000 up to 1500 DM	16 %
More than 1500 DM	8 %
No statement	9 %

TABLE 11.6. Judgement of own state of health

	Very good or good	Bad or very bad
Men, 65–67 years	29 %	21 %
Women, 65–67 years	18 %	26 %
Men, 86 years and older	21 %	29 %
Women, 86 years and older	16 %	31 %

cent of the women questioned indicated to be suffering from at least one chronic disease. Table 11.6 shows that women apparently judged their physical condition to be worse than men and that they also seem less subject to the influence of age with respect to their health state.

On the background of this demographic situation it is a matter of course that the local authorities in West Berlin make a particularly intensive effort to attend to the promotion and development of the care for the aged.

In 1972 the Freie Universität Berlin founded, for the first time in Germany a university department for gerontopsychiatry which was actually the first geriatric institution at a German university. The author took over the supervision and with it the setting-up of the department. On the ground of studies of literature and of information trips, a three-step development plan was made (Woodford-Williams, 1967). The first step in the development constitutes here the outpatient clinic which has been in operation since February 1, 1973. The second step will be achieved at the end of 1976. When the day hospital will be opened, and the third and temporarily last step provides for a clinical unit with approximately 30–40 beds. Its realization will not be possible before 1980.

This is not the place to report extensively about the work of the department. (For this see Junkers *et al.*, 1976.) Let me only give a short account in connection with the given topic about the developments so far. This will also give the opportunity to deal with a question left unanswered and mentioned at the beginning: by which principles does the provision of medical care belong to the academic commitments of gerontopsychiatry?

Research

Research planning is in accord with the research traditions of the Psychiatric Clinic of the Freie Universität Berlin, its emphasis being placed on biological psychiatry (Helmchen and Hippius, 1975), psycho-pharmacology, and methodology.

In the first step of the methodological approach a system for gerontopsychiatric diagnosis documentation has been worked out at the department in close co-operation with the Psychiatric University Clinic, Lausanne, Switzerland. It includes anamnestic, somatic, and psychopathological data and will be supplemented by a separate documentation system for gerontologically relevant social data (Hermann, 1972). Once completed, it will provide the ground for various research projects, as for instance, cost benefit studies. Further efforts are being made in clinical testing of geriatric drugs in order to improve the methodology (Coper and Kanowski, in press). In the area of biological research interest is applied to the significance of vigilance disorders within the scope of gerontopsychiatric diseases (Girke and Kanowski, 1972; Kanowski and Girke, 1975).

Teaching

Since the establishment of the department, gerontopsychiatry is an integral part of the obligatory main lecture course in psychiatry to the extent of two hours per semester. In addition the author gives lectures on the section of organic psychosis. For two semesters now the department has also been participating in carrying out the obligatory courses of instruction in psychiatry.

Its aim is the practice-orientated education of students in small groups by which they can study patients themselves under supervision and can then discuss their observations with lecturers and tutors.

Within this framework patients of the gerontopsychiatric outpatient clinic are also presented to each student group once every semester. An even greater participation of gerontopsychiatry in the instruction would certainly be desirable, however, this is, at present, not yet possible with the relatively high number of 240 students per semester. The catalogue given in the Appendix reflects the educational and learning aims which are being aspired to.

Beside the participation in obligatory courses of instruction, a seminar is being offered to those students interested in gerontopsychiatry in particular; this has, however, been only realized in three out of ten semesters due to the lack of interest by students.

Outside the university the staff members of the department participate almost constantly in educational and advanced educational courses for the various occupational groups in Berlin and the Federal Republic of Germany. Unfortunately, it is not possible to comply with all wishes in this sector.

Medical care

According to the German concept, the medical care of the ill is not the primary task of university medicine. It is only imperative here as a prerequisite for teaching and research to ensure that these remain relevant to the care of patients. Moreover, university medicine is regarded as having the commitment of safeguarding the medical care for patients in all those sectors which are not yet being considered by private or public institutions. This is usually the case with innovatory techniques. Thus the Berlin department for gerontopsychiatry is regarded as an 'experimental model'. The plan on which the development is based already corresponds to the 'psychogeriatric centre', as it was recently proposed in a report on the situation of psychiatry in the Federal Republic of Germany (*Enquete*, 1975). Neither was it a coincidence that the department became active first in the outpatient sector of care; this resulted from the supposition that improvements in care here were particularly urgent.

234

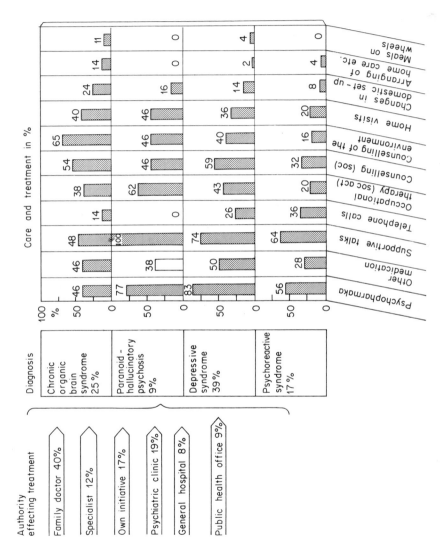

FIGURE 11.1. Survey about the allocation, diagnosis and treatment of patients of the gerontopsychiatric outpatient clinic at the Freie Universität, Berlin (n = 148)

The character of an 'experimental model' will be confirmed when one succeeds in closing therapeutic gaps, that is, in promoting new therapeutic attempts and in checking the efficiency of single procedures as well as of the entire institution—measured in terms of expenditure—by means of concurrent research. This was also the aim of the research attempts mentioned in the section on research, above. In the therapeutic field the interest is not only focused on organic and functional psychoses but also on the treatment of psychoreactive disorders. This results from the fact that for one thing its percentage is surprisingly high, being 17–25 per cent of the patients admitted, for another from our conviction that this task of gerontopsychiatry has, to a large extent, been neglected and that so far the interest has been mostly devoted to the demential and functional processes.

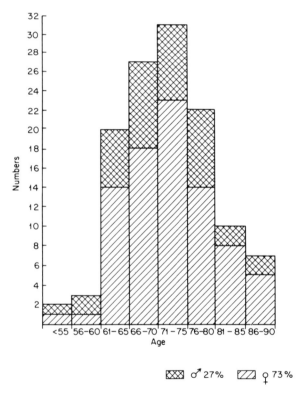

FIGURE 11.2. Age distributions of patients

Figures 11.1 and 11.2 summarize some basic data in order to briefly characterize the patients of the gerontopsychiatric outpatient clinic.

Conclusion

I hope to have demonstrated convincingly that gerontopsychiatry has to accomplish equally important and urgent tasks in the field of research, teaching, and medical care within the academic setting. Even if it may seem that the problems of education and advanced education as well as of medical care—considered merely quantitatively—should stand in the centre of efforts, one should not forget, however, that real progress in these two fields can only be achieved if research is also stimulated and allowed to advance systematically and significantly. Under the simultaneous pressure of many unresolved problems of daily practice and the increasing exhaustion of state financing funds, research threatens to get between the millstones of stagnation forced upon us by the cutting of subsidies and a scientific world controlled only by the state. It is probably one of the critical problems of our time, which must be solved so that we shall find the equilibrium between a kind of research controlled by society, that is to say by the state, and one which can be determined freely by every single scientist himself. However, this question cannot be investigated further here. The following results are of consequence for the development of gerontopsychiatry.

The abundance of the still unresolved scientific problems, of the needs for education and advanced education and for the improvement of the treatment and care of mentally ill old people urgently calls for the establishment of additional gerontopsychiatric departments (Udelman, 1973). Some of them must be installed at universities in order to stimulate particularly research and teaching, but also to develop new therapy possibilities and therapy models. With that the question which was put at the beginning, and has not yet been explicitly discussed—if gerontopsychiatry earns the rank of being a discipline of its own—has basically already been answered. Its justification does not only result from the fact that old people exist and that their number is growing constantly. To the present day there are no reliable, generally applicable criteria for the biological definition of the term 'old'. Definition according to mere calendar standards is unsatisfactory. The justification for the existence of gerontology, geriatrics, and gerontopsychiatry follows solely from the special structures, problems and models which are connected with the study of old age as a process. For medicine there is the other fact—and this is especially true for psychiatry—that diagnosis and treatment of physical and psychic disorders in old age demand specialized knowledge and experience.

Appendix

Catalogue of Teaching and Learning Aims

Social facts
(1) Basics of demography and epidemiology.
    (a) Proportions of the various age groups, classified into men and women, single, widowed, and married.
    (b) Frequency of mental disorders.
(2) Social determinants of physiological and pathological ageing.
    (a) Influence of leading concepts which are dependent on society.
    (b) Generation conflict.

(c) Change of social structure: agricultural society, industrial society, consumer society.

(d) Problems concerning occupation.

(e) Problems of sexuality and confrontation with social prejudices.

(f) Loss of friends and relatives through death: problem of the survivor.

(g) Difficulty of making new contacts.

(h) Disengagement theory and its crucial modification.

(3) Economic facts and consequences for society and the individual.

(a) Frequency of diseases in younger and older age, increase of morbidity, multimorbidity, and chronicity.

(b) Longer clinical stay with increasing age.

(c) Average income of the old, each classified according to sex.

(d) Problems of funding health care for the elderly.

(4) Social therapy.

(a) Supporting measures for the sustainment of independence.

(b) Establishment of counselling centres and outpatient clinics.

(c) Clubs for the aged and day centres.

(d) Residence homes for the aged (with separate living units).

(e) Homes for the aged.

(f) Nursing homes for the aged.

(g) Establishment of clinics for acute cases.

(h) Significance of co-ordination and co-operation of the institutions and flexibility in all directions.

(i) Negative attitudes of the aged towards institutionalization and the reasons for it.

Psychological facts

(1) Subjective assimilation of social conflicts.

(a) Problem of detachment from children.

(b) Problem of detachment from occupational process—development of new activities.

(c) Maintenance of sufficient social contacts.

(2) Personality change.

(a) Increasing gravity of personality traits.

(b) Levelling out of the personality.

(c) Increasing rigidity—decreasing ability for adaptation and renewed orientation.

(d) Retreat from social contacts.

(3) Changes in the intellectual capacity.

(a) Problem of differentiating between physiological and pathological phenomena of age.

(b) Problem: general loss of performance ability or change in the form which performance assumes.

(c) Dependency of the speed of age-dependent changes on the starting level and the practising of individual functions.

(d) Reduction of the sensory functions.

(e) Reduction of mnestic functions.

(f) Increase in reaction time: the loss of the ability to work under time pressure.

(g) Reduction in learning ability.

(h) Age-resisting functions (capacities).

(i) Change in the experiencing of time.

(4) Problem of the approaching end of life.

(a) Significance of life's balance.

(b) Psychology of dying.

(5) Individual psychological phenomena particularly characteristic of age.

(a) Development of fear and depressive reactions.

(b) Hypochondria.

(c) Worry about the material existence.

(d) Meaning of life (experiencing of guilt).

Specific old age psychiatry

(1) Biology of ageing.

(a) General theories.

(b) CNS and ageing.

(2) Influence of age on diseases already existing.

(a) Feeblemindedness.

(b) Neuroses.

(c) Schizophrenia.

(d) Manic-depressive diseases.

(c) Addiction.

(f) Suicidal tendencies.

(g) Sexual disorders.

(3) Specific diseases of old age.

(a) Psychoreactive disturbances.

(b) Involutional psychoses.

(c) Senile psychoses.

(d) Demential processes.

(4) Therapy and rehabilitation.

(a) Medical care concepts (including psychotherapy).

(b) Community service concepts.

References

Adams, G.F. (1973) 'Points of view, geriatric nursing standards', *Lancet*, **ii**, 553–555.

Bayne, J.R.D. (1974) 'Geriatrics and gerontology in medical education', *J. Am. Geriat. Soc.*, **22**, 198–202.

Bergener, M., Behrends, K., Zimmermann, R. (1974) 'Geropsychiatrische Versorgung in Nordrhein-Westfalen', *Psychiat. Prax.*, **1**, 18.

Bergmann, S. (1974) 'Nursing attitudes to psychiatry and geriatrics as preferred work areas with deviant groups', *Israel Ann. Psychiat, Re. Disc.* **12**, 156–160.

Blume, O., and Kuhlmeyer, E. (1974) *Dokumentation der Lebenssituation über 65 jähriger Bürger in Berlin*, Berlin, Senator für Arbeit und Soziales.

Bürger, M. (1965) *Altern und Krankheit als Problem der Biomorphose. IV. Aufl*, Edition Leipzig, Leipzig.

Bunzel, J.H. (1973) 'Recognition, relevance and deactivation of gerontophobia: theoretical essay', *J. Am. Geriat. Soc.*, **21**, 77–80.

Busse, E.W., and Dovenmuehle, R.H. (1960) 'Neurotic symptoms and predisposition in aging people', *J. AM. Geriat. Soc.*, **8**, 328–335.

Busse, E.W., and Pfeiffer, E. (1969) *Behavior and adaptation in late life*, Boston, Little, Brown.

Cawley, R.H., Post, F., and Whitehead, A. (1973) 'Barbiturate tolerance and psychological functioning in elderly depressed patients', *Psychol. Med.*, **3**, 39–52, in: *Excerpta Med.* **28**, section 32, 65.

Coper, H., and Kanowski, S. (1976) Geriatrika: Theoretische Grundlagen, Erwartungen, Prüfung, Kritik. *Hippokrates*, **47**, 303–319.

Dawson, D. (1965) 'Orienting the young physician to the geriatric age group and its problems', *J. Am. Geriat. Soc.*, **13**, 843–844.

Deutsches Zentrum Für Altersfragen (1975/6) *Basisinformation: Gerontologie, Gerontopsychiatrie, Experimentelle Gerontologie*, Berlin, information on request.

Enquete (1975) Bericht über die Lage der Psychiatrie in der Bundesrepublik Deutschland. Deutscher Bundestag, 7. Wahlperiode Drucksache 7/4200, Bonn, Dr. Hans Heger.

Freeman, J.T. (1971) 'A survey of geriatric education: catalogues of United States medical schools', *J. Am. Geriat. Soc.*, **19**, 746–762.

Geriscope (1967) 'Geriatrics training and the medical school', *Geriatrics*, **22**, 29–44.

Girke, W., and Kanowski, S. (1972) 'Elektroenzephalographische Untersuchungen der Vigilanz bei psychischen Störungen im höheren Alter und ihre therapeutische Bedeutung', *Act. Geront.*, **2**, 279–286.

Goldfarb, A.I. (1969) 'Institutional care of the aged', In *Behavior and adaptation in late life.* (Eds. E.W. Busse and E. Pfeiffer). Boston, Little, Brown.

Goldman, R. (1970) 'Current research in clinical gerontology: biomedical', In *Research, training and practice in clinical medicine of aging.* (Ed. L. Gitman and E. Woodford-Williams) Basel, Munich, New York, Karger.

Groh, J. (1970) 'Training for research in clinical gerontology', in: *Research, training and practice in clinical medicine of aging.* (Ed. L. Gitman and E. Woodford-Williams) Basel-Munich-New York, Karger.

Gruenberg, E.M. (1972) 'Obstacles of optimal psychiatric service delivery systems' *Psychiat. Quart.* **46**, 483–496.

Haag, G. (1967) 'Ausbildung von Mitarbeitern für die Altenhilfe', *Das Altenheim*, **6**, 187–190.

Harris, R. (1975) 'Model for a graduate geriatric programme at a university medical school', *Gerontologist*, **15**, 304–307.

Helmchen, H., and Hippius, H. (1975) *Entwicklungstendenzen biologischer Psychiatrie*, Stuttgart, Georg Thieme.

Hermann, U. (1972) 'Möglichkeiten und Grenzen der Dekumentation Gerontopsychiatrischer Sozialdaten', in *Berlin Gerontopsychiatrie 2, Janssen Symposien 9* (Ed. S. Kanowski) Düsseldorf, Janssen.

Hippius, H., and Kanowski, S. (1974) 'Zum gegenwärtigen Stand der Gerontopsychiatrie in der Bundesrepublik', *Nervenarzt*, **45**, 289–297.

Hirsch, W. (1971) 'Der Mangel an Fachkräften in der Krankenpflege', *Sozial., S. Dien. Mens.*, **2**, 10–16.

Informationsblätter (1969) Informationen aus dem Bereich der Altenhilfe, *Mangel an Altenpflegerinnen.* **11**, 5, Berlin, Deutsches Zentralinstitut für Soziale Fragen.

Isaacs, B. (1972) 'Towards a definition of geriatrics', *J. Chron. Dis.*, **25**, 425–432.

Junkers, G., Kanowski, S., and Paur, R. (1976) 'Forschung, Lehre und Krankenversorgung aus der Sicht einer Abteilung für Gerontopsychiatrie', *Z. Geront.*, **9**, 151–175.

Kaiser, H. (1973) 'Die Ausbildung des Arztes in Gerontologie und Geriatrie', *Act. Geront.*, **3**, 667–669.

Kanowski, S. (1973) 'Erfordernisse und Bedarf an Ausbildung für Arzte und nichtärztliches Personal im Bereich der Gerontopsychiatrie', *Act. Geront.*, **3**, 671–676.

240

Kanowski, S. (1974) 'Probleme der Adaptation aus psychiatrischer Sicht', *Act. Geront.*, **4**, 657–663.

Kanowski, S. (in press) 'Aufgaben, Bedarf, Lernziele und Ausbildungsprogramme im Bereich der Gerontopsychiatrie in der Bundesrepublik: aus ärztlicher Sicht', *Janssen Symposien*.

Kanowski, S., and Girke, W. (1975) 'Biologische Forschung in der Alterspsychiatrie', in *Entwicklungstendenzen Biologischer Psychiatrie*, (Ed. H. Helmchen and H. Hippius) Stuttgart, Georg Thieme.

Kay, D.W.K., Beamish, P. and Roth, M. (1964) 'Old age mental disorders in Newcastle-upon-Tyne; Part I. A study of prevalence, *Br. J. Psychiat.*, **110**, 146–158.

Kimsey, L.R., and Roberts J.L. (1969) 'Teaching geriatrics in Texas medical schools', *Texas Med.*, **65**, 35–36.

Lauter, H. (1972) 'Organisch bedingte Alterspsychosen' in *Alterspsychiatrie der Gegenwart*, vol. 2, (Ed. K.P. Kisker, J.-E. Meyer, M. Müller, and E. Stromgren) Berlin Heidelberg, New York, Springer, pp. 1103–1149.

Lauter, H. (1974) 'Epidemiologische Aspekte alterspsychiatrischer Erkrankungen', *Nervenarzt*, **45**, 277–288.

Lawton, A.H. (1971) 'Continuing postgraduate medical education in geriatrics', *J. Am. Geriat. Soc.*, **19**, 97–101.

Miller, M.B. (1975) 'Iatrogenic and nurisgenic effects of prolonged immobilization of the ill aged, *J. Am. Geriat. Soc.*, **23**, 360–369.

Müller, H. (1971) 'Beschäftigungslage und optimaler Einsatz von Arbeitskräften in Krankenanstalten', *Das Krankenhaus*, **4**, 165–170.

Pathy, M.S. (1974) 'Undergraduate teaching in geriatric medicine in the University Hospital of Wales, *Geront. Clin.*, **16**, 179–184.

Post, F. (1966) 'Somatic and psychic factors in the treatment of elderly psychiatric patients', *J. Psychosom. Res.*, **10**, 13–19.

Post, F. (1972) 'Spezielle Alterspsychiatrie', in *Alterspsychiatrie der Gegenwart*, (Ed. K.P. Kisker, J.-E. Meyer, M. Müller, and E. Stromgren) Berlin, Heidelberg, New York, Springer, pp. 1107–1101.

Radebold, H. (1976) 'Psychoanalytische Gruppenpsychotherapie mit älteren und alten Patienten (II. Mitteilung über spezifische Aspekte)', *Z. Geront.* **9**, 128–142.

Ross, C.H. (1975) 'Gero-education', *J. Am. Geriat. Soc.*, **23**, 184–189.

Rudd, T.N. (1972) 'Prescribing methods and iatrogenic situations in old age', *Geront. Clin.*, **14**, 123–128.

Sharma, K.L., and Bhandari, P. (1970) 'A study of students' stereotypes towards ageing', *Ind. J. Geront.*, **2**, 20–27.

Spence, D.L., Feigenbaum, E.M. Fitzgerald, F. and Roth, J. (1968) 'Medical student attitudes toward the geriatric patient', *J. Am. Geriat. Soc.*, **16**, 976–983.

Udelman, H.D. (1973) 'Geriatric psychiatry—a global view', *Arizona Med.*, **30**, February 1973, 89–91.

Varner, R.V., and Verwoerdt, A. (1975) 'Training of Psychogeriatricians', in *Modern perspectives in the psychiatry of old age*, (Ed. J.G. Howells) Edinburgh, London, Churchill Livingstone.

Verwoerdt, A. (1969) 'Training of geropsychiatry; in *Behavior and adaptation in late life*. (Ed. E.W. Busse and E. Pfeiffer) Boston, Little, Brown.

Williamson, J., Stokoe, I.H. Gray, S., Fischer, M., and Smith, A. (1964) 'Old people at home, their unreported needs', *Lancet*, **i**, 1117–1120.

Williamson, J. (1967) 'Detecting disease in clinical geriatrics', in *Intensive course in geriatrics for general practitioners*. (Ed. E. Woodford-Williams and A.N. Exton-Smith) Basel, New York, Karger.

Woodford-Williams, E. (1967) 'The function and structure of a geriatric department', in *Intensive course in geriatrics for general practitioners*. (Ed. E. Woodford-Williams and A.N. Exton-Smith) Basel, New York, Karger.

12

THE DEVELOPMENT OF PSYCHIATRIC SERVICES FOR THE ELDERLY IN BRITAIN

T. Arie and A.D. Isaacs

Demographic background

That the care of old people with mental disorders is likely to be the biggest challenge to health and social services of all developed countries in the remaining decades of this century is now generally recognized (WHO, 1972). In England and Wales the number of people aged 65 and over has increased more than four-fold since the beginning of the century, from over 1·5 million to over 6·5 million, and this trend will continue at least until the 1990s; in 1991 there will be a million more old people than 20 years before (Ashley, 1971).

TABLE 12.1. Population of England and Wales at successive censuses (thousands)

Year	Total all ages	Aged 65 and over	Aged 75 and over
1901	32 528	1518 (4·7%)	442 (1·4%)
1911	36 070	1878 (5·2%)	518 (1·4%)
1921	37 887	2291 (6·0%)	648 (1·7%)
1931	39 952	2963 (7·4%)	821 (2·0%)
1951	43 758	4824 (11·0%)	1567 (3·6%)
1961	46 104	5494 (11·9%)	1976 (4·3%)
1971	48 929	6496 (13·3%)	2318 (4·7%)
1974*	49 195	6865 (13·9%)	2437 (4·9%)

* 1974 figures estimated

The elderly have increased not only in numbers, but in the proportion which they form of the population (Table 12.1). This increase is due chiefly to the relative decline in the birth rate in the early part of the century, though in part of course also to higher standards of living and of medical care. The elderly (over-65s) were 4·7 per cent of the population in 1901; in 1974 the estimated proportion was 13·9 per cent. But these figures greatly understate the size of the problem, for it is not the over-65s as a whole that press so heavily upon services, but the very old among them. The number of persons aged 75 and over has increased nearly six-fold during this century, and will continue to increase into the next century even after the numbers of the elderly as a whole have levelled off. The over-75s are now 35 per cent of the elderly, and by the end of the century will be nearly 45 per cent. It should be noted that whereas the chances at birth of living to old age have increased greatly, the number of years expectation of life at the age of 65 and above has altered relatively little during this century, though the increase has been greater for women than for men. Among the very old, women outnumber men by three to one; over 80 per cent of women aged 75 and over are single, widowed, or divorced. The 'hard core' of the 'psychogeriatric problem' are these older women who are without husbands.

The social circumstances of the elderly have changed greatly (Wroe. 1973; OPCS, 1973). Old people are much more likely to live alone these days; the proportion living alone nearly doubled over the 20 years up to 1971 when 13 per cent of elderly men and 30 per cent of elderly women were living alone. And probably about half of all the very old in Britain live at the poverty line—that is to say they are either drawing, or are entitled to draw payments supplementary to the normal old age pension, or are wholly dependent on that pension. Houses in which they live are generally much older and much less well provided with basic amenities than the houses of younger people.

Contrasting with the poor conditions in which so many of the elderly live is the general increase in living standards during this century, which has brought higher expectations of relief from the burdens of old age, but especially from the burdens of caring for the elderly. Concurrently there has been a steady growth of the proportion of middle-aged women going out to work—and it is these women who have traditionally looked after the elderly and are now therefore less available.

Psychiatry and old age mental disorders

At the same time understanding of the mental disorders of old age has increased, as has the power of psychiatry to alleviate and often to cure these conditions. Chiefly through the studies of the Newcastle school of psychiatry (Roth, 1973), we have a picture of the epidemiology of these disorders.

Some 10 per cent of persons aged 65 and over living at home were found to be demented in the Newcastle studies of the early 1960s, about half of them severely (Kay et al., 1964, 1970); when figures from a subsequent cohort of old people were combined with these and reanalysed to exclude the mild cases, the prevalence was 6·2 per cent (a figure which corresponds closely with that of a more recent Scottish community survey (Gruer, 1975). The prevalence of dementia in the elderly in Newcastle increased steadily from around three per cent in persons aged 65 to 70 to over 20 per cent in those over 80; thus one in five of the very old was demented. Six out of seven of the demented were living at home, yet dementia is the main determinant of breakdown leading to institutional care; thus when two Newcastle cohorts were followed over a period of two and a half to four years, those who were found to be demented on initial examination were two and a half times as likely 'normal' old people to have been admitted to hospitals or homes, and their aggregate

TABLE 12.2. Expectation of life in England and Wales

	At birth		At 1 year		At 15 years		At 45 years		At 65 years	
	M	F	M	F	M	F	M	F	M	F
1841	40·2	42·2	46·7	47·6	43·4	44·1	23·3	24·4	10·9	11·5
1901–1910	48·5	52·4	55·7	58·3	47·3	50·1	23·3	25·5	10·8	12·0
1930–1932	58·7	62·9	62·3	65·5	51·2	54·3	25·5	28·3	11·3	13·1
1960–1962	68·1	74·0	68·0	74·4	55·3	60·9	27·1	32·1	12·0	15·3
1972	68·9	75·1	69·2	75·2	55·7	61·7	27·3	32·8	12·1	16·0

Source: Registrar General, 1974.

stay was four times as long in hospital and ten times as long in residential homes as the 'normals'—despite the shorter life expectation of the demented.

Yet despite this increased tendency of the demented to breakdown to the point of needing institutional care, dementia is probably the least recognized handicap in old people. Thus a study by Williamson and his colleagues (1964) in Edinburgh found that 80 per cent of old people living at home who had moderate or severe dementia, and 90 per cent of those with mild dementia, were unknown to their general practitioners to be demented. In the light of these findings it is not surprising that 40 per cent of the elderly in residential care in Newcastle in the late 1950s were found to have some dementia, 29 per cent to a 'developed' degree (Kay *et al.*, 1962). Some ten years later a survey of residential homes in Scotland found a prevalence of confusion and forgetfulness of 37·2 per cent (Carstairs and Morrison, 1971), and in 1970 a census of old people in residential homes in England and Wales reported that 48 per cent of women and 35 per cent of men were confused (DHSS 1976c).

In short, although most demented people are at home, the pressure of dementia on residential services is enormous. By far the biggest sector of social services expenditure is on residential care for the elderly—against which figure must be set the fact that only four per cent of the residential care staff have had any training in that field (DHSS, 1976d).

Of functional disorders of old age the Newcastle studies suggested a prevalence of around twelve per cent of neuroses and character disorders with a further two per cent or so of major functional psychoses. Forty per cent of the group of affective or neurotic disorders were of moderate or great severity, and five per cent of the old people suffering from neurotic or affective illnesses had developed them for the first time in late life (Kay *et al.*, 1964). Suicide is much more common in old age depressions (Barraclough, 1971) and indeed suicide rates (by contrast with so-called attempted suicide or parasuicide) rise with age, being much higher in old men than in old women and highest of all in old men of low social class (Registrar General, 1971).

The combined Newcastle prevalence of psychiatric morbidity amounts to some 25 per cent of old people living at home, a finding remarkably similar to that more recently found in the London Borough of Camberwell (see Chapter 9). Elderly people are as likely to consult general practitioners for such disorders as are other adults but they are much less likely to be referred to psychiatrists for further specialized help (as contrasted with institutional 'disposal') (Shepherd *et al.*, 1966); and yet the neurotic disorders of late life may present with greater intensity in the setting of deprivation which is associated with old age—lack of status, money, work, companionship—and, very importantly, poor physical health, especially cardiovascular disorders, which were found in one survey (Bergmann, 1971) to be importantly related to the development of neurotic symptoms. Marital distress in the elderly may be acute, often presenting overtly for the first time when lack of alternative social or occupational outlets, or growing infirmity and immobility may thrust the partners on to each other's resources as never before; and sexuality in old age is also a matter which is beginning to be studied in this country (Gilmore, 1973) though substantial work has been done in the United States (Pfeiffer, 1969).

Nearly 95 per cent of old people in the United Kingdom at the time of the 1971 census lived in private households; those who were in institutional settings divided approximately equally between hospitals on the one hand and residential homes on the other. Among hospital patients twice as many are in general or geriatric hospitals as in psychiatric hospitals, but the elderly account for just under one-half of all occupied beds in both types of hospital (DHSS, 1976a; OPCS, 1976). At the turn of the century old people were only one in ten of the inmates of asylums (Lewis, 1946).

During the period 1954 to 1971 the proportion of residents in psychiatric hospitals who were aged over 65 doubled, and of some 50 000 old people in these hospitals half are now over 75 years old. During that period the total number of inpatients of all ages fell by nearly 30 per cent, but the over-75s actually increased their residence rates over this period of decline of the mental hospital population. Over one half of over-75s admitted to psychiatric hospitals are first admissions, and it is likely that some 40 per cent of elderly patients in these hospitals are demented (DHSS, 1975) and in 1973 there were some 9000 admissions for senile or presenile dementia (DHSS, 1976a). Although the actual number of admissions of old people has continued to rise, in 1970 there was an unexpected fall in the first admission rate of the elderly to psychiatric hospitals, and this trend has persisted (Table 12.3). Over the years 1970–1973 the first admission rate of patients with the diagnosis of presenile or senile dementia fell by no less than 23 per cent.

TABLE 12.3. Admissions of patients aged 65 and over to psychiatric hospitals and units

	All admissions			First admissions		
	PERSONS	MALES	FEMALES	PERSONS	MALES	FEMALES
(a) Numbers						
1951	12 153	4524	7629	9275	3579	5696
1960	23 752	7888	15 864	14 932	5202	9730
1969	36 925	12 093	24 832	22 704	7768	14 936
1970*	36 901	12 177	24 724	17 109	6147	10 962
1971	36 293	11 740	24 553	16 166	5568	10 598
1972	36 867	11 778	25 089	15 665	5350	10 315
1973	37 636	11 692	25 944	15 609	5245	10 364
1974	37 718	11 760	25 958	15 416	5220	10 196
(b) Rates per 100 000 population aged 65 and over						
1951	252	230	268	193	182	200
1960	435	375	473	274	247	290
1969	591	509	641	363	327	385
1970*	581	504	628	269	254	279
1971	567	480	621	253	228	268
1972	567	472	625	241	214	257
1973	557	448	626	231	201	250
1974	549	442	617	225	196	242

* In 1970 the method of determining 1st admissions was changed
Source: England & Wales D.H.S.S., 1976a, e

The explanation of this fall is not obvious, and it has not occurred everywhere (the Goodmayes psychogeriatric service, for which one of us is responsible, has not experienced any such trend). Possible explanations include the increased availability of places in local authority residential homes over this period, the greater investment in extra-mural supportive services, or the possibility that relatively more demented patients are being admitted to geriatric rather than psychiatric hospitals. Attempts are being made to explore these possibilities, but the most likely explanation seems to be that 1969 saw the beginning of a series of reports of committees of inquiry into conditions in psychiatric hospitals, to which further reference will be made below. The attention drawn by these inquiries to the overcrowding and other shortcomings of care in these hospitals, and the criticisms made of individuals working in them, may have made many psychiatrists reluctant to admit demented patients to already often overcrowded wards.

Development of government policy

The growing pressure of old people with mental disorders on psychiatric services throughout the 1960s led on the one hand to a series of reviews of the 'psychogeriatric problem' (Scottish Home and Health Department, 1970; Society of Clinical Psychiatrists, 1971; Andrews *et al.*, 1972) and on the other to the development in a few districts of psychiatric services directed specifically towards the needs of the elderly. However the impulse towards these services came about against a background of changes in social policy in the years since the war, and these fall under three headings which it is relevant to consider briefly: (i) The development of what has come to be known as 'community care'; (ii) the move within health services towards the desegregation of the mentally ill; and (iii) the growth of the new medical specialty of geriatrics.

Community Care

We have been unable to ascertain the origins of the phrase 'community care' but these reassuring and alliterative words have become established both as part of the ideology of the caring professions, and the policy of successive governments since the war. When in 1962 the government published its hospital plan (Ministry of Health, 1962) it was made clear that the extra-mural care, alongside the development of general hospital psychiatric units, was expected to replace the large mental hospitals: and in 1963 the document which set out plans for the development of health and welfare services was subtitled 'The development of community care' (Ministry of Health, 1963). The Mental Health Act of 1959 committed the government firmly to shifting the centre of gravity of psychiatric care from hospitals to extra-mural services. The act greatly extended the responsibilities of local authorities towards the extra-mural care of the mentally ill, and resulted in rapid expansion both of numbers of social workers and of hostels, clubs, and other resources for maintaining the mentally ill outside hospitals. From the 1959 act to the further consolidation of social services in unified departments in 1971 following the recommendations of the Seebohm Committee (1968), expenditure on local authority mental health services in England and Wales increased nearly ten-fold, from some £3·7 million to £34·4 million (DHSS, 1976b). These developments were characteristically patchy between different municipalities, and in the field of services for mentally ill infirm old people it was noted by Wigley (1968) that the proportion of local authorities providing day centres, day hospitals, work centres, welfare homes or social clubs were respectively only 13, 31, 8, 26, and 12 per cent. In the intervening years expansion generally has continued, but variations in services between different localities have remained conspicuous.

The establishment of the 'Seebohm'' social services departments in 1971, and the subsequent transfer under the National Health Service Reorganization Act of 1973 of all social workers, including those employed in hospitals, to the employment of local authorities were further developments in the shift to extra-mural care. Assumptions underlying the commitment to 'community care' have recently been searchingly analysed (Hawks, 1975), and despite the many questions of feasibility, effectiveness, finance and humanity which still remain open, the current economic stringency in Britain, together with the belief that community care is necessarily cheaper than hospital care, has resulted in government policy favouring the redirection of still further resources into extra-mural services (DHSS, 1976b). The wish to avoid 'uprooting' old people and to preserve their dignity and independence in their own homes is self-evidently desirable, but there are dangers that in place of institutional care with all its common shortcomings, old people may be left at home with effectively no care at all, or their relatives and neighbours with heavy burdens to carry (Grad and Sainsbury, 1965; Hamilton and Hoenig, 1966; Sanford, 1975; Pasker *et al.*, 1976).

Desegregation of the mentally ill in the hospital service

The Regulation of Madhouses Act of 1774 initiated a sequence of legislation that was to result in the almost complete segregation of people with mental illness from those with other types of disability. This legislation was only partly retrogressive; it resulted in the development of psychiatric institutions which had many excellent qualities, and the 'single common workhouse' in which the unfortunate, the old, the crippled, the sick, and the mad were gathered together was an example of non-segregation of the mentally ill which was hardly beneficial.

Since the war a variety of factors have contributed towards the movement to desegregate the mentally ill: for instance, recognition that much mental illness was treatable by physical methods; the availability of drugs to control even the most dangerously disturbed patients; the gradual, though far from complete, destigmatization of mental illness; and the growing awareness of the importance of psychological factors in the understanding and management of physical illness. Probably experience with general ward treatment of tuberculosis—previously no less feared than mental illness—helped to establish confidence in the ability to treat the mentally ill along with the other patients. Finally the 'run-down' of mental hospitals as a result of new energetic treatments and rehabilitation, and optimistic predictions of the future trends of this run-down, consolidated the commitment to a transposition of hospital psychiatry to general hospitals.

Predictions of the run-down of mental hospitals (Tooth and Brooke, 1961) made too little allowance for the accumulation of demented old people—an underestimate which has been probably only partially corrected by the substantial increase in recommended psychiatric bed provision for the elderly which formed part of government guidance in 1972 (DHSS, 1972). In those parts of the country where general hospital psychiatry has developed most, old people are still frequently being admitted direct to large mental hospitals. The move towards general hospital units has taken place at very variable rates in different parts of the country—in the Manchester region in 1971 nearly half of all psychiatric admissions were to general and teaching hospital units, while the corresponding figure for the East Anglian region was less than five per cent. However, whereas 22 per cent of patients aged under 65 were admitted to general or teaching units in England and Wales, only 14 per cent of admissions of elderly people were to such units (DHSS, 1973). Dangers of a double standard in psychiatry, whereby mental hospitals become dumps for unwanted old people, remote from the acute treatment centres in general hospitals, are already in many places a reality and the 'scandals' which are apt to arise in such settings have become sad and familiar features of the medical landscape.

Reference has already been made to the series of official inquiries which began with the publication of the report on Ely Hospital in 1969. This revealed under-provision, demoralization and neglect in a hospital for the mentally handicapped. Since then such inquiries have become more frequent; Whittingham Hospital (National Health Service, 1972) was an example of a large mental hospital which seemed to have been largely bypassed by the tide of psychiatry into the general hospital, leaving a large stagnant pool of old people behind (and it is significant that this hospital was in the Manchester region, where general hospital psychiatry has developed most rapidly). But not all inquiries have been in mental hospitals; psychiatric units in general hospitals have had their troubles also (Northwestern Regional Health Authority, 1975), as have local authority residential homes (Oxfordshire County Council, 1974). It is not of course the shortcomings which such inquiries generally and predictably reveal that are new, but rather the climate of scrutiny which has settled over the whole sector of institutional care. The effects of this have been mixed; on the one hand they have encouraged successive governments to increase the share of resources directed to the so called 'long-stay' sector, but on the other hand staff working in these settings have come to feel more vulnerable and more threatened. Reinforcement in recent years of complaints procedures throughout the health service has compounded this, and in the opinion of many observers has contributed to the difficulties of recruitment to these hospitals, and indeed of doctors to psychiatry.

Geriatrics as a medical speciality

Writing in 1849, Dr George E. Day introduced his book on *Diseases of advanced life* with the words 'The subject is one of the highest importance and it has been strangely overlooked during the last half century by physicians of all countries'. Sir Anthony Carlisle, President of the Royal College of Surgeons in 1817 felt that ageing and disease were not synonymous and that specific diagnosis in the elderly could lead to specific and effective treatment (Livesley, 1977). Nonetheless the care of the elderly continued to take place in old stigmatized Poor Law workhouses and it was in one such ex-workhouse that Marjorie Warren started her pioneering work at the West Middlesex Hospital, demonstrating the impressive results that came from a policy of careful diagnosis and active treatment and rehabilitation (Warren, 1946). In 1947 the Medical Society for the Care of the Elderly was formed, and three years later it became the British Geriatrics Society (Adams, 1975). Sheldon's famous survey of the elderly in Wolverhampton in 1948 was another stimulus to the recognition of the extent and nature of the handicaps of old people, and following the establishment of the National Health Service in the same year, geriatrics was recognized as an official specialty. By the end of 1975 there were 317 consultants in geriatrics in England and Wales (DHSS, 1976, personal communication). Despite serious problems of recruitment of staff to geriatrics (the majority of entrants to the speciality, and currently about half of new consultant appointments in geriatrics are of doctors trained in countries other than Britain) the achievements of geriatric departments have been widely recognized and their existence has acted as a focus for the development of services for the elderly in their districts. The success of the strategy of meeting the neglected needs of the elderly by the provision of a special medical service for them has been an important stimulus to the development of psychiatric services for the elderly.

Development of special psychiatric services for the elderly

The 1950s and 1960s saw great expansion in the study of the psychiatric disorders of old age—epidemiological, pathological, and clinical. The interest was in part the consequence of the growing pressure of what is often spoken as the 'psychogeriatric problem', a pressure which had been forecast by Lewis immediately after the war (Lewis, 1946).

The development of community care and the beginnings of a shift from isolated and segregated practice largely based in menial hospitals, to a greater involvement with general practitioners, social service agencies and general hospitals, stimulated psychiatrists to reappraise the way in which hospitals should be used. It was not long before it became clear that although more effective extra-mural services enabled many patients to be looked after outside hospitals, they equally resulted in more people being referred to psychiatrists (Grad and Sainsbury, 1966).

At the same time the day hospital movement (Farndale, 1961), originally one of psychiatry's gifts to medicine, was quickly taken up and developed by geriatricians. The growing use of the domiciliary consultation service (under which as part of the National Health Service hospital consultants are able to see patients in their own homes at the request of general practitioners) further developed interest in the elderly and this service has become predominantly one for older patients (Smith and Blythe, 1971).

But the most potent factor of all was pressure on health and social services of the sheer numbers of old people, and indeed the ageing of the elderly population itself. In 1959 the World Health Organization published a review of mental health problems of the aged, with proposals for the organization of geriatric mental health services, and it was followed in 1962 by a report from Belfast which suggested that between a quarter and a third of all patients over 60 were misplaced between psychiatric and geriatric hospitals and that this misplacement increased the likelihood of death and reduced the likelihood of discharge (Kidd, 1962). Subsequent studies (Mezey et al., 1968; Langley and Simpson, 1970; Copeland et al., 1975) failed to confirm either the extent or the potential damage of such misplacement, but they had the result of focusing the attention of the need to identify the physical and mental components in the often mixed disorders of old people; the case grew for the establishment of assessment units run jointly by psychiatrists and geriatricians (Kay et al., 1966). An early unit of this sort was established in Edinburgh (Fish and Williamson, 1964), and a more comprehensive one in Nottingham where the welfare department had also the right of direct admission (Morton et al., 1968). By 1970 the establishment of 'psychogeriatric assessment units' became the official policy of the government (DHSS, 1970), and it was recommended that between 10 and 20 beds should be provided in each district hospital to provide such a joint facility. The policy of joint assessment did not at that stage derive from any evaluative studies, but it had 'face validity' which came from the obvious need for geriatricians and psychiatrists to collaborate, and from the mixed nature of so many of the disorders of the elderly. Moreover the establishment of such units seemed likely to generate foci of interest which would act as a stimulus to the improvement of local services for old people.

In practice however such units have not yet been widely established, and they have sometimes become effectively the responsibility of one rather than of both services (Prinsley, 1973).

In 1972 the government issued a further policy document on 'Services for mental illness related to old age' (DHSS, 1972), which distinguished three groups of elderly patients with mental disorders and defined the respective spheres of responsibility of geriatricians, psychiatrists, and local authority social services departments.

(1) Patients who had entered hospitals for the mentally ill before modern methods of treatment were available and who have grown old in them.
(2) Elderly patients with functional mental illness.
(3) Elderly patients with dementia, this group was further sub-divided.
   (a) The mildly to moderately demented who were not suffering from significant physical disease or illness.
   (b) The severely demented who were not suffering from other physical disease or illness.
   (c) Those with dementia whether mild or severe, who suffered from concomitant significant physical illness or disease.

Patients in category (1) were to remain the responsibility of psychiatrists though it was envisaged that their numbers would dwindle. Patients in category (2) were self-evidently the responsibility of psychiatrists. Those in category (3a) would be looked after by general practitioners and their 'primary care teams', or in local authority residential homes or day centres; those in (3b) by psychiatric services; and those in (3c) by geriatric services.

Extra bed provision (2·5 to 3 beds plus 2–3 day places per 1000 of the population aged 65 and over) was recommended, and it was envisaged that long-stay severely demented patients would be looked after in smaller 'community hospitals' serving neigbourhoods and complementing the functions of the comprehensive district general hospital.

Further stimulus to the development of psychogeriatric services had come also from the annual reports of the Hospital Advisory Service (HAS) (1970–75). This body was established as part of the government's reaction to the Ely Hospital report in 1969 (DHSS, 1969), and it has been sending mixed teams of health staff to visit geriatric and psychiatric hospitals throughout the country; the findings of these teams have each year further emphasized the need to develop services for the elderly.

The first director of the HAS on relinquishing his office joined the already growing group of psychiatrists who were making the psychiatry of old age their particular interest, and from these units a growing volume of descriptive and research studies have been appearing. Posts of consultant psychiatrist 'with a special interest in the elderly' are now often advertised, and the Royal College of Psychiatrists, through its Group for the Psychiatry of Old Age which was established under the chairmanship of Dr Felix Post in 1972, has recommended that in each health district particular psychiatrists should make the care of the elderly their special responsibility (Royal College of Psychiatrists, 1975). These posts have not always been easy to fill, because of the low prestige of work with the elderly, and because of the minimal emphasis that has been given to this work in all but a few teaching centres. However within three years membership of the Group for the Psychiatry of Old Age has risen to over a hundred, and about half of its members are working primarily in the psychiatry of old age.

There has been a wide and fruitful diversity of approach in the styles of these new psychiatric services for the elderly (e.g. Arie, 1970; Baker, 1974; Bergmann, 1972; Donovan et al., 1971; Godber, 1975; Jolley, 1976; Langley et al., 1975; Pitt, 1975; Robinson, 1975; White, 1975; Whitehead and Mankikar, 1974). Some such services are based principally on joint assessment units or day hospitals, others are concerned almost wholly with demented patients; most are active in teaching, and the best known is that at the Bethlem Royal Hospital (Bethlem Royal and Maudsley Hospitals, 1976), from which a host of publications had appeared even before the more recent developments up and down the country (e.g. Post, 1962, 1965, 1966). But against the background of this diversity, and based on the experience of those services which have developed most fully, certain general principles have made it possible to draw a profile of the type of service which seems likely increasingly to be established as a standard part of district psychiatric work (Arie, 1973).

Such a service would deal with the entire referred psychiatric morbidity, functional and organic alike, of a defined population. It would take responsibility from the first point of contact—i.e. it will not be only a 'secondary' service dealing merely with referrals from other psychiatrists. Whenever reasonable, it is always the aim of such a service to maintain old people at home, though there is no reluctance to use hospital admission for investigation and treatment where this best meets the needs of the patient, or for long-stay care where the psychiatric hospital seems the most satisfactory placement. Initial assessment is generally in the patient's home, and while the hospital is likely to be the base of the service, hospital staff and other staff located in the community (nurses, social workers, welfare assistants, physiotherapists, occupational therapists, voluntary helpers) will support patients in their homes, complementing the work of family doctors and underpinning the care given by families. Joint assessment units run by geriatrician and psychiatrist and an active day hospital complete the range of facilities.

Services more or less on this pattern are now established in about a dozen centres, and we conclude this chapter with a description of the service for which one of us is responsible, as an illustration of the way one such service has developed, and of the issues which arise in this work.

The Goodmayes psychiatric service for old people

This service was established in January 1969, and it took responsibility for all referred old people (persons aged 65 and over) in a defined catchment area; the right of referral to other psychiatrists was of course preserved, but in fact this rarely occurs. All patients are initially assessed at home by a psychiatrist—even in emergencies, in which case home assessment takes place immediately (Arie, 1970, 1976).

The unit

The hospital base is Goodmayes Hospital, a district psychiatric hospital in east London, which with its associated clinics provides a comprehensive adult psychiatric service for a population now of some 415 000 of whom about 52 000 are aged 65 and over.

In the course of time despite increasing rates of referral and admission, it proved possible rapidly to reduce the complement of beds and by the end of four years the unit's original complement of 350 beds had been reduced to 198, and it was possible greatly to diminish the crowding and to establish mixed sex 30-bed wards, and a mixed admission unit, to which all patients come regardless of diagnosis, and from which the majority are discharged home. The service is now operating just within the government's recommended bed norms and is taking well over 500 referrals a year. More detailed figures on the unit's use of beds have been reported elsewhere (Jolley and Arie, 1976).

The joint patient unit

Close collaboration between physicians and psychiatrists is fundamental to this work, but it was not felt that a formal 'psychogeriatric assessment unit', as had been recommended by the government (DHSS, 1970), was necessary, nor would it have been financially feasible. Instead of small unit of four beds (later five) was established in the neighbouring geriatric hospital (Chadwell Heath Hospital) and to this both the psychiatrists and geriatricians have the right of direct admission, and any patient so admitted becomes the joint patient of both admitting consultants (Arie and Dunn,

1973). No extra resources were involved; this development was simply a more effective use of existing resources. It was envisaged that three types of patients would be admitted. Firstly those who despite home assessment present both physical and mental components in their disorders, the relative significance of which it is not possible confidently to establish without a further period in hospital. Second, those who on home assessment appear to be suffering from disorders which require joint medical and psychiatric treatment. And finally patients who, despite suffering from a clear psychiatric illness, develop intercurrent physical problems which require urgent medical treatment prior to the implementation of the psychiatric treatment programme—for example, depressed patients who become severely dehydrated through refusal of food and drink, and who need intravenous hydration and possibly treatment of resultant infection before physical treatment of their depression can proceed.

In the unit's first 20 months 85 patients were admitted, half each by the psychiatrist and the geriatrician. The mean length of stay in the unit was 20 days and 32 per cent of the patients were discharged direct from the unit whilst 14 per cent died there. Nearly half the patients admitted by the psychiatrist were ultimately taken over by the geriatrician, or died soon after admission, indicating the high prevalence of serious physical disorders in patients referred to a psychiatric service. After the initial period of assessment and treatment in the unit, those patients who were not discharged were transferred either to the psychiatric or the geriatric unit. Three months from admission over half (54 per cent) had returned home, and 25 per cent had died in hospital.

Subsequently the initial four beds were increased to five, and they form an indispensable part of the service. This unit has eliminated any possibility of initial 'misplacement' (Kidd, 1962) of patients referred to our two departments.

Day hospital care and outpatient clinics

Day hospital care is an essential part of a psychiatric service for the elderly (Arie, 1975). Approximately 50 old people come to Goodmayes Hospital as day patients, attending from one to five days a week; with more resources, especially transport, their number could be far greater. There are three overlapping clinical groups; the largest group are patients with dementia who can be maintained in the care of their families at home provided the hospital is able to share the burden. Many of these patients have to attend each day while their familles are at work. The second group are intellectually well preserved people who have adjusted poorly to old age, and who usually first made contact through an acute psychiatric illness from which they recovered. It proves often impossible to persuade these patients to separate from the day hospital even though their attendance may be only for one or two days a week. They have a useful role among the day patients in giving continuity and acting in a sense as 'hosts and hostesses'; any attempt to discharge them is likely to cause a relapse, or the threat of one. The attendance of patients of both these groups is generally terminated only by death, or in the case of the demented patients, by the need for full institutional care as they deteriorate further.

The third group, small in terms of the number of attenders at any one time, are patients who come for investigation or short term treatment, or for whom day attendance acts as a transition between inpatient care and complete discharge or attendance at the outpatient clinic. This group is small at Goodmayes because of the policy of initial domiciliary assessment, and because follow-up of confused patients is also at home; the purpose of such follow-up is to monitor and support the function at home of the patient and his family, and this cannot satisfactorily be done at the outpatient clinic (where in any case the patient is likely to behave abnormally because of the sudden transposition into unfamiliar surroundings).

The outpatient clinic therefore exists chiefly for the continuing surveillance and support of patients with functional disorders, and for the very occasional well-preserved patient with a functional disorder whom it might be appropriate to see initially there in the same way as is traditional with younger patients (but each year less than half a dozen patients attend initially in this way).

Medical staffing

The medical team now comprises two consultants, and six trainees. The staff has expanded with the increase in the volume and scope of the work and with the unit's growing role as a training centre. In addition to the trainee psychiatrists who spend in general a year in the unit, there has been a flow of young psychiatrists and other health workers seeking periods of attachment, both from our own country and abroad, and several have gone on to establish similar services (Jolley, 1976).

But the majority of the trainee doctors have not come with a career interest in this work, but as young psychiatrists pursuing their general psychiatric training; despite the generally unattractive 'image' of geriatric work for young doctors, we are satisfied that, well done, and adequately equipped, this work should be able to compete effectively with other specialities for its share of the ablest graduates.

The nurses

Nursing is the bedrock on which psychogeriatric services (and not only psychogeriatric services) are based. Demarcation disputes about which doctors should look after the elderly with mental disorders are largely irrelevant, for the real issue is the nature of the patients' nursing needs. Very relevant is the distinction which Kushlick (1975) has made between 'hit and run' personnel, such a doctors, social workers, psychologists, and administrators, who are with the patients for periods of rarely more than ten minutes, and the direct care staff who are with the patients for hours on end, or even (as relatives) continuously.

We shall consider the work of the nursing staff in the Goodmayes unit from two points of view: first, the way in which the staff work in the inpatient unit and in the support of patients and relatives outside the hospital; and second, in terms of some more general issues of work—satisfaction and effectiveness which have arisen in the course of the unit's research.

Intra-mural and Extra-mural Nursing

This work falls into two components—indeed it might be said that it is polarized. On the one hand is the work of the acute admission and assessment unit in which the traditional model of investigation, treatment, and discharge operates for the majority of patients. Here the satisfactions of the work derive chiefly from seeing patients get better—satisfactions implicit in the goals which are defined for health workers of all sorts in the course of their education (Arie, 1971). These goals are shared in large measure by nurses working with patients extra-murally who respond in similar terms to the challenge of maintaining function in the patient's normal setting.

In the long-stay wards the role of nurses is quite different. There the task is to look after patients who have arrived after rigorous assessment culminating in the decision that they need permanent hospital care for, almost invariably, severe dependency or behaviour disorders due to irremediably gross dementia. Despite the gravity of dementia in these patients, social factors of course operate powerfully in determining the need for hospitalization, most notably the absence of relatives or their inability to tolerate the patient. Nurses working in these settings have to define their goals not in terms of cure, but of care and maximization of function in patients for whom the natural history of their disease dictates a relentlessly downhill course, which will culminate in death. The extent to which they are able to fulfil these goals depends on resources and on 'morale'; the two of course are linked.

Clarke, a sociologist supported by the Department of Health, has studied nurses on long-stay wards from the point of view of their job satisfaction in relation to their style of work and the individual characteristics of the nurses (Clarke, 1974).

The strategies which these nurses adopt to accommodate to giving 'care-terminated-only-by-death' are various, and give rise to the question whether this work should not more appropriately be done in a setting defined as residential rather than hospital care, for the former is explicitly committed to 'care' rather than to the traditional medical model based on 'cure'.

Yet despite the strategies for redefining goals away from the traditional one of cure, the nurses in the long-stay wards frequently see themselves as working in a 'dumping ground', where the 'failures' of the hospital accumulate; and despite emphasis by the medical staff on supporting the care of patients in the long-stay wards, the nurses see the time, interest, and the energies of the doctors spent mostly in the acute unit and on extra-mural care. In part this grumbling is one way of sustaining morale, but the perceptions by these nurses of the concern for their work and the willingness of the senior members of the medical, nursing, and administrative hierarchies to listen to and deal with their problems are important determinants of job satisfaction; in this the observations are in accord with those of Revans (1964), which were made in a variety of settings including hospitals.

Clarke also made detailed observations of the techniques for coping with certain traditionally difficult aspects of behaviour, and in particular with incontinence; these have been reported in detail elsewhere (Arie, *et al.*, 1976), and the techniques adopted are often complex and their consequences unplanned and unmeasured. Thus an excellently organized cheerful ward in which the majority of patients were incontinent appeared by the diligence of its regimes for preventing patients remaining wet and smells developing, actually make it harder for patients to be continent. The issues of long-stay care and the very question whether the long-stay component and the acute treatment component should realistically be undertaken by one common team, and in the same hospital setting, remain open and deserve closer study; it is a fruitful field for 'action research' in the form of varied solutions and their evaluation.

Extra-mural nursing—the use of nurses to intervene and support patients in their homes—is characteristic of almost all psychogeriatric services. In Goodmayes three nursing networks concerned predominantly with patients outside the hospital have been established. On the one hand a 'community nursing unit' is based within the hospital and serves the whole hospital including the psychogeriatric unit, which is its main single client. This team of trained nurses is available around-the-clock both to intervene in crises in patients' homes, and to give continuing support and make available nursing procedures. Each month the team takes some 20 new referrals from the psychogeriatric unit and makes well over 100 visits to elderly patients. Initial assessment is always by a psychiatrist, but thereafter the community nursing unit may, together with the general practitioner, take over the care of the patient at home. Great store is set on the regularity of reporting back by the nurses on all contacts with patients, and the often brief but relevant notes which complement personal discussion emphasize the importance of good communication and record-keeping on which such teamwork depends.

Complementing the work of the hospital-based community nursing unit are two groups of nurses based outside the hospital. On the one hand are 'community psychiatric nurses' working from a district health centre, and taking referrals not only from the hospital but direct from family doctors and relating to whichever physician initiates the referral. On the other hand there is a liaison system with health visitors and district nurses—a category of staff who have a long tradition in Britain, but hitherto the former have been chiefly concerned with the care of mothers and babies, while the latter have tended to confine themselves to practical nursing procedures in the home. Both groups are increasingly willing now to undertake both the surveillance and the support of elderly people, and their ability to detect and report mental disturbance palpably increasing as they become more involved in the work; studies elsewhere (Harwin, 1973) show that nursing personnel with relatively simple training can be enabled to detect the bulk of significant psychiatric morbidity in old people at home. The extra-murally based nurses work closely with the unit, attending its meetings (in the case of the health visitors and district nurses in the person of a senior nurse who acts as liaison officer), bringing problems for discussion, taking referrals reporting back and indentifying closely with the whole enterprise.

Other members of the team

A full-time social worker is seconded from the local authority, by whom following the recent reorganization of social services and of the National Health Service all social workers are now employed (DHSS, 1974); she is a crucial member of the team and has become very skilful in work with the elderly, and especially confused people—a field of skill too little emphasized, in our experience, in the training of social workers. Other social workers are extra-murally based, and liaise with varying degrees of closeness and effectiveness.

Voluntary work, under a district co-ordinator, takes many forms, from specific tasks—such as entertainment or escort—to general support and befriending. This work is capable of, and indeed urgently requires, development both in identification of services which can appropriately be performed by individual volunteers and in stimulating neighbourhood projects, not least by mobilization of the 'young-olds'. There must be many analogous possibilities to the scheme which has recently been reported for the rehabilitation of dysphasic patients entirely through the mobilization of groups of volunteers (Griffiths, 1975).

Psychologists who are only minimally involved with testing, have begun to explore the scope for behavioural modification techniques and psychotherapy with the elderly, and to conduct groups for patients and for relatives.

As with all elderly patients *occupational therapy* and *physiotherapy* is essential and both these tasks are undertaken at Goodmayes largely by 'untrained' local housewives who are employed as occupational therapy or physiotherapy 'helpers'. These ladies work in pairs on the wards, after an initial induction course and with continuing supervision and support by professional staff of the departments concerned.

Conclusion

Psychiatric morbidity in the elderly poses clinical and organizational problems which are beginning to be solved, though growing numbers of the very old, and increasing public expectations, are likely to present formidable difficulties in the remaining years of this century and beyond. Work with the elderly has until now been of low prestige, and even stigmatized, in the health services of those highly developed countries which need it most. There is encouraging evidence that such attitudes may be capable of change, and the last decade has seen such changes clearly developing in Britain.

References

Adams, G. (1975) 'Eld health: origins and destiny of British geriatrics', *Age and Ageing*, **4**, 65–68.

Andrews, J., Bardon, D., Gander, D.R., Gibson, K.B., Mallett, B.L., and Robinson, K.V. (1972) 'Planning psychogeriatric care', *Gerontologia Clinica*, **14**, 100–109.

Arie, T. (1970) 'The first year of the Goodmayes psychiatric service for old people', *Lancet*, **ii**, 1175–1178.

Arie, T. (1971) 'Morale and the planning of psychogeriatric services', *British Medical Journal*, **iii**, 166–170.

Arie, T. (1973) 'Psychiatric needs of the elderly', in *Needs of the elderly for health and welfare services* (Ed. R.W. Canvin and N.G. Pearson) Exeter, Institute of Biometry and Community Medicine Publication No. 2.

Arie, T. (1975) 'Day care in geriatric psychiatry', *Gerontologia Clinica*, **17**, 31–39.

Arie, T. (1976) 'The Goodmayes psychiatric service for old people', *The Gerontologist*, **3**, 280–281.

Arie, T., Clarke, M., and Slattery, Z. (1976) 'Incontinence in geriatric psychiatry', in *Incontinence in the elderly* (Ed. F.L. Willington) London, Academic Press.

Arie, T., and Dunn, T. (1973) 'A "do-it-yourself" psychiatricgeriatric joint patient unit', *Lancet*, **ii**, 313–316.

Ashley, J.S.A. (1971) 'The challenge of another million by 1991', *Modern Geriatrics*, 320–329.

Baker, A.A. (1974) 'Why psychogeriatrics?' *Lancet*, **i**, 795–796.

Barraclough, B. (1971) 'Suicide in the elderly', in *Recent developments in psychogeriatrics*, (Ed. D.W.K. Kay and A. Walk) Royal Medico-psychological Association, Ashford, Headley Brothers.

Bergmann, K. (1971) 'The neuroses of old age', in *Recent development in psychogeriatrics*, (Ed. D.W.K. Kay and A. Walk) Royal Medico-Psychological Association, Ashford, Headley Brothers.

Bergmann, K. (1972) 'Psychogeriatric care in Great Britain, with special reference to the place of the day hospital', Janssen Symposium. *Gerontopsychiatrie*. **2**.

Bethlem Royal and Maudsley Hospitals *Report 1970–1975*. See also *Institute of Psychiatry Report for 1972–3*, pp. 33–36.

Carstairs, V., and Morrison, M. (1971) *The elderly in residential care*. Scottish Health Service Studies, 19, Edinburgh, Scottish Home and Health Department.

Clarke, M. (1974) Research Reports to DHSS.

Copeland, J.R.M., Kelleher, M.J., Kellett, J.M., Barron, G., Cowan, D.W.F., and Gourlay, A.J. (1975) 'Evaluation of a psychogeriatric service: the distinction between psychogeriatric and geriatric patients', *British Journal of Psychiatry*, **126**, 21–29.

Day, G.E. (1849) *Diseases of advanced life*, London, T.S.W. Boone.

DHSS (1969) (Department of Health and Social Security) *Report of the committee of enquiry into allegations of ill treatment of patients and other irregularities at the Ely Hospital, Cardiff*, Comnd. 3975, London, Her Majesty's Stationery Office.

DHSS (1970) *National Health Service psychogeriatric assessment units*, Memorandum with Circular HM(70)11, London, Her Majesty's Stationery Office.

DHSS (1972) *Services for mental illness related to old age*, Memorandum with Circular HM(72)71, London, Her Majesty's Stationery Office.

DHSS (1973) *Psychiatric hospitals and units in England and Wales, 1971*, Statistical and Research Report Series No. 6. London, Her Majesty's Stationery Office (and personal communications).

DHSS (1974) *Social work support for the health service*, Report of the Working Party, London, Her Majesty's Stationery Office.

DHSS (1975) *Censuses of patients in mental illness hospitals, 1971, and mental illness day patients, 1972*, Statistical and Research Report Series No. 10, London, Her Majesty's Stationery Office.

DHSS (1976a) *Psychiatric hospitals and units in England, 1973*, Statistical and Research Report Series No. 12, London, Her Majesty's Stationery Office.

DHSS (1976b) *Health and personal social services statistics for England, 1975*, London, Her Majesty's Stationery Office.

DHSS (1976c) *The census of residential accommodation*, London, Her Majesty's Stationery Office.

DHSS (1976d) *Report of the working party on manpower and training for the social services*, London, Her Majesty's Stationery Office.

Donovan, J.F., Williams, I.E.I., and Wilson, T.S. (1971) in *Recent developments in psychogeriatrics*, (Ed. D.W.K. Kay and A. Walk) Royal Medico-Psychological Association, Ashford, Headley Brothers.

Farndale, J. (1961) *The day hospital movement in Great Britain*, Oxford, Pergamon.

Fish, F., and Williamson, J. (1964) 'A delirium unit in an acute geriatric hospital', *Gerontologia Clinica*, **6**, 71–80.

Gilmore, A. (1973) 'Attitudes of the elderly to marriage', *Gerontologia Clinica*, **15**, 124–132.

Godber, C. (1975) 'The psychiatry of old age', in *Doctors and old age*, London, British Geriatrics Society.

Grad, J., and Sainsbury, P. (1965) 'An evaluation of the effects of caring for the aged at home', in *Psychiatric disorders in the aged*, World Psychiatric Association Symposium, Manchester, Geigy.

Grad, J., and Sainsbury, P. (1966) *Evaluating the effectiveness of community mental health services*, (Ed., E.M. Gruenberg) New York, Milbank Memorial Fund.

Griffiths, V.E. (1975) 'Volunteer scheme for dysphasia and allied problems in stroke patients', *British Medical Journal*, iii, 633–635.

Gruer, R. (1975) 'Needs of the elderly in the Scottish borders', *Scottish Health Service Studies, No. 33*, Edinburgh, Scottish Home and Health Department.

Hamilton, M.W., and Hoenig, J. (1966) 'The elderly psychiatric patient and the medical and social services', *The Medical Officer*, **15**, 193–196.

Harwin, B. (1973) 'Psychiatric morbidity among the physically impaired elderly in the community: a preliminary report', in *Roots of evaluation* (Ed. J.K. Wing and H. Hafner) London, Oxford University Press for Nuffield Provincial Hospitals Trust.

Hawks, D. (1975) 'Community care: an analysis of assumptions', *British Journal of Psychiatry*, **127**, 276–285.

Hospital Advisory Service (1970–1975) *Annual reports*, London, Her Majesty's Stationery Office.

Jolley, D.J. (1976) 'Psychiatrist to psychogeriatrician: a conversion experience', *British Journal of Psychiatry* (Supplement) Nov. 11–13.

Jolley, D.J., and Arie, T. (1976) 'A psychiatric service for old people: how many beds?' *British Journal of Psychiatry*: **129**, 418–423.

Kay, D.W.K., Beamish, P., and Roth, M. (1962) 'Some medical and social characteristics of elderly people under state care', *Sociological Review Monograph No. 5*, (Ed. P. Halmos) Keele, University of Keele.

Kay, D.W.K., Beamish, P., and Roth, M. (1964) 'Old age mental disorders in Newcastle upon Tyne: I', *British Journal of Psychiatry*, **110**, 146–158.

Kay, D.W.K., Roth, M., and Hall, M.R.P. (1966) 'Special problems of the aged and the organization of hospital services', *British Medical Journal*, **ii**, 967–972.

Kay, D.W.K., Bergmann, K., Foster, E.M., McKechnie, A.A., and Roth, M. (1970) 'Mental illness and hospital usage in the elderly: a random sample followed up', *Comprehensive Psychiatry*, **1**, 26–35.

Kidd, C.B. (1962) 'Misplacement of the elderly in hospital', *British Medical Journal*, **ii**, 1491–1495.

Kushlick, A. (1975) *Some ways of setting, monitoring and attaining objectives for services for disabled people*, Winchester, Health Care Evaluation Research Team, Research Report No. 116.

Langley, G.E., and Simpson, J.H. (1970) 'Misplacement of the elderly in geriatric and psychiatric hospitals', *Gerontologia Clinica*, **12**, 149–163.

Langley, G.E., Wright, W.B., Sowden, R.R., and Cobby, J.M. (1975) 'The Exe Vale joint psychogeriatric assessment clinic (Hallett Clinic)', *Age and Ageing*, **3**, 125–128.

Lewis, A.J. (1946) 'Ageing and senility: a major problem of psychiatry', *Journal of Mental Science*, **92**, 150–170.

Livesley, B. (1977) 'The climacteric disease', *J. Amer. Geriatrics Society*, **xxv**, 4, 162–166.

Mezey, A., Hodkinson, H.M., and Evans, G.J. (1968) 'The elderly in the wrong unit', *British Medical Journal*, **iii**, 16–18.

Ministry of Health (1962) *A hospital plan for England and Wales*, Comnd. 1604, London, Her Majesty's Stationery Office.

Ministry of Health (1963) *Health and welfare: the development of community care*, Comnd.

1973, London, Her Majesty's Stationery Office.

Morton, E.V.B., Barker, M.E., and MacMillan, D. (1968) 'The joint assessment and early treatment unit in psychogeriatric care', *Gerontologia Clinica*, **10,** 65.

National Health Service (1972) *'Report of the committee of inquiry into Whittingham Hospital'*, Comnd. 4861, London, Her Majesty's Stationery Office.

Northwestern Regional Health Authority (1975) *Committee of inquiry into the transfer of patients from Fairfield to Rossendale Hospital'*, Manchester, Northwestern Regional Health Authority.

OPCS (1973) (Office of Population Censuses and Surveys) *The general household survey. Introductory report*, London, Her Majesty's Stationery Office.

OPCS (1976) *Report of the hospital inpatient enquiry: preliminary tables, 1973*, London, Her Majesty's Stationery Office.

Oxfordshire County Council (1974) *Orchard House*, Report to Social Services Committee, Oxford, Oxford County Council.

Pasker, P., Thomas, J.P.R., and Ashley, J.S.A. (1976) 'The elderly mentally ill—whose responsibility?', *British Medical Journal*, **ii,** 164–166.

Pfeiffer, E. (1969) 'Sexual behaviour in old age', in *Behaviour and Adaptation in late life*, (Ed. E.W. Busse and E. Pfeiffer) Boston, Little, Brown.

Pitt, B. (1975) *Psychogeriatrics*, London, Churchill–Livingstone.

Post, F. (1962) *The significance of affective symptoms in old age*, Maudsley Monograph 10, London, Oxford University Press.

Post, F. (1965) *The clinical psychiatry of late life*, London, Pergamon.

Post, F. (1966) *Persistent persecutory states of the elderly*, London, Pergamon.

Prinsley, D. (1973) 'Psychogeriatric ward for mentally disturbed elderly patients', *British Medical Journal*, **iii,** 575–577.

Registrar General (1971). *Occupational mortality tables, England and Wales, 1961*, London, Her Majesty's Stationery Office.

Registrar General (1974) *Statistical review for England and Wales, 1972*, London, Her Majesty's Stationery Office.

Revans, R.W. (1964) *Standards for morale: cause and effect in hospitals*. London, Oxford University Press for Nuffield Provincial Hospitals Trust.

Robinson, R.A. (1975) 'The assessment centre', in *Modern perspectives on the psychiatry of old age* (Ed. J.G. Howells) London, Churchill–Livingstone.

Roth, M. (1973) 'Providing a service for psychogeriatric patients', in *Roots of evaluation*, (Ed. J.K. Wing and H. Hafner) London, Oxford University Press for Nuffield Provincial Hospitals Trust.

Royal College of Psychiatrists (1975) 'Norms for Medical Staffing of a Psychogeriatric Service', *News and Notes*, supplement to *British Journal of Psychiatry*, July.

Sanford, J.R.A. (1975) 'Tolerance of debility in elderly dependents by supporters at home', *British Medical Journal*, **iii,** 471–473.

Scottish Home and Health Department (1970) *Services for the elderly with mental disorders*, Edinburgh, Her Majesty's Stationery Office.

Seebohm Committee (1968) *Report of the committee on local authority and allied personal social services*, Comnd. 3703, London, Her Majesty's Stationery Office.

Sheldon, J.H. (1948) *The social medicine of old age*, London, Oxford University Press.

Shepherd, M., Cooper, B., Brown, A.C., and Kalton, G.W. (1966) *Psychiatric morbidity in general practice*, London, Oxford University Press.

Smith, M.V., and Blythe, J.D. (1971) Domiciliary consultations, *Update plus*, February, 135–140.

Society of Clinical Psychiatrists (1971) *The organization of psychogeriatrics*, Ipswich, Society of Clinical Psychiatrists.

Tooth, G.C., and Brooke, E.M. (1961) 'Trends in the mental hospital population', *Lancet*, **i,** 710–713.

Warren, M.W. (1946) 'Care of the chronic sick', *Lancet*, **i,** 841–843.

White, D.M.D. (1975) 'Psychogeriatrics and community Care', *Lancet*, **i**, 27–29.

Whitehead, T., and Mankikar, G. (1974) 'Geriatric psychiatry in the general hospital', *Lancet*, **i**, 1213–1215.

Wigley, G. (1968) 'Community services for mentally ill old people', *Lancet*, **ii**, 963–966.

Williamson, J., Stokoe, I.H., Gray, S., Fisher, M., Smith, A., McGhee, A., and Stephenson, E. (1964) 'Old people at home: their unreported needs', *Lancet*, **i**, 1117–1120.

WHO (1972) (World Health Organization) *Psychogeriatrics*, Report of a WHO Scientific Group, Geneva, World Health Organization.

Wroe, D.C. (1973) 'The elderly', in *Social trends, 1973*, London, Her Majesty's Stationery Office.

INDEX